Vascular Complications of Surgery and Intervention

Ramyar Gilani • Joseph L. Mills Sr.
Editors

Vascular Complications of Surgery and Intervention

A Practical Guide

Springer

Editors
Ramyar Gilani
Michael E. DeBakey Department of Surgery
Baylor College of Medicine
Houston, TX, USA

Joseph L. Mills Sr.
Michael E. DeBakey Department of Surgery
Baylor College of Medicine
Houston, TX, USA

ISBN 978-3-030-86712-6 ISBN 978-3-030-86713-3 (eBook)
https://doi.org/10.1007/978-3-030-86713-3

This Springer imprint is published by the registered company Springer Nature Switzerland AG
The registered company address is: Gewerbestrasse 11, 6330 Cham, Switzerland

Introduction

We welcome the reader to the inaugural edition of *Vascular Complications of Surgery and Intervention – A Practical Guide*. Complications are an unpleasant topic, but they are best anticipated, recognized, and promptly addressed should they occur. As vascular specialists, much of our daily thought and attention is committed to preventing, diagnosing, mitigating, and rescuing vascular complications. We are not alone in this quest. The concept for this book developed through daily clinical practice over many years of real-world experience connected with patients experiencing the breadth of challenges covered in this text. The words expressed in the following pages describe the efforts by experts in the field as they commit to advancing healthcare quality by all professionals.

Unintended vascular complications resulting from derangement and manipulation are well known to providers and impact patients in various ways and degrees. The vascular system is a ubiquitous, interconnected network that encompasses all regions of the body and is vital to the viability of its organs and structures. Therefore, the range of possibility for unintended consequence is vast. In addition, a wide variety of medical professionals and personnel encounter this robust, yet delicate system in the scope of their practice. Levels of familiarity and training remain widely variable particularly in modern times due in part to the increasing sub-specialization of medicine. However, the range of potential complications and their management can be described in a succinct and practical manner for all providers to guide prevention and management. Lastly, given the potential for serious harm and even death, understanding the medicolegal landscape surrounding these untoward occurrences will foster self-awareness and culture of safety.

The content of this text is directed towards dedicated healthcare professionals managing patients affected by undesired complications of vascular derangement and for those providers performing interventions either directly upon the vascular system or procedures that have potential for collateral impact. It should be noted that the book does not discuss the wide range of potential non-vascular specific complications of patients undergoing vascular interventions such as myocardial infarction or respiratory failure. The content will be divided into four separate parts. The material begins with an introduction to vascular anatomy and function. There follows a part that aims to cover specific complications of the vascular system that can occur in any patient even without intervention. The third part addresses complications encountered during intervention and surgery. The fourth and final part is dedicated to the delayed and long-term sequelae attributable to vascular complications.

The general principles section is targeted toward any level of provider wishing to become more familiar with the basic anatomy and physiology of the vascular system. This unit covers topics such as regional vascular anatomy encountered for access and exposure. A brief discussion of thrombosis, hemorrhage, and ischemia has been included. A short segment on vascular imaging is included to raise awareness of its important applications and utility. This introduction will be useful as a reference for subsequent sections.

The section on non-intervention related complications is intended for any and all providers managing patients who may have suffered any of a set of complications that relate to common derangements of the vascular system. Topics covered in this section include thromboembolic events, stroke and spinal paralysis, and a special discussion on approaches to pediatric patients. The goal is to provide the reader with practical and actionable concepts rather than offer an extensive review of medical literature. For example, suspect PE in the following situations; make the diagnosis by performing this study; and treat with these medications.

Interventions and manipulation of the vascular system are performed by a wide range of generalists and specialists, none of whom is immune to experiencing resulting complications. The section on performing interventions is targeted toward a wide range of specialists who may potentially encounter a direct or indirect complication as a result of the intervention. The content covers accepted principles on how to perform procedures safely. This includes discussion on access, exposure, and incorporation of a procedural checklist. For example, how does one safely access the common femoral artery? This is followed by a discussion covering situations where the risk of inadvertent collateral sequelae of potentially life-threatening hemorrhage and ischemia is significant. Chapters provide tips and techniques to stay clear of complications and, should one occur, how to navigate back to safety. The final element of this procedural emphasis section covers the occcult complications from interventions, the so-called "I didn't think it was possible, but it certainly is" list. Emphasis is placed upon unrecognized hemorrhage and ischemia particularly during specialized surgery such as neurosurgical, orthopedic, gynecologic, and urologic interventions.

Vascular complications may present distant to any particular point in time as a delayed presentation is certainly possible. It is important to address the topics of infection and erosion involving native vessels and grafts that are well-known but often have more delayed complications, which can wreak substantial limb and life-threatening havoc. Strategies for re-operative surgery aim to provide specific practical approaches to formulate a plan when dealing with potentially hostile anatomic situations. Certainly no discussion would be complete without touching on the medicolegal ramifications of undesired vascular complications. Our aim is to promote awareness, anticipation, and surveillance as the best tools to guard against complications.

"The eternal providence has appointed me to watch over the life and health of Thy creatures. May the love for my art actuate me at all times; may neither avarice nor miserliness, nor thirst for glory or for a great reputation engage my mind; for the enemies of truth and philanthropy could easily deceive me and make me forgetful of my lofty aim of doing good to Thy children.

May I never see in the patient anything but a fellow creature in pain.

Grant me the strength, time and opportunity always to correct what I have acquired, always to extend its domain; for knowledge is immense and the spirit of man can extend indefinitely to enrich itself daily with new requirements. Today he can discover his errors of yesterday and tomorrow he can obtain a new light on what he thinks himself sure of today.

Oh, God, Thou has appointed me to watch over the life and death of Thy creatures; here am I ready for my vocation and now I turn unto my calling." —Moses Maimonides

Houston, TX, USA

Ramyar Gilani
Joseph L. Mills Sr.

Contents

Contributors

Arsalan Amin Micahel E. DeBakey Department of Surgery, Baylor College of Medicine, Houston, TX, USA

George E. Anton Department of Vascular Surgery, Cleveland Clinic, Heart, Vascular and Thoracic Institute, Mayfield Heights, OH, USA

Cleveland Clinic, Department of Vascular Surgery, Heart, Vascular and Thoracic Institute, Mayfield Heights, OH, USA

Kristofer M. Charlton-Ouw HCA Gulf Coast Division, Vascular Surgery, Gulf Coast Vascular, HCA Houston Healthcare, Departments of Clinical and Biomedical Sciences, University of Houston College of Medicine, Houston, TX, USA

Stephen R. Chen Department of Interventional Radiology, University of Texas M.D. Anderson Cancer Center, Houston, TX, USA

Jayer Chung Division of Vascular Surgery and Endovascular Therapy, Michael E DeBakey Department of Surgery, Baylor College of Medicine, Houston, TX, USA

Sara C. Fallon Pediatric Surgery, Texas Children's Hospital/Baylor College of Medicine, Houston, TX, USA

Ravi K. Ghanta Division of Cardiothoracic Surgery, Michael E. DeBakey Department of Surgery, Baylor College of Medicine, Houston, TX, USA

Ramyar Gilani Michael E. DeBakey Department of Surgery, Baylor College of Medicine, Houston, TX, USA

Courtney Grant Division of Vascular and Endovascular Therapy, Michael E DeBakey Department of Surgery, Baylor College of Medicine, Houston, TX, USA

Nawar Hudefi Division of Vascular Surgery and Endovascular Therapy, Michael E DeBakey Department of Surgery, Baylor College of Medicine, Houston, TX, USA

Brian C. Imada Department of Radiology, Baylor College of Medicine, Houston, TX, USA

Rebecca Kelso Novant Health Heart and Vascular Institute, Presbyterian Hospital, Charlotte, NC, USA

Ahmed F. Khouqeer Michael E. DeBakey Department of Surgery, Baylor College of Medicine, Houston, TX, USA

Juan E. Marcano Division of Cardiothoracic Surgery, Michael E. DeBakey Department of Surgery, Baylor College of Medicine, Houston, TX, USA

Jessica M. Mayor Division of Vascular Surgery and Endovascular Therapy, Michael E DeBakey Department of Surgery, Baylor College of Medicine, Houston, TX, USA

Joseph L. Mills Sr. Division of Vascular Surgery and Endovascular Therapy, Michael E DeBakey Department of Surgery, Baylor College of Medicine, Houston, TX, USA

Bindi Naik-Mathuria Pediatric Surgery, Texas Children's Hospital/Baylor College of Medicine, Houston, TX, USA

Zachary S. Pallister Division of Vascular and Endovascular Therapy, Michael E DeBakey Department of Surgery, Baylor College of Medicine, Houston, TX, USA

Michael E. DeBakey Department of Surgery, Baylor College of Medicine, Houston, TX, USA

Xin Peng Division of Vascular Diseases and Surgery, Wexner Medical Center, The Ohio State University, Columbus, OH, USA

Amir Pezeshkmehr Division of Interventional Radiology, Department of Radiology, Texas Children's Hospital/Baylor College of Medicine, Houston, TX, USA

Ravi R. Rajani Division of Vascular and Endovascular Surgery, Emory University School of Medicine, Atlanta, GA, USA

Christopher R. Ramos Division of Vascular and Endovascular Surgery, Emory University School of Medicine, Atlanta, GA, USA

Veronica Lenge de Rosen Department of Radiology, Department of Internal Medicine, Baylor College of Medicine, Houston, TX, USA

Robbin S. Sabo Cleveland Clinic, Heart & Vascular Institute Regional Vascular Lab, Mayfield Heights, OH, USA

Eric Silberfein Baylor College of Medicine, Houston, TX, USA

Ben Taub Hospital, Division of Surgical Oncology, Michael E. DeBakey Department of Surgery, Houston, TX, USA

Bruce L. Tjaden Division of Vascular and Endovascular Surgery, Cooper University Health Care, Camden, NJ, USA

Mathew J. Wall Jr. Division of Cardiothoracic Surgery, Michael E. DeBakey Department of Surgery, Baylor College of Medicine, Houston, TX, USA

Jeremy Ward Micahel E. DeBakey Department of Surgery, Baylor College of Medicine, Houston, TX, USA

Part I

General Principles

Regional Vascular Anatomy

1

Brian C. Imada and Stephen R. Chen

Embryologic Development of Vascular Tree

The vasculature is divided into the arterial system, venous system, and lymphatic system. The arterial system carries blood away from the heart via progressively smaller arteries, arterioles, and capillaries of distal organs. The venous system returns blood from the body via progressively larger venules and veins back to the heart. The lymphatic system collects interstitial fluid from tissues and organs and drains into the bilateral subclavian veins [1].

The vascular system is essential to the development of the embryo, delivering oxygen to and metabolic waste away from cells of the developing embryo. Consequently, the cardiovascular system is the first functional organ system that develops in the embryo.

In embryonic development, the epiblast (a precursor to ectoderm) invaginates to form the primitive streak. The germ layer is seen in the earliest stages of embryonic development and consists of an inner layer (endoderm), middle layer (mesoderm), and an outer layer (ectoderm). In the mesoderm, mesodermal cells, known as hemangioblasts, cluster into blood islands, which then differentiate into angioblasts. These angioblasts develop into the endothelium and blood cells. Blood island cell clusters continue to form and coalesce to develop into long channels that fill with blood cells.

Concurrently, cells from the proximal lateral intraembryonic mesoderm assemble around the body axis into endocardial tubes. These tubes fuse and elongate

B. C. Imada
Department of Radiology, Baylor College of Medicine, Houston, TX, USA
e-mail: Brain.Imada@bcm.edu

S. R. Chen (✉)
Department of Interventional Radiology, University of Texas M.D. Anderson Cancer Center, Houston, TX, USA
e-mail: srchen@mdanderson.org

R. Gilani, J. L. Mills Sr. (eds.), *Vascular Complications of Surgery and Intervention*, https://doi.org/10.1007/978-3-030-86713-3_1

anteriorly. The tubes then split into ventral aortae, loop, and further extend posteriorly as two symmetrically paired dorsal aortae. These dorsal aortae merge to develop into a single tube. Cardinal veins develop from differentiated migratory angioblastic precursor cells.

The dorsal aorta forms ventral to the notochord and the posterior cardinal vein forms dorsal to trunk endoderm.

Blood flows caudally from the heart through the dorsal aorta and returns rostrally through the cardiac vein.

During early embryonic angiogenesis, angioblasts are the precursors of endothelial cells. As the embryo continues to develop, endothelial cells develop from precursor cells, as well as from endothelial cells already integrated into the developing vascular bed of the embryo. In further stages of development, endothelial cells develop solely from the already existing endothelial cells. Throughout development, vascular smooth muscle cells known as pericytes are recruited to the primitive endothelial cells to promote mature blood vessel formation [1].

Vasculogenesis describes the de novo formation of blood vessels by angioblasts, mesodermal precursors, during the early stages of vascular development. These angioblasts relocate to specific areas of the embryo and coalesce with other angioblasts to form loose cords, which then differentiate into endothelial cells. An important contributor in this initiation of vasculogenesis is basic fibroblast growth factor (bFGF). These primitive structures then form the basis for subsequent expansion of vessels. The dorsal aorta develops through the first groups of angioblasts arising at the site of vessel formation. The endocardium, ventral aortae, and posterior cardinal veins form through the second mechanism of angioblast migration to the different sites of vessel formation.

Other genes essential to vascular system development include vascular endothelial growth factor (VEGF), VEGF receptor-2 (VEGFR-2), and VEGFR-1.

Endothelial cells also produce signals to induce the earliest stages of organogenesis, as can be seen in liver and pancreatic development.

Over time, the vascular tree branches and establishes new connections via cell division, migration, and assembly of endothelial cells from preexisting vessels via angiogenesis. Angiogenesis describes the process in which a group of cells migrate in an outward direction from a parent vessel. These endothelial cells extend from the tip via reorganization of the cells in response to angiogenic growth factors such as VEGF, transforming growth factor beta (TGF-β), platelet-derived growth factor (PDGF), and angiopoietin-1. These tip cells migrate to form new sprouts, while cells behind, named stalk cells, proliferate. The cells at the tip eventually fuse with other cells to form a bridge and establish new branches. These new connections then form a patent lumen to form a channel for blood flow [2].

The bifurcation of blood vessels occurs with arteriogenesis, which is the development of collateral arteries from preexisting arteriolar connections by growth. This process involves active proliferation and remodeling of smooth muscle cells and endothelial cells.

Pruning and remodeling of the vasculature occurs throughout embryologic development, which involves numerous cycles of angiogenesis and vasculogenesis with concurrent apoptosis. Cells divide or die based on the growing needs of the embryo, and this pruning and remodeling is induced by different hemodynamics, metabolic demands, and growth factor secretions. The embryologic vascular plexus initially starts out as homogenous, equal-sized vessels. These vessels then become smaller or larger, forming a variety of vascular connections throughout the embryo. Hemodynamic stress plays a key role in the circumferential growth of the blood vessels.

In early development, arteries and veins are indistinguishable from one another. The differentiation into arteries and veins is determined by endothelial cells at a molecular level, with arterial- and venous-specific markers localized in a posterior-arterial and anterior-venous pole [3].

Head and Neck

Intracranial

Arteries

The arterial supply to the head and neck arises from the three branches of the aortic arch and consists of the common carotid arteries and the vertebral arteries.

The common carotid arteries ascend obliquely and bifurcate into the external and internal carotid arteries at the level of the thyroid cartilage. The left common carotid artery consists of a thoracic and cervical portion. The thoracic portion arises in the mediastinum directly from the aortic arch, and the cervical portion begins at the level of the left sternoclavicular joint. The right common carotid artery does not have a thoracic portion.

The internal carotid artery usually arises between the C3 and C5 vertebral level. The origins of the right and left internal carotid arteries are highly variable relative to each other, with the majority of the population with asymmetric origins bilaterally.

The Bouthillier classification is a system used to classify the divisions of the internal carotid artery into seven segments. The segments are the cervical (C1), petrous (horizontal, C2), lacerum (C3), cavernous (C4), clinoid (C5), ophthalmic (supraclinoid, C6), and communicating (terminal, C7) segments (Fig. 1.1).

The cervical segment has no significant branches within the neck. The branches of the petrous segment are the caroticotympanic artery and the vidian artery. A notable attribute of the petrous segment is that it is fixed to the bone as the internal carotid artery enters the skull base, which prevents the cervical carotid from extending intracranially. The lacerum segment has no branches.

The cavernous segment gives off a meningohypophyseal trunk and inferolateral trunk. The meningohypophyseal trunk further branches into the inferior hypophyseal artery, tentorial artery, and clival artery. The inferior hypophyseal artery perfuses the pituitary, the tentorial artery supplies the tentorium, and the clival artery supplies the dura of the clivus. The inferolateral trunk supplies CN III, CN IV, CN VI, and the trigeminal ganglion.

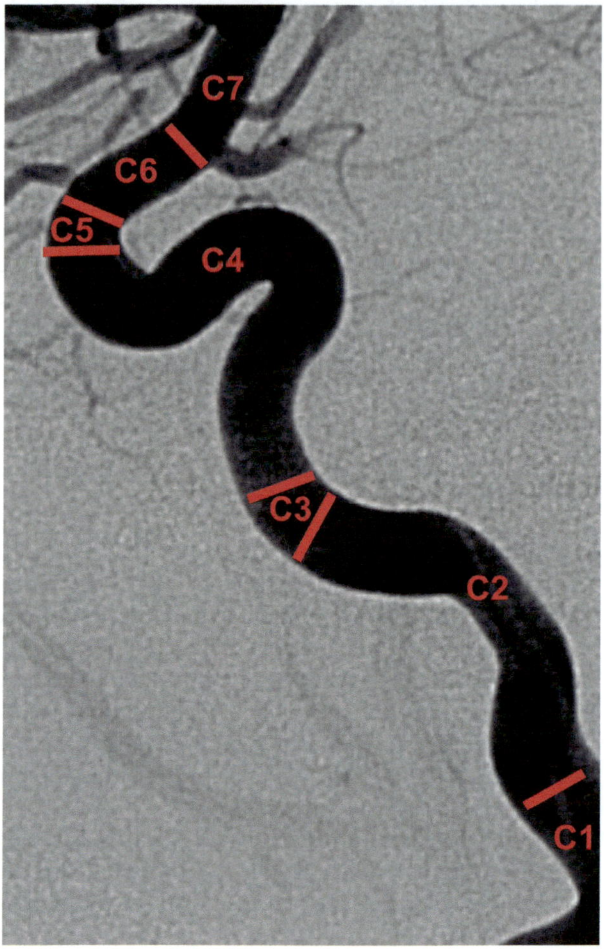

Fig. 1.1 Bouthillier classification of the internal carotid artery. C1, cervical segment; C2, petrous/horizontal segment; C3, lacerum segment; C4, cavernous segment; C5, clinoid segment; C6, ophthalmic/supraclinoid segment; C7, communicating/terminal segment

The two carotid rings demarcate the proximal and distal portions of the clinoid segment. These carotid rings are important in preventing an intracranial subarachnoid hemorrhage from the rupture of an inferiorly located aneurysm. The branches of the ophthalmic segment include the ophthalmic artery and superior hypophyseal artery. The ophthalmic artery supplies the optic nerve, and the superior hypophyseal artery has branches that supply the optic nerve, optic chiasm, pituitary stalk, and pars tuberalis (anterior lobe of the pituitary gland). The ophthalmic artery is clinically significant and can serve as an anatomic landmark for the distal carotid dural ring, as the takeoff of the ophthalmic artery is just distal to the distal carotid ring. Aneurysms located superior to the distal carotid dural ring can cause subarachnoid hemorrhage, so they are usually treated more aggressively than aneurysms located proximal to this ring.

The branches of the communicating segment include the posterior communicating artery (P-comm), anterior choroidal artery, anterior cerebral artery, and middle cerebral artery. The posterior communicating artery is an anastomosis to the posterior circulation and courses between the optic tract and CN III. This anatomic relationship is clinically important in that an aneurysm of the posterior communicating artery can cause a CN III palsy secondary to mass effect. The posterior communicating artery gives off the anterior thalamoperforator vessels. The anterior choroidal artery is the most distal branch of the internal carotid artery and supplies the optic chiasm, hippocampus, and posterior limb of the internal capsule.

There are three segments of the anterior cerebral artery (Figs. 1.2 and 1.3). The A1 segment (horizontal/pre-communicating segment) courses over the ipsilateral optic chiasm and optic nerve. The A2 segment (vertical/post-communicating segment) enters the interhemispheric fissure anterior to the lamina terminalis. The A3 segment consists of the distal anterior communicating artery and cortical branches. The anterior cerebral artery ends in the choroid plexus in the roof of the third ventricle after coursing around the splenium of the corpus callosum [4].

The A1 segment of the anterior cerebral artery gives off the recurrent artery of Heubner, an artery that supplies the caudate head and anterior limb of the internal capsule. This artery arises proximal to the anterior communicating artery. The A1 segment also gives rise to the medial lenticulostriate perforator arteries, which perfuse the medial basal ganglia.

The middle cerebral artery consists of four segments (Figs. 1.2 and 1.3). The M1 segment is the horizontal segment of the middle cerebral artery and extends from the internal carotid terminus to the origin of the sylvian fissure. This segment gives off the lateral lenticulostriate perforator arteries, which perfuse the lateral basal ganglia [5]. The M2 segment consists of the sylvian segment of the middle cerebral artery to the bottom of the sylvian fissure. Branches of this segment supply the

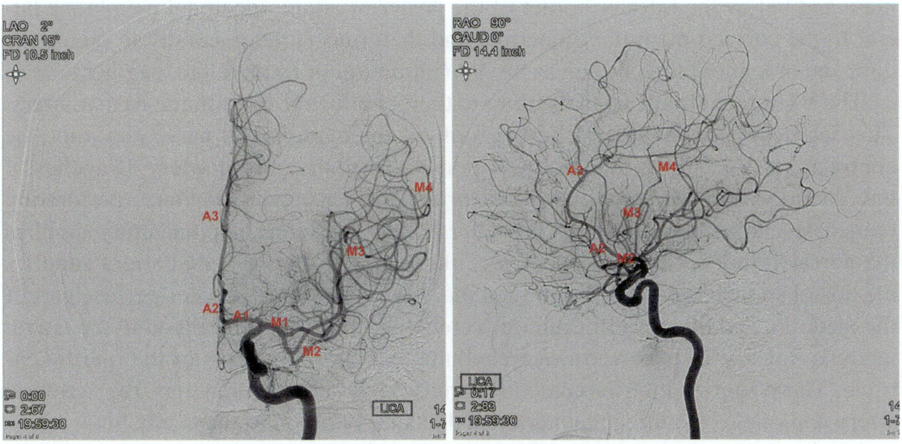

Figs. 1.2 (left) and **1.3** (right) Cerebral internal carotid artery angiogram. A1, horizontal/pre-communicating segment of the anterior cerebral artery (ACA); A2, vertical/post-communicating segment of the ACA; A3, distal anterior communicating artery and cortical branches of the ACA; M1, horizontal segment of the middle cerebral artery (MCA); M2, sylvian segment of the MCA

temporal lobe and insular cortex (Wernicke's speech area), parietal lobe (cortical sensory area), and inferolateral frontal lobe. The M3 segment is the cortical segment and extends from the top of the sylvian fissure to the cortical surface. Branches of the M3 segment supply the lateral cerebral cortex. The small cortical branches of the middle cerebral artery make up the M4 segment.

The other major pair of arteries that supply the head and neck are the vertebral arteries. The vertebral arteries branch off the first part of the subclavian artery and ascend within the transverse foramina of the cervical vertebrae, posterior to the internal carotid artery and anterior to the hypoglossal nerve (CN XII) roots. The vertebral artery supplies the blood supply to the posterior fossa, occipital lobes, the portions of the vertebrae, and spinal column.

The vertebral artery is divided into four segments. The V1 (perforaminal, extraosseous) segment begins at its origin to the transverse foramen of C6. This segment angles posteriorly between the longus colli muscle medially and anterior scalene laterally, then through the colliscalene triangle, behind the common carotid artery, then entering the transverse foramen of the C6 vertebral body. The branches of the V1 segment include segmental cervical muscular branches and spinal branches.

The V2 (foraminal) segment runs from the transverse foramen of the C6 vertebral body to the transverse foramen of the C2 vertebral body. The V2 segment ascends through the transverse foramen of the C6 vertebral body to the transverse foramen of C3; then the artery turns superolaterally through the L-shaped transverse foramen of the C2 vertebral body. The V2 branches are the muscular and spinal branches and the anterior meningeal artery.

The V3 (atlantic, extradural, or extraspinal) segment is the segment from the transverse foramen of the C2 vertebral body to the dura. The V3 segment exits the transverse process of the C2 vertebral body, then sweeps laterally to pass through the transverse foramen of C1, then runs past the posterior border of the C1 lateral mass and below the inferior border of the posterior atlanto-occipital membrane lateral to the cervico-medullary junction, and then runs superomedially to pierce the dura and arachnoid to continue as the V4 (intradural or intracranial) segment.

The V4 segment runs from the dura to their confluence to form the basilar artery. This segment ascends anterior to the roots of the hypoglossal nerve and joins the contralateral V4 segment at the lower pons to form the basilar artery. Branches of the V4 artery are the anterior spinal artery, posterior spinal artery, perforating branches, and posterior inferior cerebellar artery. The anterior spinal artery supplies the dorsal spinal cord to the conus medullaris, the posterior spinal artery supplies the dorsal spinal cord and inferior medulla, the perforating branches perfuse part of the medulla, and the posterior inferior cerebellar artery supplies blood to the lateral medulla, tonsils, inferior vermis/cerebellum, and choroid plexus of the fourth ventricle. The posterior inferior cerebellar artery is the largest branch of the vertebral artery and one of the three main arteries that supply blood to the cerebellum.

The basilar artery continues as the posterior cerebral artery, which gives off thalamoperforators that supply the thalamus. There are four segments of the posterior cerebral artery (Figs. 1.4 and 1.5). The P1 and P2 segments are deep segments of the posterior cerebral artery. The P1 segment lies between the end of the basilar artery and the posterior communicating artery. The branches of the P1 segment include the

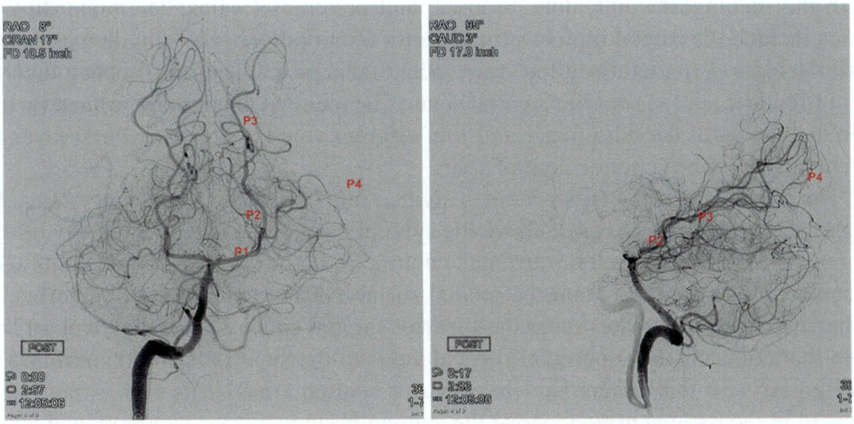

Figs. 1.4 (left) and **1.5** (right) Posterior cerebral artery angiograms. P1, thalamic-subthalamic arteries of the posterior cerebral artery (PCA); P2, thalamogeniculate and posterior choroidal arteries of the PCA; P3, quadrigeminal segment of the PCA; P4, cortical segment of the PCA

thalamic-subthalamic arteries which supply the paramedial portions of the upper midbrain and thalamus [6]. The artery of Percheron is a vascular anatomic variant that arises from the P1 segment. This artery is a dominant thalamic perforator that supplies the bilateral ventromedial thalami and rostral midbrain. This artery is clinically significant, as an infarct of this artery would cause bilateral ventromedial thalamic infarction. Patients present with altered mental status, vertical gaze palsy, memory impairment, hemiplegia, cerebellar ataxia, and deranged movement.

The P2 segment branches are the thalamogeniculate arteries and posterior choroidal arteries. The thalamogeniculate arteries perfuse the ventrolateral thalamus, while the posterior choroidal arteries perfuse the lateral geniculate body, pulvinar, posterior thalamus, hippocampus, and parahippocampal gyrus [6].

The P3 and P4 are the superficial segments of the posterior cerebral artery. The P3 segment is the quadrigeminal segment and gives rise to the anterior and posterior inferior temporal arteries, which supply a portion of the temporal lobe. The P4 segment is the cortical segment located within the calcarine fissure, and its branches include the occipitotemporal artery, occipitoparietal artery, and calcarine artery [6]. The P4 segment terminates as the calcarine artery.

The circle of Willis is a central intracranial anastomosis that links the internal carotid arteries to the vertebrobasilar circulation. The circle of Willis is located in the cisterna interpeduncularis. Anteriorly, the anterior cerebral arteries are joined by the anterior communicating artery. Posteriorly, the basilar artery continues as the posterior cerebral artery and joins the ipsilateral internal carotid artery by the posterior communicating artery.

Veins/Sinuses

The cranial veins include diploic veins and meningeal veins. The diploic veins run through channels in the diploe of the bones of the cranium. These veins anastomose with the meningeal veins, dural sinuses, and pericranial veins. The main diploic veins include the frontal diploic vein, anterior temporal (parietal) diploic vein, posterior temporal (parietal) diploic vein, occipital diploic vein, and smaller diploic vein tributaries of the superior sagittal sinus. The meningeal veins are formed by the venous plexus of the dura mater and join efferent veins in the outer dural layer to eventually join the superior sagittal sinus.

The supratentorial venous system is divided into superficial and deep systems. In regard to the superficial veins, above the sylvian fissure, the lateral convexity of the brain is drained by the anterior, frontal, central, and parietal veins. These veins also receive venous drainage from the medial surface of the brain from the interhemispheric fissure, before they enter the superior sagittal sinus. The vein of Trolard is a vein that connects the superficial cortical veins to the superior sagittal sinus and is the largest vein that drains into the superior sagittal sinus. This vein is normally located in the parietal region, above the sylvian fissure.

The superficial middle cerebral vein drains the lateral aspect of the brain close to the sylvian fissure. This vein usually drains posteriorly into the transverse sinus but may also drain anteriorly into the deep middle cerebral vein.

The superficial portions of the brain under the sylvian fissure and inferior aspect of the temporal and occipital lobes drain into the transverse sinus. The vein of Labbe is the vein that drains the temporal convexity into the transverse or sigmoid sinus. This vein is the largest lateral vein under the sylvian fissure. It is important to identify this vein during surgery, as a retraction injury to the vein of Labbe could lead to venous infarction and aphasia.

The deep cerebral veins consist of the paired internal cerebral veins, the basal veins of Rosenthal, and the thalamic veins. The internal cerebral veins are paired veins that course approximately two millimeters from the midline. These veins drain the deep white matter of the frontal horns and the body of the lateral ventricles via the medial and lateral subependymal veins. The basal veins of Rosenthal are formed in the medial portion of the lateral cerebral fissures after joining the deep middle cerebral veins. The veins then leave the lateral cerebral fissures and course around the superior aspect of the uncus to pass posteriorly in the perimesencephalic cisterns to drain posteriorly into the vein of Galen.

The thalamostriate veins are deep veins that outline the inferolateral wall of the body of the lateral ventricle. The intersection of the septal vein and the thalamostriate vein is also known as the *venous angle*. This is the angiographic landmark used for identifying the foramen of Monro.

The site of drainage of the deep veins is the vein of Galen. The vein of Galen receives blood from the internal cerebral veins, basal veins of Rosenthal pericallosal veins, and the veins that drain the superior aspect of the posterior fossa. The vein of Galen courses beneath the splenium of the corpus callosum and then drains into the straight sinus.

The dural venous sinuses also drain intracranial venous blood. The superior sagittal sinus is located within the dura at its junction with the falx cerebri and drains the motor and sensory cortices. The transverse sinuses are paired sinuses that drain into the sigmoid sinus, which then drains into the jugular bulb. The torcula herophili is the confluence of the superior sagittal sinus, transverse sinus, and straight sinus.

The cavernous sinus is the lateral border of the sella turcica and contains the oculomotor nerve, trochlear nerve, ophthalmic nerve, abducens nerve, and the cavernous portion of the internal carotid artery. The superior and inferior ophthalmic veins drain into the cavernous sinus anteriorly, and sphenoparietal sinus drains into the cavernous sinus anterolaterally. The superficial sylvian veins and the uncal veins also occasionally drain into the cavernous sinus.

The cavernous sinus drains posteriorly into the superior petrosal sinus, posteroinferiorly into the inferior petrosal sinus, and inferiorly into the pterygoid plexus. The right and left cavernous sinuses are connected by the sinus intercavernous anterior and the sinus intercavernous posterior. The facial vein connects to the cavernous sinus via the angular vein.

In terms of the venous drainage of the pituitary gland, small hypophyseal veins drain the anterior lobe of the pituitary and drain into lateral adenohypophyseal veins to converge into the confluent pituitary veins on the surface of the gland. The confluent pituitary veins then travel laterally to join the ipsilateral cavernous sinus.

The venous drainage of the posterior fossa is made up of three major groups. The superior group is made up of the drain precentral cerebellar vein, posterior mesencephalic veins, and superior vermian veins and drains into the vein of Galen. The anterior group is made up of the anterior pontomesencephalic vein and petrosal veins and drains into the petrosal sinus. The posterior group is made up of inferior vermian veins formed by the superior and inferior retrotonsillar tributaries and drains into the torcula herophili and transverse sinus.

Extracranial

Arteries

The superficial arteries of the head and neck are mainly supplied by the external carotid artery. The external carotid artery begins at the C4 vertebral level, around the upper border of the thyroid cartilage. The artery arises medial and anterior to the internal carotid artery, ascending upward and anteriorly before curving slightly posteriorly to the space behind the neck of the mandible. Throughout its course, the external carotid artery narrows in size.

The external carotid artery can be divided into anterior and posterior branches. The anterior branches are the superior thyroid, lingual, and facial arteries. The superior thyroid artery is the first anterior branch of the external carotid artery, at around the level of the hyoid bone [5]. This artery branches into terminal branches at the apex of the thyroid gland. The superior thyroid artery supplies the structures of the larynx and thyroid gland. Its branches include the superior marginal arcade, posterior glandular arcade, lateral glandular arcade, hyoid branch, sternocleidomastoid artery, superior laryngeal artery, and cricothyroid artery [5].

The lingual artery is the second branch of the external carotid artery. The lingual artery supplies the floor of the mouth and muscles of the tongue [5]. It originates from the external carotid artery anteromedially, between the origins of the superior thyroid artery and facial artery. The artery travels upward obliquely and medially and then curves down and anteriorly to form a loop. From there, it courses anterior horizontally and then ascends to the inferior surface of the tongue. The branches of the lingual artery include the suprahyoid branch, dorsal artery of the tongue, and sublingual artery.

The facial artery arises from the external carotid artery anteriorly. It runs medial to the mandibular ramus to eventually reach the lower border of the mandible to take a superficial course. This artery supplies blood to the structures of the face, including the muscles, skin, submandibular gland, tonsils, and soft palate. The branches of the facial artery are the cervical branches, ascending palatine artery, tonsillar artery, glandular branches, submental artery, facial branches, inferior labial artery, superior labial artery, lateral nasal branch (angular artery), inferior masseteric artery, jugal trunk artery, middle mental artery, and anterior jugal artery [5].

The posterior branches of the external carotid artery include the ascending pharyngeal artery, occipital artery, posterior auricular artery, superficial temporal artery, and internal maxillary artery [5].

The ascending pharyngeal artery has an anterior division and a posterior division and supplies the base of the skull. The branches of the anterior division include pharyngeal branches and the inferior tympanic artery. The branches of the posterior division are a jugular branch and a hypoglossal nerve branch [5].

The occipital artery arises at the level of the facial artery and courses in the opposite direction, coursing backward and superiorly. The branches of the occipital artery include sternocleidomastoid branches, a mastoid branch, an auricular branch, muscular branches, and meningeal branches [5].

The posterior auricular artery is a small artery of the external carotid artery that supplies the auricle and the scalp posterior to the auricle. Its three main branches include the stylomastoid artery, an auricular branch, and an occipital branch [5].

As the external carotid artery enters the parotid gland, it gives rise to its terminal branches, the superficial temporal and internal maxillary arteries.

The superficial temporal artery arises close to the parotid gland, behind the neck of the mandible. The superficial temporal artery supplies a portion of the face and scalp. The branches of the superficial temporal artery include the transverse facial artery, an anterior auricular branch, the zygomatico-orbital artery, middle temporal artery, a frontal branch, and a parietal branch [5].

The internal maxillary artery is the larger of the two terminal branches of the external carotid artery. This artery arises from behind the neck of the mandible, passes the lower head of the lateral pterygoid muscle, and distally enters the pterygopalatine fossa. This artery can be subdivided into three segments: the mandibular segment, pterygoid segment, and pterygopalatine segment [5].

The mandibular segment is the portion of the maxillary artery that lies behind the neck of the mandible. The branches of the mandibular segment include the deep auricular artery, anterior tympanic artery, middle meningeal artery, frontal branch, parieto-occipital branch, petrosquamosal trunk, accessory meningeal artery, and inferior alveolar (dental) artery [5]. The middle meningeal artery enters intracranially via the foramen spinosum of the sphenoid bone and is the largest meningeal artery [5]. The middle meningeal artery is clinically significant. It can commonly rupture at the pterion, which can cause an epidural hematoma [7]. Additionally, damage to this artery can lead to the development of aneurysms or arteriovenous fistulas [7].

The pterygoid segment runs superficial or deep to the lateral pterygoid muscle in the temporal fossa. Its branches include the deep temporal branches, pterygoid branches, masseteric arteries, and buccal artery [5].

The pterygopalatine segment enters the pterygopalatine fossa and divides into several branches named based on the direction which they exit the fossa. These branches include the superior alveolar artery, infraorbital artery, greater palatine artery, pharyngeal branch, artery of the pterygoid canal, and sphenopalatine artery [5]. The sphenopalatine artery is the terminal branch of the maxillary artery and supplies the nasal cavity. This artery is commonly responsible for causing epistaxis.

Veins

There is significant variation observed regarding the superficial veins of the head and neck. This chapter will cover the most common pattern observed.

The supratrochlear vein originates in the anterior head and connects to tributaries of the frontal superficial temporal vein. The vein then travels close to midline to reach the surface of the nose, joined by the nasal arch and supraorbital vein, and then collectively courses laterally to form the facial vein near the medial canthus [5]. The supraorbital vein originates near the zygomatic process of the frontal bone and then travels medially above the orbit. The supraorbital vein then joins the supratrochlear vein to form the facial vein. A branch of the supraorbital vein goes through the supraorbital notch to anastomose with the superior ophthalmic vein [5].

The facial vein is formed by the combination of the supratrochlear and supraorbital veins. The facial vein travels obliquely near the side of the nose, where it is also known as the angular vein. The vein then courses posterolaterally under the orbit, then down and posterior to the facial artery until it reaches the angle of the mandible. At the angle of the mandible, it is joined by the retromandibular vein. The facial vein eventually drains into the internal jugular vein at the level of the greater horn of the hyoid bone. The facial vein is connected to the cavernous sinus via the superior ophthalmic vein [5].

The superficial temporal vein originates in the venous network of the scalp. The pterygoid venous plexus is made up of tributaries from the sphenopalatine, deep temporal, pterygoid, masseteric, buccal, dental, greater palatine, and middle meningeal veins. The pterygoid plexus connects to the facial vein via the deep facial vein and with the cavernous sinus via the sphenoidal emissary foramen, foramen ovale, and foramen lacerum [5].

The maxillary vein is a short vein that accompanies the first portion of the maxillary artery. The retromandibular vein lies within the parotid gland, between the external carotid nerve and facial nerve, and is made up of two divisions. The anterior division joins the facial vein, while the posterior division forms the external jugular vein after joining with the posterior auricular vein. The posterior auricular vein is formed in the parieto-occipital network and also receives blood from the occipital and superficial temporal veins while also occasionally receiving tributaries from the auricle and stylomastoid veins. The posterior auricular vein travels inferiorly behind the auricle to join the posterior branch of the retromandibular vein to form the external jugular vein [5].

The occipital vein originates in the posterior venous network of the scalp and joins the deep cervical and vertebral veins to eventually drain into the internal jugular vein [5].

The external jugular vein is formed by the posterior division of the retromandibular vein and the posterior auricular vein near the angle of the mandible. The external jugular vein drains blood from the scalp, face, and subcutaneous tissue. The external jugular vein has a superficial course inferiorly, covered by the platysma, superficial fascia, and skin. Its main tributaries include the posterior external cervical vein, transverse cervical vein, suprascapular vein, and anterior jugular vein. The external jugular vein eventually joins the subclavian vein [5].

The posterior external jugular vein originates in the occipital scalp and drains the skin and muscles to join the middle part of the external jugular vein. The anterior jugular vein originates near the hyoid bone at the junction of the superficial submandibular veins and descends parallel to midline, turning lateral and deep distally to join the external jugular vein. This vein also receives drainage from the laryngeal vein and small thyroid vein. The anterior jugular vein usually connects to the contralateral anterior jugular vein distally by the jugular arch [5].

The internal jugular vein drains blood from the skull, brain, and superficial and deep parts of the neck and face. The vein originates at the jugular foramen at the cranial base as the continuation of the sigmoid sinuses and then descends down the neck in the carotid sheath to eventually join the subclavian vein posterior to the sternal end of the clavicle to form the brachiocephalic vein. The internal jugular vein is located anterior and lateral to the internal carotid artery. Its main tributaries include the inferior petrosal sinus and the facial, lingual, pharyngeal, and superior and middle thyroid veins [5].

The inferior petrosal sinus exits the skull through the anterior part of the jugular foramen and joins the superior jugular bulb (origin of the internal jugular vein). The lingual veins are made up of a dorsal lingual vein that drains the sides and dorsum of the tongue and a deep lingual vein that begins at the tip of the tongue and runs posteriorly along the inferior surface of the tongue [5].

The pharyngeal veins begin at the pharyngeal plexus external to the pharynx, where they join the meningeal veins and eventually drain into the internal jugular vein.

The superior thyroid vein is formed by deep and superficial tributary veins and is joined by the superior laryngeal and cricothyroid veins. The branches of the superior thyroid vein correspond to the branches of the superior thyroid artery and eventually drain into the internal jugular vein.

The middle thyroid vein drains the inferior thyroid gland. The laryngeal and tracheal veins join the middle thyroid vein to drain into the internal jugular vein.

The inferior thyroid vein arises from the venous plexus that also communicates with the middle and superior thyroid veins. The left inferior thyroid vein arises from the plexus and joins the left brachiocephalic vein. The right inferior thyroid vein joins the right brachiocephalic vein at the junction of the origin of the superior vena cava.

The vertebral veins are formed from small tributaries from the internal vertebral plexuses, which arise from the vertebral canal above the posterior arch of the atlas. Small muscular veins form a plexus around the vertebral artery that ends as the vertebral vein, which then emerges from the transverse foramen of the sixth cervical vertebra, descends posterior to the artery, and drains into the posterior aspect of the brachiocephalic vein. Its main tributaries are the occipital vein, muscular veins, veins from the internal and external vertebral plexus, and the anterior vertebral and deep cervical veins [5].

The anterior vertebral vein arises from a plexus around the transverse processes of the upper cervical vertebra. This vein travels and descends parallel to the ascending cervical artery and joins the terminal vertebral vein. The deep cervical vein originates in the suboccipital region as communicating branches from the occipital vein and small muscular venous branches from the posterior neck. This vein receives tributaries from the plexuses around the cervical vertebrae and ends in the lower part of the vertebral veins [5].

Normal Variants

Vertebral artery anatomy may be asymmetric due to vertebral arterial hypoplasia. The absence or termination of the posterior inferior cerebellar artery of one of the vertebral arteries is commonly seen, with a left-dominant vertebral artery the most common variant. Variable origin of the vertebral arteries may also occasionally be seen, with the left vertebral artery originating directly from the aortic arch.

A complete circle of Willis is an arterial vascular circuit in which no component is absent or hypoplastic. Although this is described in the literature, a complete circle of Willis is only seen in a minority of cases. Commonly variants are hypoplasia of one or both posterior communicating arteries, absent or fenestrated anterior communicating artery, hypoplastic or absent A1 segment of the anterior communicating artery, and a fetal origin of the posterior communicating artery. Fetal origin of the posterior communicating artery is seen when the origin of the posterior communicating artery is from the internal carotid artery (instead of originating from the posterior cerebral artery) with an absent or hypoplastic P1 segment of the posterior cerebral artery. In this variant, the posterior circulation is supplied entirely by the ipsilateral internal carotid artery via an enlarged posterior communicating artery.

Congenital absence of one or both internal carotid arteries can occur, but is rare. If one internal carotid artery is absent, intrasellar intercarotid communicating arteries are common. In these individuals, there is a high incidence of associated aneurysms.

Persistent carotid-vertebrobasilar anastomotic connections are commonly seen. During embryogenesis, a number of carotid to basilar connections are formed. However, these connections normally regress soon after birth. However, sometimes these connections persist after birth. They are named for the structures adjacent to its course in the head and neck.

A persistent primitive trigeminal artery is the most common persistent carotid-basilar connection. It represents a persistent embryonic vessel that connects the precavernous segment of the internal carotid artery with the basilar artery. This artery courses adjacent to the trigeminal nerve before joining the basilar artery. This artery is associated with an increased incidence of aneurysms and arteriovenous malformations.

Other less common carotid-basilar connections include a persistent hypoglossal artery, which connects the cervical segment of the internal carotid artery with the basilar artery (Fig. 1.6), and a proatlantal intersegmental artery, which connects the internal carotid artery with the vertebral artery.

The external carotid artery does display variant branching patterns. Commonly seen variants are a common origin of the lingual and facial arteries (linguofacial trunk), common origin of the occipital and posterior auricular arteries, and common origin of the occipital and posterior auricular arteries.

There are some normal dural venous sinus variants, including absence of the hypoplastic transverse sinus. Also seen are hypoplastic sigmoid sinuses or internal jugular veins. A common variant of the torcula herophili is the diversion of the superior sagittal sinus directly into the right transverse sinus and the straight sinus directly into the left transverse sinus.

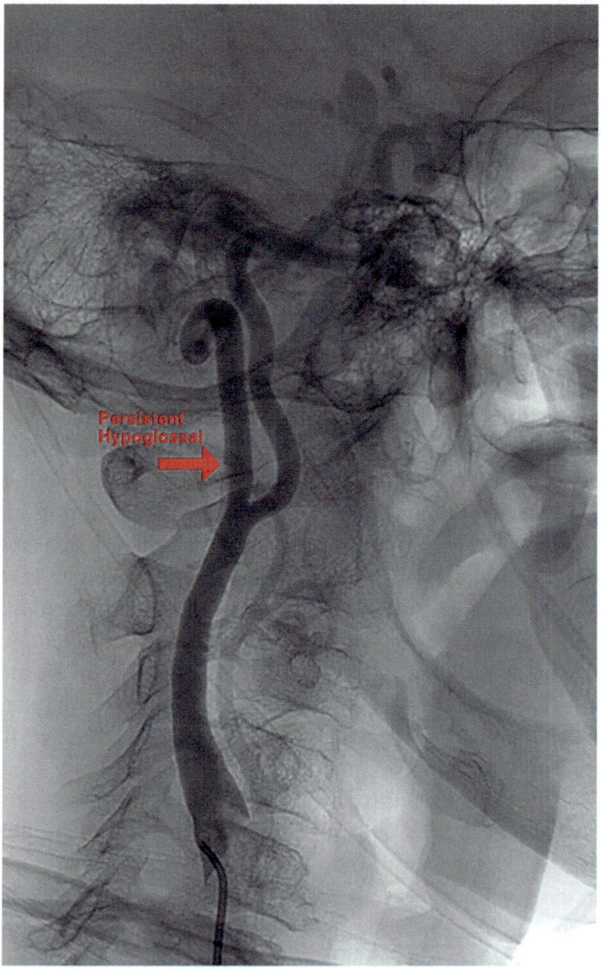

Fig. 1.6 Persistent hypoglossal artery. A persistent carotid-basilar connection connecting the cervical segment of the internal carotid artery with the basilar artery

Chest

The thoracic aorta is divided anatomically into four regions: the root, ascending aorta, transverse aorta (aortic arch), and the descending aorta. The aortic root is the segment of the aorta from the aortic valve annulus to the sinotubular junction. The sinuses of Valsalva are composed of three cusps located above the annulus and terminate at the sinotubular junction. The left and right coronary arteries arise from the left and right sinuses of Valsalva, respectively, while the posterior cusp/sinus is not associated with a coronary artery, and is therefore sometimes referred to as the non-coronary cusp.

The ascending aorta begins at the base of the left ventricle and usually lies approximately 6 cm posterior in relation to the sternum [8].

The aortic arch/transverse aorta originates at the upper border of the right second sternocostal joint. The arch initially courses superoposteriorly, then leftward and anterior to the trachea, and subsequently posteriorly to the left of the trachea. The arch eventually passes inferiorly on the left of the T4 vertebra to continue inferiorly as the descending aorta.

In the majority of the population, there are three branches of the aortic arch, which include (from right to left) the brachiocephalic (innominate) artery, the left common carotid artery, and the left subclavian artery. The brachiocephalic artery then divides into the right subclavian and right common carotid arteries. The segment of the arch between the left subclavian origin and the ligamentum arteriosum is referred to as the isthmus. Just distal to the isthmus, a contour bulge along the lesser curvature can be seen, known as the ductus bump. It should be noted that this is a normal anatomic structure and should not be confused for a pseudoaneurysm.

The aortic arch is categorized into three different types based on the angle between the branches and the aortic arch. The criterion is the vertical distance from the origin of the brachiocephalic artery to the top of the aortic arch. If the distance is less than the diameter of the brachiocephalic artery, the arch is classified as type I. If the distance is between 1 and 2 diameters, it is a type II arch. If the distance is greater than 2 diameters, it is a type III arch [9].

The brachiocephalic artery is the first and largest branch of the aortic arch. It divides into the right subclavian and right common carotid arteries. The right subclavian artery perfuses the upper limb, while the right common carotid artery perfuses the neck and brain. The right vertebral artery arises from the right subclavian artery.

The left common carotid artery is the second branch of the aortic arch. The left subclavian artery arises from the aortic arch shortly after the left common carotid artery.

The descending thoracic aorta begins at the lower level of the T4 vertebral body, descends to the left of the spine, approaches midline, then subsequently travels anterior to the vertebral column as it becomes the abdominal aorta. The descending aorta provides visceral arterial branches to the pericardium, lungs, bronchi, esophagus, and parietal branches to the thoracic wall.

The walls of the descending aorta are perfused by a network of small vessels known as the vasa vasorum, which arise from the intercostal arteries of the thoracic aorta and lumbar arteries from the abdominal aorta [5].

The pulmonary circulation consists of the pulmonary arteries and pulmonary veins. The right and left pulmonary arteries arise from the pulmonary trunk, which originates from the right ventricle of the heart. The pulmonary arteries deliver deoxygenated blood to the lungs. Newly oxygenated blood is then brought back to the heart via the left atrium by the right and left pulmonary veins.

Veins

The brachiocephalic veins are large bilateral veins in the upper thorax formed by the confluence of the internal jugular and subclavian veins. The left subclavian vein lies anterior to the left subclavian and common carotid arteries, following an oblique rightward path to join the right brachiocephalic vein. The right brachiocephalic vein lies anterior to the right brachiocephalic artery and then joins the left brachiocephalic vein to form the superior vena cava. The main tributaries of the left brachiocephalic vein are the left vertebral, internal thoracic, inferior thyroid, superior intercostal, thymic, and pericardiophrenic veins. The tributaries of the right brachiocephalic vein are the right vertebral vein, internal thoracic vein, inferior thyroid vein, and occasionally the first right intercostal vein [5].

The superior vena cava is the main vein for venous drainage of the superior body and drains into the right atrium. The superior vena cava has direct contact with the right lung, pleura, trachea, right pulmonary hilum, and aorta [5]. Its main tributaries include the azygos vein and small mediastinal veins.

The azygos vein is formed by the confluence of the ascending lumbar veins, subcostal veins, and lumbar azygos vein. The azygos vein ascends in the posterior mediastinum to the level of the T4 vertebral body and then subsequently arches anteriorly above the right pulmonary hilum to drain into the superior vena cava. Its main tributaries are the posterior intercostal veins, the hemiazygos vein, the accessory hemiazygos vein, and esophageal, mediastinal, and pericardial veins. The right bronchial veins also drain into the azygos vein near the right hilum [5].

The hemiazygos vein originates on the left side, ascends anteriorly to the spine, and then crosses the vertebral column to the right to reach the azygos vein. Its main tributaries include the lower three posterior intercostal veins, a common venous trunk formed by the left ascending lumbar vein, and the subcostal vein. The accessory hemiazygos vein results from the confluence of numerous posterior intercostal veins and descends laterally to the thoracic spine to drain into the azygos vein. In some instances, the accessory hemiazygos vein drains into the hemiazygos vein instead.

In regard to the spine and spinal cord, numerous venous plexuses freely anastomose with each other to eventually connect with the intervertebral veins [5].

Normal Variants

The aortic arch has a number of variants, including a right aortic arch, cervical aortic arch, or a double aortic arch. A right aortic arch exists if the right fourth primitive arch persists instead of the left fourth arch persisting. The branch vessel origins of the right-sided aortic arch are a mirror image of the left-sided aortic arch. The double aortic arch represents persistent primitive arches. Cervical arches are aortic arches that are unusually high, seen in the thoracic outlet or even in the neck, and represent persistence of the third arch instead of the fourth arch during development.

The normal aortic arch branch pattern is seen in the majority of the population; however, variants do exist. The most common variant seen is the common origin of the brachiocephalic and left common carotid arteries. This is erroneously referred to as a "bovine arch," as a true bovine arch is a single vessel coming from the aortic arch, which then divides into the bilateral subclavian arteries and a bicarotid trunk. Other possible variants include the brachiocephalic artery giving off the left common carotid artery or four branches directly off the aortic arch. Two common scenarios exist for four branches arising from the aortic arch, an aberrant right subclavian artery or direct origin of the left vertebral artery. An aberrant right subclavian artery has its origin directly off the aortic arch distal to the left subclavian artery and then courses behind the esophagus on its way to the right arm. In most cases, patients are asymptomatic. However, in some cases, patients can experience dysphagia secondary to esophageal compression by the right subclavian artery, a clinical scenario known as *dysphagia lusoria* [10]. An aberrant right subclavian artery is clinically important to know for thyroid surgery planning, as the recurrent laryngeal nerve would not be in its usual location [11], which normally loops under the right subclavian artery. Aberrant right subclavian arteries may also become aneurysmal.

Abdomen and Pelvis

Abdominal Aorta

The abdominal aorta starts at the level of the diaphragm as it passes through the aortic hiatus at approximately the T12 vertebral level. The aorta descends slightly lateral to midline in close proximity to the vertebral column. The abdominal aorta bifurcates into the common iliac arteries, at approximately the L4 vertebral level, at the level of the umbilicus [5].

Anteriorly, the abdominal aorta is in close anatomical proximity to the celiac plexus, lesser sac/omental bursa, pancreatic body, and splenic vein. The left renal vein is in close proximity to the anterior aortic wall behind the superior mesenteric vein. On the right of the aorta are the cisterna chyli, thoracic duct, and azygos vein. The right crus of the diaphragm separates the aorta from the inferior vena cava.

More inferiorly, the aorta and inferior vena cava come in contact at around the L2 vertebral level. On the left of the aorta lies the celiac ganglion at the diaphragmatic crus and the duodenojejunal flexure, sympathetic trunk, ascending duodenum, and inferior mesenteric vasculature at the L2 vertebral level.

As the abdominal aorta descends, its diameter decreases as it gives off numerous visceral branches. The ventral branches of the abdominal aorta include the celiac artery, superior mesenteric artery, and inferior mesenteric artery. The celiac artery, also known as the celiac trunk or celiac axis, is the first ventral branch off of the abdominal aorta (Fig. 1.7). It most commonly courses anteriorly in a horizontal direction, but can course cranially or caudally [5]. The three main branches of the celiac trunk are the left gastric artery, common hepatic artery, and splenic artery.

The left gastric artery is the smallest branch of the celiac trunk. It courses cranially to the left behind the omental bursa to the superior portion of the stomach while giving off distal esophageal branches and branches to the gastric fundus. The artery then turns anterior and inferior to run along the lesser curvature of the gastric body, reaches the pylorus, and terminates by forming anastomotic connections with the right gastric artery. The left gastric artery also anastomoses with the splenic artery via short gastric arteries [5].

The common hepatic artery courses anteriorly and to the right toward the porta hepatis. After the takeoff of the gastroduodenal artery, the common hepatic artery becomes the proper hepatic artery. The gastroduodenal artery travels inferiorly between the duodenum and neck of the pancreas and has three branches: anterior and posterior pancreaticoduodenal arcades, the terminal branch, and the right gastroepiploic artery. The pancreaticoduodenal arcades supply the head of the pancreas, pancreatic uncinate process, and duodenal bulb. The anterior pancreaticoduodenal arcade is also called the superior pancreaticoduodenal artery and is a terminal branch of the gastroduodenal artery. This artery forms anastomotic connections with the superior mesenteric artery or inferior pancreaticoduodenal artery [5].

The right gastroepiploic artery is another terminal branch of the gastroduodenal artery. The right gastroepiploic artery courses along the greater curvature of the gastric body and provides the main blood supply to the stomach. This artery anastomoses with branches of the right and left gastric arteries and terminates as it anastomoses with the left gastroepiploic artery along the greater curvature.

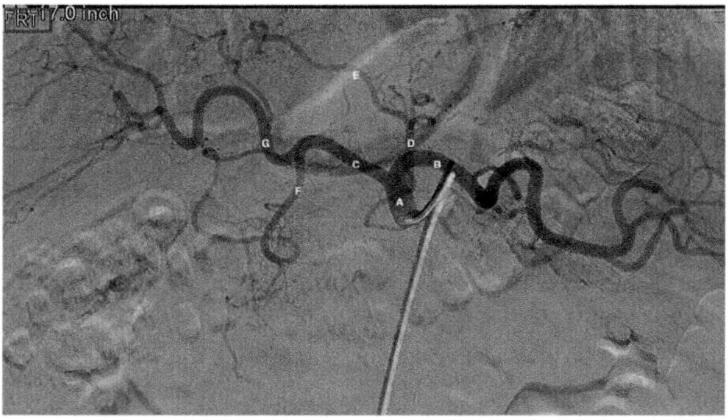

Fig. 1.7 Celiac artery angiogram. A, celiac artery; B, splenic artery; C, common hepatic artery; D, left gastric artery; E, replaced left hepatic artery; F, gastroduodenal artery; G, proper hepatic artery

The hepatic artery also gives rise to the right gastric artery, which can arise from any part of the hepatic artery, and anastomoses with the left gastric artery.

As the proper hepatic artery enters the porta hepatis, the artery bifurcates into the right and left hepatic arteries. The cystic artery usually arises from the right hepatic artery and supplies the gallbladder. The right and left hepatic arteries further subdivide to supply arterial blood to the hepatic parenchyma.

The splenic artery is the largest branch of the celiac trunk and provides branches to the pancreas, stomach, and spleen. Branches of the splenic artery include the dorsal pancreatic artery, short gastric arteries, posterior gastric artery, left gastroepiploic artery, and terminal and segmental splenic branches. The dorsal pancreatic artery usually arises from the splenic artery and supplies the majority of blood to the neck and proximal body of the pancreas. This artery commonly forms anastomotic connections with the gastroduodenal artery.

The short gastric arteries arise from the splenic artery to supply blood to the cranial portion of the greater curvature of the stomach. They can range in number from one artery to up to nine [5]. These arteries anastomose with other gastric branches. The posterior gastric artery arises from the splenic artery to supply the left stomach and omentum.

The splenic artery eventually enters the splenic hilum and divides into multiple segments to supply the splenic parenchyma.

The superior mesenteric artery is the second ventral branch off the abdominal aorta and provides blood to the small intestine, right colon, and majority of the transverse colon (Fig. 1.8). Its origin is approximately 1 centimeter below the takeoff of the celiac trunk, at the T12–L1 level. The branches of the superior mesenteric artery include the inferior pancreaticoduodenal artery, jejunal and ileal branches, ileocolic artery, right colic artery, and middle colic artery [5].

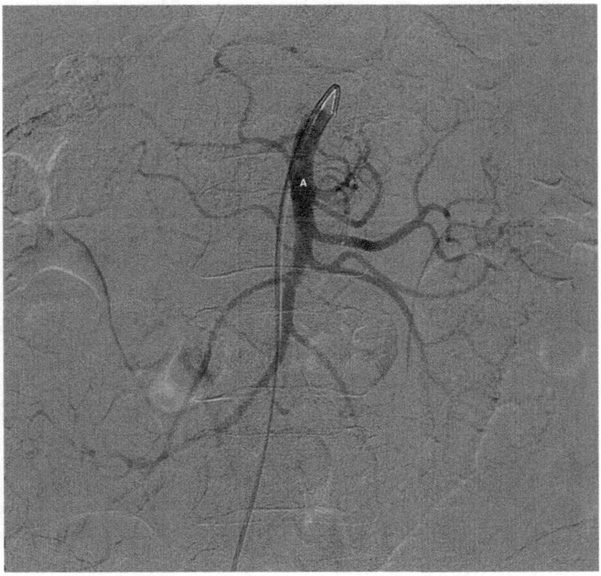

Fig. 1.8 Superior mesenteric artery angiogram. A: superior mesenteric artery

The inferior pancreaticoduodenal artery is the first branch of the superior mesenteric artery from the right side and divides into an anterior and posterior branch. The anterior branch joins the anterior pancreaticoduodenal arcade formed in conjunction with the superior pancreaticoduodenal artery of the gastroduodenal artery and the posterior branch anastomoses with the posterior pancreaticoduodenal arcade. The right colic artery has a retroperitoneal course and supplies the right ascending colon and hepatic flexure. The middle colic artery supplies the majority of the transverse colon. The ileocolic artery is the terminal branch of the superior mesenteric artery and perfuses the terminal ileum, right colon, cecum, and appendix (via the appendicular artery).

The inferior mesenteric artery provides the blood supply to the left third of the transverse colon, descending colon, sigmoid colon, and most of the rectum (Fig. 1.9). Its origin is a few centimeters above the aortic bifurcation, to the left of midline at the L2–L3 vertebral level, and has a significantly smaller diameter when compared to the superior mesenteric artery. The major branches include the left colic artery, which supplies the descending colon; the sigmoid arteries, which run in the sigmoid mesocolon to supply the sigmoid colon; and the superior rectal artery, which supplies the superior rectum.

The lateral branches of the abdominal aorta are the inferior phrenic, middle suprarenal, renal, and gonadal arteries. The inferior phrenic arteries arise from the aorta at or just above the celiac trunk and ascend along the diaphragmatic crura to supply the diaphragm. The arteries give off smaller superior suprarenal branches to partially supply the superior portions of the adrenal glands. The middle suprarenal arteries arise at roughly the same level as the superior mesenteric artery and supply the adrenal glands. The inferior suprarenal artery arises from the renal arteries.

The renal arteries arise laterally at the L1–L2 vertebral level, approximately 1–2 centimeters below the origin of the superior mesenteric artery. Each renal artery gives off one or more inferior suprarenal arteries to perfuse the adrenal gland. The

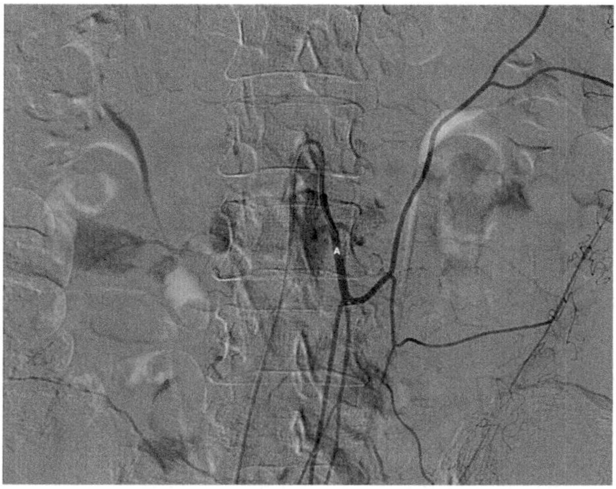

Fig. 1.9 Inferior mesenteric artery angiogram. A: inferior mesenteric artery

renal artery then divides into an anterior and a posterior branch and further subdivides into segmental branches to supply the renal vascular segments.

The gonadal arteries are composed of the testicular arteries in males and ovarian arteries in females. These arteries arise anterolaterally from the abdominal aorta, within a few centimeters below the renal arteries. The arteries descend parallel to their companion gonadal veins, anterior to the inferior vena cava. The right gonadal artery descends anterior to the right ureter, while the left gonadal artery initially descends posterior to the left gonadal vein and then turns anteriorly to the ureter distally [5].

The ovarian arteries course down to the pelvis to supply the ovaries and uterine broad ligament. The ovarian arteries supply the ureters and fallopian tubes and have anastomotic connections with the uterine arteries. The bilateral testicular arteries course into the deep inguinal ring and enter the spermatic cord, into the inguinal canal, and ultimately into the scrotum. The testicular artery supplies blood to the ureter, perirenal fat, iliac lymph nodes, and cremaster muscle.

The dorsal branches of the abdominal aorta include the lumbar and median sacral arteries. Normally, there are four lumbar arteries on each side of the aorta. The branches of these arteries include the dorsal ramus that supplies the dorsal muscles, joints, and integument and spinal and muscular branches. The median sacral artery origin is just above the abdominal aortic bifurcation and descends at midline, anterior to the L4 and L5 vertebra, sacrum, and coccyx. This artery forms anastomotic connections with the rectum, iliolumbar artery, and lateral sacral arteries.

The terminal branches of the abdominal aorta are the common iliac arteries, which start at the L4 vertebral level. The common iliac arteries then bifurcate into the external iliac and internal iliac arteries. The common iliac arteries supply the surrounding tissues and muscles in the pelvis, peritoneum, ureter, and nerves. The common iliac arteries normally do not have branches before they bifurcate.

The internal iliac artery divides into an anterior division and a posterior division. The anterior division perfuses most of the pelvic viscera, while the posterior division perfuses the musculature of the pelvic and gluteal regions. The branches of the anterior division include the superior and inferior vesical arteries, middle rectal artery, uterine artery, vaginal artery, obturator artery, and internal pudendal artery.

The superior vesical artery provides blood to the vesical fundus, ductus deferens, and ureteral arteries, while the inferior vesical artery supplies the vesical fundus, prostate, seminal vesicle, lower ureter, and ductus deferens. The middle rectal artery anastomoses with the superior and inferior rectal arteries and supplies the lower rectum, seminal vesicle, prostate, and walls of the bladder [5].

The uterine artery supplies blood to the ureter, vagina, uterus, broad ligament, and round ligament and generally supplies the medial half of the ovary and medial two thirds of the fallopian tube. The ovarian artery supplies the other portions of the ovary and fallopian tube not supplied by the uterine artery. The vaginal artery provides blood supply to the vagina, vesical fundus, and rectum. The internal pudendal artery is made up of the inferior rectal and inferior gluteal arteries and supplies the external genitalia and muscles of the buttock and thigh.

The branches of the posterior division of the internal iliac artery include the iliolumbar artery, lateral sacral arteries, and superior gluteal artery. The iliolumbar artery consists of an iliac branch that supplies the iliac bone and iliacus muscle and a lumbar branch that supplies the ventral rami of the L5, S1, and S2 nerves, and the psoas major, quadratus lumborum, and erector spinae muscles. The lateral sacral arteries supply the sacral vertebrae, sacral canal, and dorsal sacral muscle and skin. The superior gluteal artery is the largest branch of the internal iliac artery that supplies the gluteal and pelvic structures.

The external iliac artery is the continuation of the common iliac artery as it descends laterally along the psoas major to enter the thigh as it passes posterior to the inguinal ligament to become the femoral artery to perfuse the leg. The branches of the external iliac artery are the inferior epigastric artery and deep circumflex iliac artery. The inferior epigastric artery originates medially from the external iliac artery just above the inguinal ligament. This artery anastomoses with the superior epigastric and lower posterior intercostal arteries [5].

A number of arterial collateral pathways in the abdomen and pelvis exist. The celiac artery forms an anastomosis with the superior mesenteric artery via the superior pancreaticoduodenal artery, off the gastroduodenal artery, and the inferior pancreaticoduodenal artery. A rare short-segment direct connection between the celiac artery and the superior mesenteric artery exists that represents a persistent embryologic remnant, known as the arc of Buhler.

The superior mesenteric artery forms collaterals with the inferior mesenteric artery in a number of anastomotic connections. The arc of Riolan is an anastomosis between the middle colic artery from the superior mesenteric artery and left colic artery from the inferior mesenteric artery. The marginal artery of Drummond is an anastomosis made up of the terminal branches of the ileocolic, right colic, and middle colic arteries of the superior mesenteric artery and the left colic and sigmoid arteries of the inferior mesenteric artery. The artery of Drummond is normally small in diameter but can become prominent in the setting of superior mesenteric or inferior mesenteric artery pathology/disease.

The iliac artery also forms a number of collateral pathways. The external iliac artery forms an anastomotic connection with the thoracic aorta via the inferior epigastric artery from the external iliac artery and the internal thoracic artery from the thoracic aorta. The external iliac artery also anastomoses with the internal iliac artery via the deep circumflex artery and iliolumbar artery. The Winslow pathway is a collateral pathway that connects the intercostal and internal mammary arteries to the external iliac artery via the superior and inferior epigastric arteries, which is commonly seen in the setting of aortoiliac occlusive disease.

Veins

The femoral vein continues superiorly as the external iliac vein. The external iliac vein's main tributaries are the superior gluteal veins, inferior gluteal veins, internal pudendal veins, obturator vein, lateral sacral veins, middle rectal vein, rectal venous plexus, vesical plexus, prostatic venous plexus and dorsal veins of the penis and penile venous plexus (in males), and uterine and vaginal plexuses (in females) [5].

The external iliac vein then joins the internal iliac vein to become the common iliac vein at the level of the sacroiliac joint. The common iliac vein receives tributaries from the iliolumbar vein, lateral sacral vein, inferior epigastric vein, deep circumflex iliac vein, and pubic vein.

The right and left common iliac veins converge at the L4–L5 vertebral level to form the inferior vena cava. The left common iliac vein crosses posterior to the right common iliac artery. This anatomic relationship can be clinically significant, as the left common iliac vein can be compressed by the overlying right common iliac artery, causing a swollen left leg due to venous congestion, a condition known as May-Thurner syndrome.

The inferior vena cava then ascends up the abdomen parallel to the right of the abdominal aorta to carry venous blood from the lower extremities, pelvis, and abdominal structures and organs. In the abdomen, the inferior vena cava receives tributaries from the lumbar veins, ascending lumbar veins, right gonadal vein, right and left renal veins, suprarenal veins, inferior phrenic veins, and right, middle, and left hepatic veins.

The gonadal veins consist of the testicular veins (in males) and ovarian veins (in females). The testicular veins drain the testis and epididymis, while the ovarian veins drain the ovaries. The right gonadal vein drains directly into the inferior vena cava, inferior to the right renal vein, while the left gonadal vein drains directly into the left renal vein.

The hepatic veins drain the hepatic parenchyma via three main hepatic veins: the right, middle, and left hepatic veins. An individual vein separately drains the caudate lobe. The right hepatic vein courses through the right hepatic fissure and divides the right hepatic lobe into anterior segments (segments VIII and V) and posterior segments (segments VI and VII). The middle hepatic vein courses through the middle hepatic fissure and divides the right hepatic lobe from the left hepatic lobe. The middle hepatic lobe drains the medial portion of the left hepatic lobe (segment IV) and also receives some blood from hepatic segment V. The left hepatic vein courses partially at the fissure for the ligamentum teres and at the left hepatic fissure between segments II and III. The left hepatic vein drains the lateral portion of the left hepatic lobe (segments II and III) and receives tributaries from hepatic segment IV. The caudate lobe vein drains the caudate lobe and drains directly into the inferior vena cava at a lower position in relation to the three main hepatic veins. All three main hepatic veins converge into to drain into the inferior vena cava [5].

The portal vein is formed by the splenic vein and the mesenteric vein. The portal vein is anatomically positioned posterior to the pancreatic head and anterior to the inferior vena cava. The portal vein carries visceral blood to the liver, where it reaches the sinusoids, and then subsequently drains into the hepatic veins and ultimately the inferior vena cava. At the porta hepatis, the portal vein lies posterior to the bile duct and hepatic artery. The bile duct lies anterolateral to the portal vein, while the hepatic artery is situated medially.

The portal vein divides into right and left branches at the porta hepatis. The right portal vein receives the cystic vein and then enters the right hepatic lobe, where it divides into the four segments of the right hepatic lobe (segments V, VI, VII, and VIII). The left portal vein enters the right hepatic lobe and then branches into the four segments of the left hepatic lobe (segments I, IV, II, and III).

The main tributaries of the portal vein include the paraumbilical veins, ligamentum teres, right and left gastric veins, and cystic veins. The right gastric vein courses along the lesser curvature of the stomach to eventually join the portal vein, while the left gastric vein courses upward in the lesser curvature of the stomach and through the lesser omentum to eventually reach the portal vein. The left gastric vein shares numerous anastomoses with the lower esophageal veins. The paraumbilical veins extend along the ligamentum teres and medial umbilical ligament to connect veins of the anterior abdominal wall to the left portal vein, which provides a potential portosystemic shunt.

The splenic vein is a large vein (measuring approximately 1 cm) that forms from multiple smaller segmental veins at the splenic hilum to travel posterior to the pancreatic body and tail while receiving numerous pancreatic venous branches and tributaries such as the short gastric veins, left gastroepiploic vein, and pancreatic veins. The short gastric veins drain the gastric fundus and part of the greater curvature and share anastomotic connections with the lower esophageal veins, which can become enlarged in the setting of portal hypertension. The left gastroepiploic vein runs along the greater curvature of the stomach to reach the splenic vein, while the pancreatic veins drain the pancreatic body and tail then drain into the splenic vein.

The superior mesenteric vein drains portions of the stomach, pancreas, small intestine, cecum, ascending colon, and transverse colon. It is formed by the tributaries of the jejunal and ileal veins, ileocolic vein, right and middle colic veins, right gastroepiploic vein, and pancreaticoduodenal veins. The superior mesenteric vein courses behind the pancreatic head and horizontal portion of the duodenum and anterior to the inferior vena cava to join the splenic vein.

The inferior mesenteric vein drains the rectum, sigmoid colon, and left colon. Its main tributaries include the superior rectal vein, sigmoid veins, and left colic vein. The inferior mesenteric vein usually drains into the splenic vein and then eventually into the portal vein.

The inferior vena cava eventually converges with the superior vena cava, azygos vein, and coronary sinus in the thoracic cavity to empty into the right atrium.

Normal Variants

As noted above, the anatomy of the celiac trunk is highly variable. The normal celiac artery branches are seen in approximately 75% of the population, but in the other cases, the right and left hepatic arteries may be duplicated ("accessory" hepatic artery) or originate from a vessel other than the proper hepatic artery ("replaced" hepatic artery) [5]. In a replaced or accessory right hepatic artery, the right hepatic artery arises from the superior mesenteric artery. In a replaced or accessory left hepatic artery, the left hepatic artery arises from the left gastric artery (Fig. 1.10). A replaced right hepatic artery can be clinically significant in the setting of abdominal surgery, superior mesenteric artery pathology, or transarterial hepatic intervention. A replaced left hepatic artery can be clinically significant in the setting of a surgical gastrectomy, when resection of this artery can predispose to left hepatic lobe ischemia/injury.

In regard to renal arteries, the majority of the population have single renal arteries supplying both kidneys. However, accessory renal arteries are occasionally seen (Fig. 1.11). These accessory arteries can arise from the abdominal aorta either above or below the main renal artery, following it into the renal hilum.

A persistent sciatic artery is a rare vascular embryological anomaly where the fetal sciatic artery persists to supply the majority of the blood supply to the leg

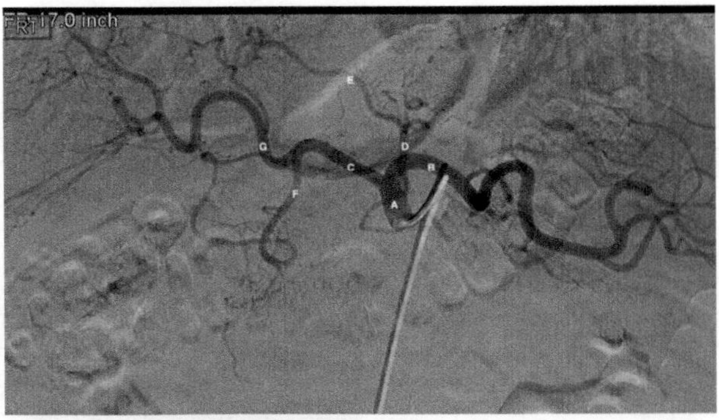

Fig. 1.10 Celiac artery angiogram. Celiac artery angiogram demonstrates a replaced left hepatic artery (E) from the left gastric artery (D), an anatomic variant. A, celiac artery; B, splenic artery; C, common hepatic artery; D, left gastric artery; E, replaced left gastric artery; F, gastroduodenal artery; G, proper hepatic artery

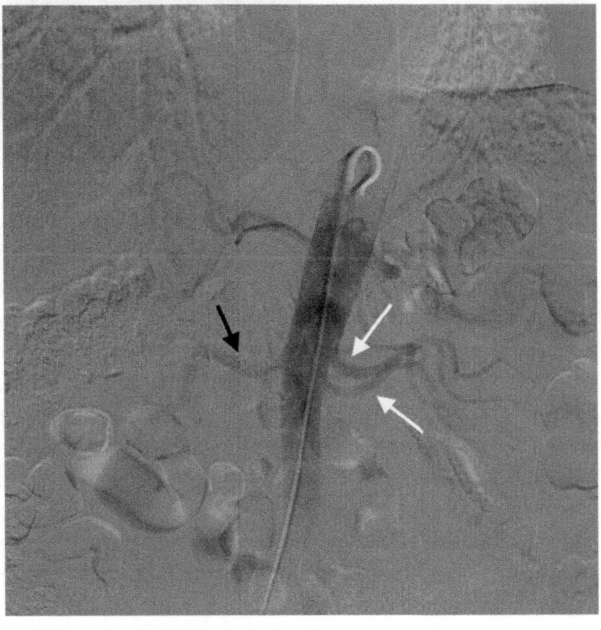

Fig. 1.11 Abdominal aorta angiogram. Abdominal aortic angiogram performed demonstrates a single right renal artery (black arrow) and two left renal arteries (white arrows)

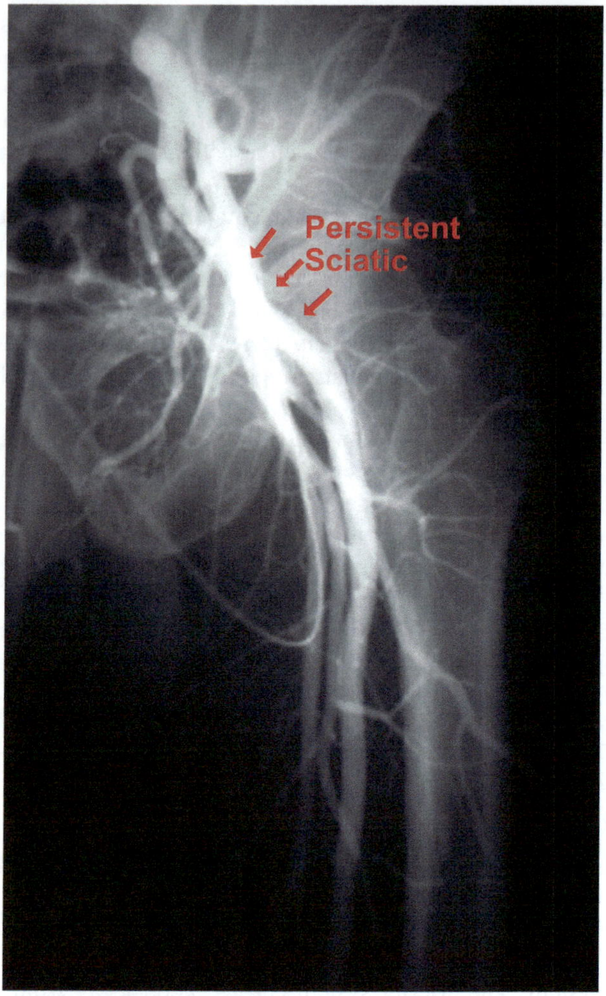

Fig. 1.12 Left lower extremity arterial angiogram. Angiography of the left lower extremity arterial system demonstrates a persistent sciatic artery (red arrows)

(Fig. 1.12) [5, 12]. This variant represents a continuation of the internal iliac artery with continuation distally to the popliteal artery. During early fetal development, this artery supplies the majority of the blood to the lower limb. The sciatic artery normally regresses around the third month of embryologic life, after the superficial femoral artery develops from the external iliac artery and connects to the popliteal artery. If the femoral vascular system does not develop, the sciatic artery becomes dominant, and a rudimentary femoral artery remains. The persistent sciatic artery passes posterior to the femur in the thigh to eventually anastomose with the distal vasculature in the leg. Individuals with a persistent sciatic artery may be predisposed to aneurysm formation [12], early atherosclerotic changes within the vessel, and critical limb ischemia. Furthermore, this persistent artery can have clinical significance, as not identifying this vascular anomaly can lead to inappropriate surgical bypass of assumed occlusive disease of the superficial femoral artery.

Upper Extremities

Arteries

The right subclavian artery originates from the brachiocephalic artery and is divided into three segments by the anterior scalene muscle. The first segment part of the artery is immediately after its origin off the brachiocephalic artery to the medial border of the anterior scalene muscle. This first segment gives off three of the branches of the subclavian artery: the vertebral artery, internal mammary/thoracic artery, and thyrocervical trunk. The second segment of the subclavian artery courses behind the right sternoclavicular joint and passes superiorly behind the anterior scalene muscle. The segment gives off the costocervical trunk. The third segment of the artery courses horizontally and slightly inferiorly from the lateral border of the anterior scalene muscle to the outer border of the first rib at the origin of the superior thoracic artery. The dorsal scapular artery arises from the third segment of the subclavian artery.

The left subclavian artery originates from the aortic arch, after the origin of the left common carotid artery. The first segment ascends in the direction of the neck and then turns laterally to cross behind the left anterior scalene muscle. The second and third segments follow the same course as the right subclavian artery. Unlike the right subclavian artery, the costovertebral trunk arises from the second segment of the left subclavian artery.

The branches of the internal mammary/thoracic artery include the pericardiophrenic artery, mediastinal artery, pericardial branches, intercostal branches, perforating branches, musculophrenic artery, and superior epigastric artery. The thyrocervical trunk produces three branches: the inferior thyroid artery, suprascapular artery, and superficial cervical artery. The branches of the costovertebral trunk are the superior intercostal artery, which supplies the first two intercostal spaces, and the deep cervical artery, which supplies the deep posterior cervical muscles.

As the subclavian artery travels down the arm, its name changes. As the subclavian artery passes the outer border of the first rib, it becomes the axillary artery. The branches of the axillary artery are the superior thoracic artery, thoracoacromial artery, lateral thoracic artery, subscapular artery, and anterior and posterior circumflex humeral arteries.

As the axillary artery passes the lower border of the teres major muscle, the artery becomes the brachial artery. The brachial artery courses down the arm, medially to the humerus and then eventually anterior to the humerus. The branches of the brachial artery include the profunda brachial artery, the main nutrient artery of the humerus, muscular branches (coracobrachialis, biceps, brachialis), and the superior and inferior ulnar collateral arteries.

At the radial head, the brachial artery bifurcates into the ulnar and radial arteries. The ulnar artery gives off the common interosseous artery, which then bifurcates into the anterior and posterior interosseous arteries. The radial artery runs through the forearm and wrist, until it reaches the hand. The branches of the radial artery are the radial recurrent artery, muscular branches, and palmar carpal branch. The ulnar artery begins at the radial neck, passing down and medial to reach the ulnar side of the forearm, and then crosses lateral to the pisiform bone at the wrist. The ulnar artery typically supplies the superficial palmar arch in the hand, while the radial artery supplies the deep palmar arch.

Veins

In the hand laterally, the dorsal venous network joins with the dorsal digital vein from the radial side of the index finger and both dorsal digital veins of the thumb to continue proximally as the cephalic vein. Medially, the dorsal venous network is joined by the dorsal digital vein from the ulnar side of the fifth finger and continues proximally as the basilic vein.

In the upper limb, the veins can be categorized into the superficial and deep venous systems. The superficial veins of the forearm are the cephalic vein, basilic vein, and median vein of the forearm. The cephalic and basilic veins drain blood from the superficial tissues of the upper arm. The cephalic vein ascends subcutaneously lateral to the biceps to drain into the axillary vein just below the level of the clavicle in the infraclavicular fossa. The basilic vein ascends subcutaneously in the dorsal side of the forearm and then moves forward to the ventral surface. It is joined proximally by the median cubital vein and then ascends between the biceps and pronator teres muscles. At the shoulder level, the basilic vein perforates the deep fascia to continue as the axillary vein. The median vein of the forearm is formed by the superficial palmar venous plexus and ends in the basilic or median cubital vein [5].

The deep veins of the hand and upper arm are companions of the arteries and follow their respective courses up the forearm. The superficial and palmar arterial arches are accompanied by the superficial and deep palmar venous arches. The common palmar digital veins open into the superficial palmar venous arch, and the palmar metacarpal veins drain into the deep palmar venous arch.

In the forearm, the radial, interosseous, and ulnar veins accompany their companion arteries and eventually connect at the elbow to form the brachial vein. The brachial vein receives venous tributaries in the forearm and travels proximally to join the basilic vein to form the axillary vein at the shoulder.

The axillary vein begins at the lower border of the teres major muscle as the continuation of the basilic vein. The major tributary of the axillary vein is the cephalic vein. The axillary vein continues up to the outer border of the first rib, where it becomes the subclavian vein. The subclavian vein courses from the outer border of the first rib to the medial border of the anterior scalene muscle. The subclavian vein is located anterior and inferior to the subclavian artery and is protected by the clavicle. The subclavian vein receives tributaries from the external jugular and dorsal scapular veins. The subclavian vein continues medially, where it eventually joins the internal jugular vein to form the brachiocephalic vein. The bilateral brachiocephalic veins coalesce together on the right side of the thorax to form the superior vena cava.

Normal Variants

The subscapular, circumflex humeral, and profunda brachii can arise at a common origin. The axillary artery may divide into the ulnar and radial arteries instead of the brachial artery. Occasionally, the anterior interosseous artery persists and supplies the deep palmar arch of the hand instead of the radial artery. Also, in some instances, the radial artery can originate from either the axillary artery or at the proximal brachial artery, known as a high origin of the radial artery.

An accessory cephalic vein may be present in some cases.

Lower Extremities

Arteries

The external iliac artery becomes the common femoral artery as it gives off the inferior epigastric artery usually around the level of the inguinal ligament. Branches of the common femoral artery include the superficial epigastric artery, superficial circumflex iliac artery, and superficial and deep external pudendal arteries.

The common femoral artery then bifurcates into the deep femoral (profunda femoris) artery and the superficial femoral artery (Fig. 1.13). The deep femoral artery supplies the deep muscles of the thigh, while the superficial femoral artery continues down the leg to supply the leg and foot.

The superficial femoral artery descends anteriorly and medially into the flexor muscle compartment known as the adductor hiatus (Hunter's canal) and then emerges from the canal as the popliteal artery. At the distal border of the popliteus muscle, the popliteal artery divides into the anterior tibial artery and the tibioperoneal trunk (Fig. 1.14). The tibioperoneal trunk further divides into the posterior tibial and peroneal (fibular) arteries. The posterior tibial artery is the most medial artery in the calf and the anterior tibial artery is the most lateral.

The anterior tibial artery is the only anterior artery of the lower leg and courses anterior and lateral down the leg, traverses the interosseous membrane, and then runs down the front of the anterior tibia to terminate as the dorsalis pedis artery at the dorsum of the foot. The posterior tibial artery terminates into the medial and lateral plantar arteries in the foot. The lateral plantar artery anastomoses with the dorsalis pedis artery to complete the plantar arch [5].

Veins

The veins of the lower extremity are divided into three main divisions: deep, superficial, and perforating. These veins are located in two compartments, deep and superficial, with the deep compartment separated by muscular fascia and the superficial component separated by the muscular fascia below and by the dermis above [13].

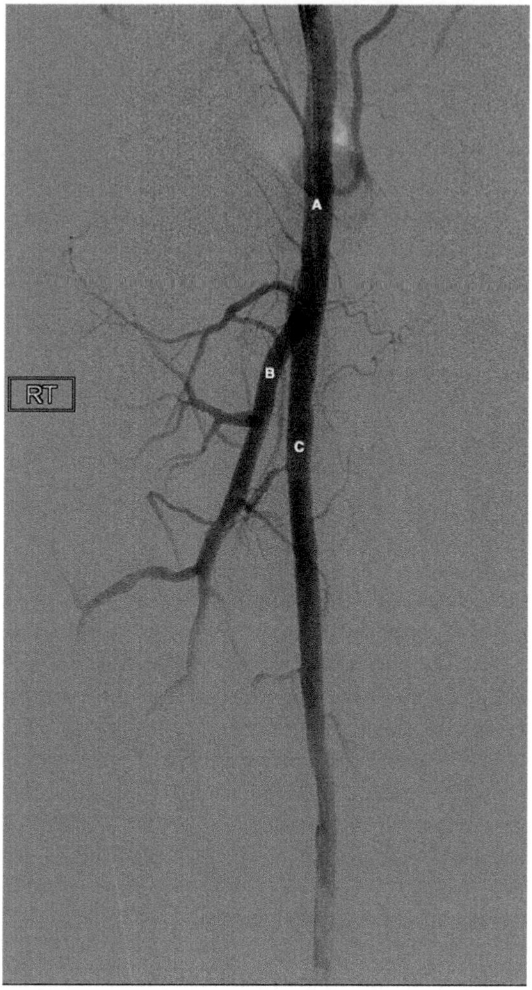

Fig. 1.13 Common femoral artery angiogram. A, common femoral artery; B, deep femoral (profunda femoris) artery; C, superficial femoral artery

The deep venous system in the calf is composed of six paired veins that are in close proximity to their corresponding artery and are named the anterior tibial, posterior tibial, and peroneal veins. These veins ascend individually to eventually join together in the lower popliteal space to form the popliteal vein. The posterior tibial vein is the most medial vein in the calf, with the anterior tibial being the most lateral.

The superficial venous system is composed of the great and small saphenous veins. The great saphenous vein originates at the medial aspect of the foot as the continuation of the medial marginal vein of the foot and receives deep pedal tributaries as it ascends anteromedially within the calf. The great saphenous vein then continues medially to the knee and into the thigh. The great saphenous vein eventually drains into the common femoral vein at the saphenofemoral junction,

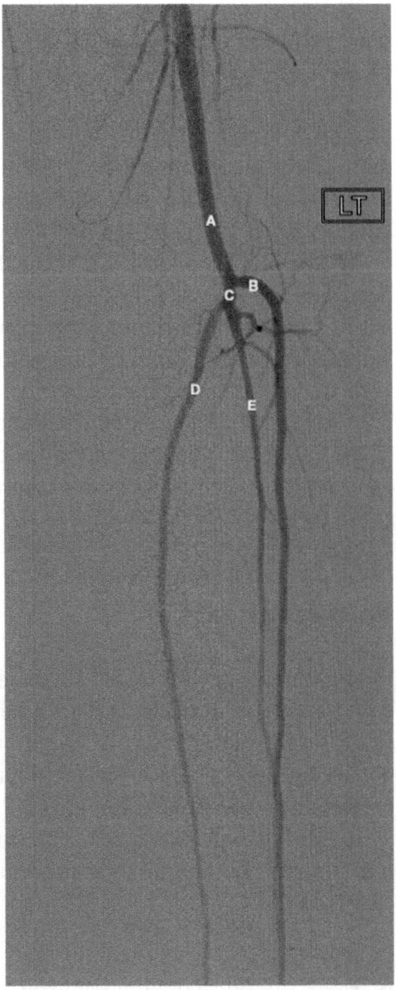

Fig. 1.14 Lower extremity angiogram. A, popliteal artery; B, anterior tibial artery; C, tibioperoneal trunk; D, posterior tibial artery; E, peroneal artery

a confluence located just below the inguinal ligament. At the groin, the great saphenous vein receives tributaries from the external pudendal vein, superficial epigastric vein, and external circumflex veins before entering the saphenofemoral junction.

The great saphenous vein is the longest vein in the body and is clinically significant, as it is frequently used for cardiac and peripheral vascular procedures. Anterior and posterior accessory saphenous veins are veins that run parallel anteriorly and posteriorly, respectively, to the great saphenous vein.

The small saphenous vein originates in the lateral foot as the continuation of the lateral marginal vein of the foot and ascends posterolaterally in the lower calf. In the upper calf, the vein courses through the two heads of the gastrocnemius muscle and travels superiorly until it enters the popliteal space to drain into the popliteal vein.

The popliteal vein receives tributaries from the small saphenous vein, gastrocnemius vein, and other muscular veins. Above the adductor canal, at the upper margin of the popliteal fossa, the popliteal vein becomes the femoral vein. The name "superficial femoral vein" is now not commonly used as it is actually a deep vein. The deep femoral (profunda femoris) vein drains the deep muscles of the lateral thigh and then connects with the popliteal vein. In clinical situations where the femoral vein occludes with thrombus, the deep femoral vein serves as a critical collateral vessel. The deep femoral vein lies anterior to the profunda femoris artery.

The common femoral vein forms from the confluence of the femoral vein and the deep femoral vein and then becomes the external iliac vein at the level of the inguinal ligament. The common femoral vein lies medial to the common femoral artery. Tributaries of the common femoral vein are the muscular veins, profunda femoris vein, and great saphenous vein [5].

Above the inguinal ligament, the external iliac vein is the final common pathway of the venous drainage of the lower extremity. The internal iliac vein then joins the external iliac vein to form the common iliac vein, where it joins the contralateral common iliac vein at the level of the L4 vertebra to form the inferior vena cava.

Normal Variants

In two thirds of patients, the small saphenous vein drains entirely into the popliteal vein just above the knee at the saphenopopliteal junction. In a third of patients, the small saphenous vein can drain into a posterior medial tributary of the great saphenous vein, directly into the great saphenous vein, or into the femoral vein via a perforating vein in the thigh [13].

In other variant drainage of the small saphenous vein, the saphenopopliteal junction may not be present, and the small saphenous vein can be duplicated in 4% of cases [13].

References

1. Udan RS, Culver JC, Dickinson ME. Understanding vascular development. Wiley Interdiscip Rev Dev Biol. 2013;2(3):327–46.
2. Chappell JC, Bautch VL. Chapter 2: Vascular development: genetic mechanisms and links to vascular disease. In: Koopman P, editor. Current topics in developmental biology, vol. 90. Amsterdam: Academic Press; 2010. p. 43–72.
3. Ribatti D, Nico B, Crivellato E. The development of the vascular system: a historical overview. In: Walker JM, Ribatti D, editors. Vascular morphogenesis: methods and protocols. New York: Springer New York; 2015. p. 1–14.
4. Tahir RA, Haider S, Kole M, Griffith B, Marin H. Anterior cerebral artery: variant anatomy and pathology. J Vasc Interv Neurol. 2019;10(3):16–22.
5. Uflacker R. Atlas of vascular anatomy: an angiographic approach. 2nd ed. Philadelphia: Lippincott Williams & Wilkins; 2006.
6. Kuybu O, Tadi P, Dossani RH. Posterior cerebral artery stroke. StatPearls. Treasure Island: StatPearls Publishing LLC; 2020.

7. Natali AL, Leo JT. Neuroanatomy, middle meningeal arteries. StatPearls. Treasure Island: StatPearls Publishing LLC; 2020.
8. Bavry AA, Kumbhani DJ. Indications and techniques of percutaneous procedures: coronary, peripheral and structural heart disease. Springer; 2012.
9. Madhwal S, Rajagopal V, Bhatt DL, Bajzer CT, Whitlow P, Kapadia SR. Predictors of difficult carotid stenting as determined by aortic arch angiography. J Invasive Cardiol. 2008;20(5):200–4.
10. Whitley A. Dysphagia lusoria: a case study. J Vasc Nurs. 2001;19(1):14–7; quiz 8-9.
11. Polednak AP. Anatomical variation in the right non-recurrent laryngeal nerve reported from studies using pre-operative arterial imaging. Surg Radiol Anat. 2019;41(8):943–9.
12. Brantley SK, Rigdon EE, Raju S. Persistent sciatic artery: embryology, pathology, and treatment. J Vasc Surg. 1993;18(2):242–8.
13. Almeida JI. Chapter 1: Venous anatomy. In: Almeida JI, editor. Atlas of endovascular venous surgery. 2nd ed. Philadelphia: Content Repository Only! 2019. p. 1–20.

Impact of Hemorrhage, Thrombosis, and Ischemia

2

Jeremy Ward and Arsalan Amin

Abbreviations

α	Alpha angle
AD	Autosomal dominant
ADP	Adenosine diphosphate
ALI	Acute limb ischemia
AR	Autosomal recessive
ATLS	Advanced trauma life support
ATP	Adenosine triphosphate
CABG	Coronary artery bypass graft
CLI	Chronic limb ischemia
CO	Cardiac output
COX	Cyclooxygenase
Cr	Creatinine
CT	Computed tomography
CTA	Computed tomography angiography
CVP	Central venous pressure
DAPT	Dual antiplatelet therapy
DDAVP	Desmopressin
DIC	Disseminated intravascular coagulation
DOAC	Direct oral anticoagulant
DVT	Deep vein thrombosis
FFP	Fresh frozen plasma
FIO_2	Fraction of inspired oxygen
GCS	Glasgow coma scale

J. Ward (✉) · A. Amin
Micahel E. DeBakey Department of Surgery, Baylor College of Medicine, Houston, TX, USA
e-mail: Jeremy.Ward@bcm.edu; Arsalan.Amin@bcm.edu

R. Gilani, J. L. Mills Sr. (eds.), *Vascular Complications of Surgery and Intervention*, https://doi.org/10.1007/978-3-030-86713-3_2

Gp1b	Glycoprotein Ib
GPIIb–IIIa	Glycoprotein IIb–IIIa
Hb	Hemoglobin
Hct	Hematocrit
Hep-PF4	Heparin-platelet factor 4
HIT	Heparin-induced thrombocytopenia
HITT	Heparin-induced thrombocytopenia and thrombosis
INR	International normalized ratio
IVC	Inferior vena cava
LMWH	Low-molecular-weight heparin
LY30	Fibrinolysis at 30 min
MA	Maximum amplitude
MAP	Mean arterial pressure
MTP	Massive transfusion protocol
NOAC	Novel oral anticoagulant
NOMI	Nonocclusive mesenteric ischemia
P_aO_2	arterial partial oxygen pressure
PCWP	Pulmonary capillary wedge pressure
PE	Pulmonary embolism
PLTs	Platelets
PT	Prothrombin time
PTT	Partial thromboplastin time
RoS	Reactive oxygen species
SMA	Superior mesenteric artery
SOFA	Sequential Organ Failure Assessment
SvO_2	Venous oxygen saturation
SVR	Systemic vascular resistance
TB	Total bilirubin
TBI	Traumatic brain injury
TEG	Thromboelastography
tPA	Tissue plasminogen activator
TXA	Tranexamic acid
TxA_2	Thromboxane A_2
V/Q	Ventilation/perfusion
VTE	Venous thromboembolism
vWD	von Willebrand disease
vWF	von Willebrand factor

Introduction

Surgical patients are often afflicted by coagulopathy and hemorrhage, both of which can serve to limit adequate tissue perfusion resulting in ischemic injury. While some patients maybe at increased risk of thrombosis or hemorrhage due to inherent disorders or medications, those who are critically ill are at an increased risk of ischemic insults caused by derangements in the mechanisms involved in maintaining homeostasis. Thus hemorrhage, thrombosis, and ischemia are intimately related conditions.

Hemorrhage

Before delving into various etiologies of hemorrhage, one must begin with a basic understanding of the mechanisms required to achieve hemostasis [1–3]. Initial response to injury involves a transient vasoconstrictive period followed by endothelial expression of von Willebrand factor (vWF). Platelet adherence to vWF at the site of injury is mediated by glycoprotein Ib (GpIb) receptors with ensuing platelet activation to release adenosine diphosphate (ADP) and thromboxane A_2 (TxA_2). These factors induce further platelet chemoattraction to assist in primary hemostasis through the formation of a platelet plug, as aggregated platelets bind one another via glycoprotein IIb–IIIa (GpIIb–IIIa) receptors. Following the formation of a platelet plug, tissue factor (factor III) mediates the activation of the coagulation cascade, resulting in the formation of a stabilized fibrin clot. The extrinsic pathway is triggered by exposure of tissue factor in response to injury and defined by measurement of the prothrombin time (PT). The intrinsic pathway is triggered by surface contact activation of coagulation factor XII (Hageman factor), prekallikrein, and high-molecular-weight kininogen and is monitored via the partial thromboplastin time (PTT). The extrinsic pathway is dependent upon factor VII, while the intrinsic pathway involves factors VIII, IX, XI, and XI. The extrinsic and intrinsic pathways converge into the common pathway which involves factors X, V, II (prothrombin) and I (fibrinogen) and results in the formation of cross-linked fibrin. Thrombin (factor IIa) is crucial in the coagulation cascade for its role in activating multiple other clotting factors and promoting platelet activation and aggregation. The coagulation cascade is a highly autoregulated process through the activation of inhibitory mechanisms, including the expression of tissue plasminogen activator (tPA) and thrombomodulin, to confine the hemostatic process at the site of tissue injury.

Although several mechanisms exist through which cells and tissues suffer ischemic insults, common etiologies observed in surgical patients involve the loss of circulatory blood volume as a result of hemorrhage. Clinically, the effects of hemorrhage are dependent upon the underlying etiology and source of blood loss, the volume and rate of blood loss, and the body's ability to achieve hemostasis [1]. The etiology of hemorrhage is typically related to traumatic injuries, surgical blood loss, vascular injury complicating surgery, or postoperative hemorrhage. This can be further complicated through the use of antiplatelet or anticoagulation medications. Additionally, it has been well established that uncontrollable bleeding is the most common cause of preventable death due to trauma. Furthermore, the physiologic and hemodynamic manifestations associated with hemorrhage correlate with the degree of blood loss.

A key principle in the management of hemorrhage, whether traumatic or perioperative, involves a rapid yet thorough assessment of the patient to identify and subsequently control the source of the bleeding. Hemorrhage from external wounds or that associated with extremity trauma can be controlled through the application of direct manual pressure and/or the use of a tourniquet [4]. Patients with blunt or penetrating trauma presenting in extremis with hemodynamic instability or hard signs of vascular injury should be taken emergently to the operating room for resuscitation and damage control surgery [4, 5]. Otherwise, blunt or penetrating trauma injuries without indications for emergent exploration require further diagnostic workup. This typically includes contrast-enhanced computed tomography (CT) or CT angiography (CTA) imaging. Intraoperative hemorrhage is generally easily recognized; however, difficulty gaining control of the source may result in significant blood loss. Blood loss may be exacerbated when the bleeding is not in the immediate operative field, or when a minimally invasive approach must be converted to an open one for management. Similarly, postoperative hemorrhage may be complicated by delay in diagnosis and the need to return to the operating room for control.

While there exist several etiologies which drive hemorrhagic diatheses, several are more frequently encountered in the clinical setting of surgical or trauma patients [6]. It is imperative to keep in mind that some hemorrhagic disorders also exhibit a simultaneous component of thrombosis.

The most common inherited bleeding disorders include von Willebrand disease (vWD) and hemophilia A, with vWD being the more prevalent and vWD type I being the most common of the subtypes. Interestingly, vWF and factor VIII are synthesized and secreted by endothelial cells, unlike the other clotting factors which are produced by hepatocytes [7]. vWD types I (AD) and III (AR) are characterized by a quantitative deficiency of vWF, while vWD type II (AD) is characterized by a qualitative defect in vWF. The consequence of vWD lies within deficient platelet adhesion and subsequent clot formation. Desmopressin (DDAVP) is the mainstay of treatment for vWD types I and II, stimulating the release of vWF from endothelial cells; however, vWD type III is characterized by the complete absence of vWF, rendering DDAVP ineffective. Hemophilia A is an X-linked recessive disorder resulting in varying degrees of factor VIII deficiency. Characterized by severe hemorrhage in association with traumatic injuries or operative procedures, patients additionally suffer from problematic joints caused by repeat bouts of spontaneous joint space hemorrhage (hemarthrosis). The predominant treatment of hemophilia A involves the transfusion of recombinant factor VIII.

Heparin-induced thrombocytopenia (HIT) is driven by the formation of antibodies against the heparin-platelet factor 4 (Hep-PF4) complex with the potential for paradoxical development of thrombosis (HITT). Patients suspected to have HITT are screened by calculating a 4 T score and an ELISA to detect the antibody; however, confirmatory testing relies on a serotonin release assay. HITT should be treated by stopping all heparin use (including flushes) and starting a non-heparin-based anticoagulant (e.g., bivalirudin); however, in the setting of hemorrhage, this can propose a serious predicament.

Disseminated intravascular coagulation (DIC) is a thrombohemorrhagic disorder characterized by widespread activation of the clotting cascade with consequent microvascular thrombi formation and a consumptive coagulopathy. A combination of these derangements contributes to tissue hypoxia and ischemic injury. DIC is triggered by the release of tissue factor and thromboplastic substances or through TNF-mediated endothelial injury; the primary etiologies responsible for DIC include severe trauma, sepsis, obstetric complications, or malignant neoplasms. The diagnosis is characterized by a prolonged PT and PTT, thrombocytopenia, decreased levels of fibrinogen, and increased levels of fibrin degradation products. Treatment of DIC involves addressing the underlying etiology and providing supportive care.

Although not characterized as intrinsic disorders, the use of antiplatelet or anticoagulation medications often complicates the management of hemorrhage; this situation is most frequently encountered in patients with atherosclerotic disease, history of blood clots, arrhythmias (e.g., atrial fibrillation), or mechanical heart valves. Aspirin irreversibly binds to cyclooxygenase (COX-1 and COX-2) enzymes, inhibiting the production of TxA_2 and consequently inhibiting platelet aggregation. Clopidogrel (Plavix) is also an antiplatelet agent, often used to reduce rates of myocardial infarctions and cerebrovascular accidents, as well as to increase patency rates of coronary and vascular stents as part of dual antiplatelet therapy (DAPT) modality with concurrent use of aspirin. Similar to the end result of aspirin, clopidogrel irreversibly prevents platelet aggregation through inhibition of ADP receptors. Although they have different mechanisms of action, aspirin and clopidogrel render platelets ineffective for approximately 7 days. A commonly utilized anticoagulant, warfarin (Coumadin) disrupts the coagulation cascade by inhibiting vitamin K-dependent clotting factors (II, VII, IX, and X). Warfarin also inhibits proteins C and S (anticoagulant regulatory proteins) resulting in an initial period of transient hypercoagulability with an associated link to an adverse phenomenon recognized as warfarin-induced skin necrosis. This unfavorable effect is often avoided through the concurrent use of heparin, until therapeutic effects of warfarin are achieved, in a practice recognized as "bridging therapy." The anticoagulation effects of warfarin can be negated in emergent situations by the administration of prothrombin complex concentrate (PCC; KCentra), the transfusion of fresh frozen plasma (FFP), or administration of intravenous phytomenadione (vitamin K). Although relatively inexpensive, a drawback to the use of warfarin is the requirement to regularly monitor the prothrombin time (PT)/international normalized ratio (INR) to maintain therapeutic levels of anticoagulation [7]. In response to this cumbersome detail, a newer class of drugs has emerged, known as the novel oral anticoagulants or direct oral anticoagulants (NOAC/DOAC). Most commonly encountered are apixaban (Eliquis) or rivaroxaban (Xarelto) which selectively inhibit factor Xa, or dabigatran (Pradaxa) which selectively inhibits factor IIa (thrombin) [8]. The anticoagulant properties of apixaban or rivaroxaban can be reversed through the administration of PCC, while dabigatran can be reversed with a specific monoclonal antibody, idarucizumab (Praxbind), or hemodialysis.

In the critically ill surgical patient, concurrent dysfunction of multiple organ systems often exists which can also contribute to derangements in achieving hemostasis. Nutritionally deficient patients and those with the inability to absorb fat-soluble vitamins have increased propensity for deficiency of vitamin K-dependent clotting factors II, VII, IX, and X. The liver is also responsible for the production of the majority of procoagulant and anticoagulant factors; thus hepatic dysfunction may be associated with both hemorrhage and thrombosis [7]. An elevated PT/INR is the most specific measure of hepatocyte dysfunction with regard to coagulation. Renal derangements can also interfere with the normal processes of clot formation; however, hemodialysis and the administration of DDAVP can serve to counteract the negative effects of uremic platelet dysfunction.

It is important to have a grounded approach to evaluating and treating patients suffering from significant hemorrhage [2]. In the setting of traumatic injuries or recent surgical procedures complicated by subsequent rapid large volume blood loss, anatomic defects should primarily be considered, as laboratory abnormalities may present in a delayed fashion and emergent surgical intervention may be warranted. Complicating the scenario can be the residual effects of intraoperative heparin use with inadequate reversal using protamine sulfate, specifically after cardiovascular surgical procedures. Similarly, therapeutic anticoagulation for deep vein thrombosis, atrial fibrillation, or valvular disease or antiplatelet therapy for coronary disease or stents often complicates the perioperative period with intraoperative or postoperative hemorrhage. Initial evaluation of hemorrhage should include laboratory workup to assess the patient's hemoglobin and hematocrit (Hb/Hct), platelet (PLT) count, coagulation factors (PT/INR and PTT), chemistries (evaluation of renal function), and fibrinogen levels. Thrombocytopenia or elevated bleeding times are indicative of platelet dysfunction, while elevated PT/INR and PTT represent disruptions of the extrinsic or intrinsic coagulation pathways, respectively. Elevated PT/INR and/or PTT can also signal disruptions of the common coagulation cascade. Additionally, PT/INR and PTT are utilized to monitor the anticoagulant effects of warfarin and heparin, respectively; therefore, elevated levels may be representative of pharmaceutical hemostatic derangements. Fibrinogen levels not only exhibit a directly proportional relationship with time to clot formation, they also are less sensitive to the effects of heparin and direct thrombin inhibitors. Thromboelastography (TEG) allows for a more specific evaluation of the underlying cause of the disruption in the normal processes of hemostasis, including analysis of both coagulation and fibrinolysis [2, 9, 10]. The primary components of thromboelastography (Fig. 2.1) include the R-time (latency period to initiation of clot formation), α-angle (rate of fibrin accumulation), maximum amplitude (MA; clot strength), and LY30 (rate of fibrinolysis after reaching maximum clot strength). Prolongation of the R-time is indicative of coagulation factor deficiency and can be addressed through the transfusion of FFP, while an abnormal α-angle represents inadequate fibrinogen levels and is corrected through administration of cryoprecipitate. Decreased clot strength can be corrected through platelet transfusion or administration of DDAVP, while increased fibrinolysis can be counteracted with the use of tranexamic acid (TXA) or aminocaproic acid (Amicar). TXA was shown in the CRASH-2 trial to offer a survival benefit in patients with traumatic hemorrhaging [10, 11].

Although the previous discussion has described various entities individually, it is important to remember that quite often there are multiple factors simultaneously at

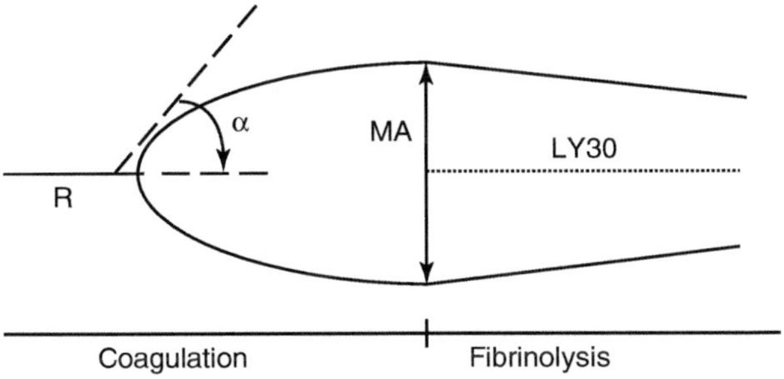

Fig. 2.1 Thromboelastography (TEG). R = R-time, MA = maximum amplitude, LY30 = fibrinolysis at 30 min, α = alpha angle

play, which further increase the complexity of diagnosis and management. One such example, often seen in critically ill patients, is deemed the lethal triad. The triad consists of acidosis, hypothermia, and coagulopathy [9, 12]. A vicious cycle of inadequate perfusion resulting in tissue ischemia and acidosis, with subsequent decreased production of ATP consequently disrupts the body's natural ability to maintain homeostatic temperatures, thus promotes coagulopathy through dysfunction of key enzymes involved in regulating the coagulation cascade. Adequate resuscitation and addressing the underlying etiology of hemorrhage are crucial in interrupting the progression of the lethal triad cycle. Initial resuscitation efforts involve targeting a goal systolic blood pressure of 90 mmHg and typically include the administration of two liters of crystalloid prior to initiating transfusion of blood products. In regard to packed red blood cells, a restrictive strategy (Hb goal 7–9 g/dL) provides an equal survival benefit as compared to a more liberal transfusion strategy (Hb goal 10–12 g/dL) as was most notably demonstrated in the 1999 TRICC trial [10, 13]. Another cornerstone of treating severe hemorrhage is the activation of massive transfusion protocol (MTP), which involves transfusing pRBCs, FFP, and PLTs in a 1:1:1 ratio and was shown in the PROPPR trial to more effectively achieve hemostasis and reduce hemorrhage-associated mortality [10, 14]. Finally, the concept of permissive hypotension advocates for delaying resuscitation by avoiding excess crystalloid administration prior to control of hemorrhage [10]. Excess crystalloid transfusion can exacerbate the lethal triad by causing a dilutional deficiency of clotting factors and exacerbating acidosis. With ongoing resuscitation of the bleeding patient, it is important to understand the contents of the available components. FFP contains vWF, fibrinogen, and coagulation factors I, VII, VII, IX, X, and XIII, while cryoprecipitate contains vWF, fibrinogen, and clotting factors VIII and XIII [10]. PCC exists as three-factor (II, IX, and X) PCC or four-factor (II, VII, IX, and X) PCC, while TXA and Amicar act similarly as antifibrinolytics through the inhibition of plasminogen or plasmin, respectively, consequently preventing downstream breakdown of the fibrin clot [10].

Thromboembolic Disease

Thrombosis involves the formation of a platelet plug with subsequent activation of the clotting cascade for clot stabilization. However, there is also the simultaneous activation of inhibitory mechanisms to limit clotting to the site of injury [3].

The predominant mediators of inhibiting clot formation include protein C (degradation of factors Va and VIIIa), antithrombin (inactivation of factors IIa, IXa, and Xa), and plasmin (breakdown of fibrin) [3]. Disturbances to these counterbalancing forces can promote uncontrolled thromboembolism or severe hemorrhage. The following is a discussion regarding venous thromboembolism (VTE) disease which typically encompasses deep vein thrombosis (DVT) or pulmonary embolism (PE) as well as manifestations of arterial thromboembolic disease.

Critically ill injured or surgical patients have increased risk of thrombosis secondary to factors collectively recognized as Virchow's triad (endothelial injury, venous stasis, and hypercoagulability) [1, 3, 15]. A higher propensity for thrombus formation has also been recognized as associated with factors (e.g., prolonged surgery, severe trauma, spinal cord injury, and cardiac or respiratory failure) which augment the derangements of Virchow's triad. Calculation of the Caprini score can aid in risk stratifying patients for development of venous thromboembolism and guide the management of prophylaxis [15–17]. VTE risk can be mitigated through both mechanical prophylaxis (i.e., sequential compression) and chemoprophylaxis with subcutaneous low-molecular-weight heparin (LMWH; enoxaparin, Lovenox) or unfractionated heparin [17]. Rarely, some high-risk patients with contraindications to chemoprophylaxis (e.g., intracranial hemorrhage, high risk of uncontrolled hemorrhage) may warrant placement of an inferior vena cava (IVC) filter to reduce the risk of DVT embolization to the pulmonary circuit, resulting in a PE. Clinical symptoms of acute onset extremity pain and swelling should prompt consideration of DVT and the need for diagnostic evaluation beginning with venous duplex ultrasonography. Acute PE is typically heralded by new onset of tachycardia, dyspnea, hypoxia, and possibly signs of anxiety or right heart failure. The diagnosis of pulmonary embolism is made predominately via chest CTA (some institutions may have specific imaging orders for CT PE Protocol); however, diagnosis can also be suggested by a ventilation/perfusion (V/Q) scan or echocardiogram findings of right heart strain and pulmonary hypertension [15]. The mainstay of treatment for DVT and PE involves anticoagulation, initially with intravenous heparin or low-molecular-weight heparin and subsequent transition to either oral anticoagulants (i.e., Warfarin versus NOAC/DOAC) or continued LMWH. Treatment duration is dependent upon the etiology associated with thrombus formation: provoked (e.g., traumatic, postop, etc.; $t = 3$ months), spontaneous ($t = 3$–6 months), or high-risk (e.g., recurrent VTE, malignancy, or hypercoagulability; t = lifetime/indefinite therapy) [15]. Hemodynamically significant pulmonary embolism can cause worsening cardiogenic shock or cardiopulmonary collapse and require more aggressive therapy with systemic fibrinolysis using tPA or thromboembolectomy (mechanical or surgical) in patients with contraindications to anticoagulation. Aside from embolization to the pulmonary vasculature, additional serious sequelae of DVT include worsening venous obstruction resulting in phlegmasia alba dolens and subsequently phlegmasia cerulea dolens [15, 18]. Phlegmasia alba dolens is the result of complete occlusion of the deep venous outflow tract resulting in an edematous, painful, and milky white-appearing lower extremity and can be treated with systemic anticoagulation, thrombectomy, or catheter-based thrombolysis. Further progression of venous obstruction involving the superficial system results in phlegmasia cerulea dolens, characterized by severe pain, swelling, and cyanosis of the lower limb, requiring catheter-directed pharmaco-mechanical thrombolysis therapy in an effort to prevent development of venous gangrene [18]. Long-term sequelae include chronic venous insufficiency and post-thrombotic syndrome.

While cigarette smoking and increased circulating levels of estrogen can increase the risk of VTE formation, a handful of disorders directly impact the balancing forces of the coagulation cascade. Additionally, as mentioned in the discussion of hemorrhagic diatheses, certain diagnoses are characterized by simultaneous coagulopathy and thrombus formation (e.g., DIC or HIT). Factor V Leiden and prothrombin G20210A are genetic disorders caused by single nucleotide mutations, resulting in a hypercoagulable state [1]. Mutation of the factor V gene renders it resistant to the counter-regulatory inactivation by protein C, while mutation of the prothrombin gene caused increased circulating levels of prothrombin (factor II). Genetic mutations are also responsible for deficiencies in antithrombin III, protein C, or protein S and consequently affect the inhibitory mechanisms of the coagulation cascade [1]. Antiphospholipid antibody syndrome (previously recognized as lupus anticoagulant syndrome) induces a state of hypercoagulability by causing endothelial injury, activating platelets, and promoting upregulation of certain clotting factors [1].

Although the preceding discussion was limited to the venous system, thromboembolic disease can also affect arterial circulation and is the basis of myocardial infarctions, cerebrovascular accidents, and peripheral vascular disease. Arterial thromboembolic disease is predominately associated with underlying atherosclerotic plaques, intracardiac mural thrombi, arrhythmias such as atrial fibrillation, or valvular vegetations; however, VTE can paradoxically affect the arterial system in the presence of a patent foramen ovale or atrial septal defect [1].

A chronical inflammatory process is responsible for the formation of macrophage-based foam cells, which coalesce to form atherosclerotic plaques. Accumulation of plaque results in varying grades of stenosis with consequent arterial insufficiency; furthermore, fragments of ulcerated plaque may become dislodged and consequently serve as atherosclerotic emboli. Additionally, it is important to note that arterial thrombus/plaque formation typically occurs at branch points of the arterial tree, whereas arterial emboli become lodged distal to the origin of the vessel. The presence of significant atherosclerotic plaque perpetuates clinical disease, most notably affecting the carotid arteries (transient ischemic attacks or cerebrovascular accidents), coronaries (myocardial infarctions), mesenteric arteries (mesenteric ischemia), aortoiliac disease, femoropopliteal disease, and tibioperoneal disease (claudication, rest pain, and tissue loss). In response to atherosclerotic disease, aside from medical management and lifestyle modification, there are a variety of surgical options designed to restore perfusion to once ischemic tissues. Although well-established procedures such as carotid endarterectomy (as guided by the NASCET and ACAS trials), coronary artery bypass grafts (CABG), aortoiliac and femoral endarterectomies, and anatomical versus extraanatomical bypass procedures have long been practiced, there has also been the increasing use of percutaneous endovascular interventions such as balloon angioplasty and stenting. Despite these well-established practices, surgeons are often faced with the challenge of acute ischemia as a consequence of embolic disease. It is important to note that emboli can cause an acute infarction of any organ(s) or tissues; however, two of the more commonly recognized examples include acute mesenteric ischemia and limb ischemia and are discussed below. Although arterial thromboembolic events classically present in postoperative cardiac surgery patients, given the hypercoagulable state present in surgical patients, the presence of either preexisting or new-onset arrhythmias such as postoperative atrial fibrillation, or the diagnosis of HITT, arterial thromboembolic disease can occur in any postoperative patient.

There exist four variants of mesenteric ischemia: acute (embolic obstruction of superior mesenteric artery, SMA), chronic (SMA atherosclerotic disease), acute venous thrombosis (decreased perfusion secondary to decreased venous outflow), and nonocclusive mesenteric ischemia (NOMI; a state of decreased perfusion associated with cardiogenic shock or use of vasopressors) [19]. An underlying principle which limits the extent of tissue ischemia with chronic mesenteric ischemia is perfusion via collateral circulation through the pancreaticoduodenal arteries, arch of Riolan, and marginal artery of Drummond. Acute mesenteric ischemia is typically characterized by abdominal pain disproportionate to physical exam findings and bloody diarrhea, while chronic mesenteric disease manifests with postprandial abdominal pain, "food fear," and consequently weight loss. Treatment of embolic disease involves surgical or percutaneous embolectomy, revascularization with a prosthetic bypass graft, and resection of nonviable bowel, while atherosclerotic disease can be treated with either autologous venous or prosthetic bypass grafting (dependent upon the absence of nonviable bowel) or endovascular intervention. Similar to VTE, mesenteric venous thrombosis is treated with anticoagulation, but may also require catheter-based thrombolytic therapy.

Similar to mesenteric ischemia, acute limb ischemia (ALI) is a consequence of interrupted perfusion to one or more limbs, primarily affecting the lower extremity as a consequence of arterial emboli [20]. Chronic limb-threatening ischemia (CLTI) is differentiated from ALI, such that CLTI typically affects patients with long-standing peripheral vascular disease and is associated with symptoms of claudication, rest pain, and nonhealing wounds or tissue loss [21, 22]. ALI is often characterized by the "six Ps" (pain, pulselessness, poikilothermia, paresthesia, pallor, and paralysis); however, these findings are often not all present simultaneously, nor do they all need to be for confirmation of the diagnosis. Acute and chronic limb ischemia were further categorized by Rutherford in Tables 2.1 and 2.2, respectively, based on clinical findings and objective data [20, 22]. Patients with suspected Rutherford Class I or II acute limb ischemia should promptly be started on intravenous anticoagulation with either unfractionated heparin or a direct thrombin inhibitor such as bivalirudin or argatroban [20–22]. Furthermore, patients with a threatened limb should be considered for surgical thromboembolectomy or catheter-directed thrombolytic therapy, whereas amputation should be considered in patients with irreversible ischemia to prevent systemic consequences of tissue necrosis [20–22].

Table 2.1 Acute limb ischemia Rutherford classification

–	–	Clinical findings		Doppler signals	
Classification	Description	Sensory deficits	Motor deficits	Arterial	Venous
I: Viable	Viable limb, no immediate threat	None	None	Audible	Audible
IIa: Marginally threatened	Salvageable if treated promptly	Minimal	None	Inaudible	Audible
IIb: Immediately threatened	Salvageable with immediate revascularizations	Rest pain	Mild-moderate	Inaudible	Audible
III: Irreversible	Permanent tissue loss	Anesthetic	Paralysis	Inaudible	Inaudible

Table 2.2 Chronic limb ischemia Rutherford classification

Fontaine grade	Rutherford classification	Clinical presentation	Objective criteria
I	0	Asymptomatic	Normal treadmill or reactive hyperemia test
IIa	1	Mild claudication	Ankle pressure >50 mmHg after exercise, but at least 20 mmHg lower than resting value
IIb	2	Moderate claudication	Between Rutherford 1–3
	3	Severe claudication	Unable to complete treadmill test, ankle pressure <50 mmHg after exercise
III	4	Ischemic rest pain	Resting ankle pressure <30–50 mmHg; ankle or metatarsal pulse volume flat or barely pulsatile; toe pressure <30 mmHg
IV	5	Minor tissue loss	Resting ankle pressure <50–70 mmHg; ankle or metatarsal pulse volume flat or barely pulsatile; toe pressure <40 mmHg (nondiabetics) vs <50 mmHg (diabetics); transcutaneous oxygen pressure <30 mmHg
	6	Major tissue loss (nonhealing ulcer, focal gangrene with diffuse pedal ischemia, wound extension beyond metatarsals, foot non-salvageable)	

Although the diagnosis should be confirmed on CTA, therapeutic intervention, specifically the initiation of systemic anticoagulation, should not be delayed in the setting of high suspicion for acute ischemia secondary to embolic disease. Additionally, patients should be resuscitated with intravenous fluids, and underlying metabolic derangements such as acidosis which occur with tissue malperfusion should be corrected. The risk of acute embolic events can also be reduced with the use of oral anticoagulation therapy. As with the use of the Caprini score to risk stratify patients for VTE, the CHA_2DS_2-VASc score can risk stratify patients with underlying atrial fibrillation for an arterial embolic event [23]. Analogous to hemorrhage, arterial or venous thromboembolic disease may also limit adequate tissue perfusion, resulting in ischemic injury which can extend beyond a single organ or body part and manifest with systemic consequences.

Ischemic Injury

Having considered both hemorrhage and thromboembolic disease, it is now pertinent to conclude with a discussion of the ultimate consequence of both, ischemic injury. A basic yet essential component of all living organisms, the cell, is dependent upon the delivery of oxygen and nutrients in order to carry out the functions of cellular metabolism. While hypoxia impairs aerobic metabolism, ischemia disrupts both aerobic and anaerobic metabolisms, precipitating a quicker onset and more severe state of tissue injury [24]. Broadly categorized into one or more categories (i.e., hypovolemic or hemorrhagic, cardiogenic, distributive: septic or neurogenic, or obstructive), shock is a state of inadequate perfusion, resulting initially in reversible ischemic injury with subsequent progression to irreversible multiorgan failure [9, 24]. Unlike the previously discussed examples of isolated tissue ischemia (e.g., acute mesenteric or limb ischemia) caused by embolic disease, shock manifests systemically, affecting multiple body systems simultaneously.

The fundamental derangement which defines shock is cellular hypoxia, resulting from either isolated or any combination of the following: decreased oxygen delivery, increased oxygen consumption, and/or poor oxygen utilization [25]. Furthermore, aside from insufficient end-organ perfusion, hypoxia may also be a result of hypoxemia secondary to decreased pulmonary gas exchange or increased dead space ventilation. Hypovolemia, the most common etiology of shock, is associated with low circulating blood volume most often secondary to hemorrhage. The advanced trauma life support (ATLS) guidelines categorize hemorrhagic shock into four classes (Table 2.3) based on the volume percentage of blood loss and subsequent physiologic symptoms, which do not become apparent until greater than 15% blood loss [26]. Sepsis is a life-threatening organ dysfunction caused by a dysregulated host response to infection, as determined by a Sequential Organ Failure Assessment (SOFA) score (Table 2.4) of two or more. The combination of these two entities results in septic shock, defined as the inability to maintain a mean arterial pressure (MAP) of at least 65 mmHg without the use of vasopressors and a serum lactate level greater than 2 mmol/L despite adequate resuscitation [27]. Cardiogenic shock is caused by intracardiac pump failure, resulting in decreased cardiac output;

Table 2.3 Categories of hemorrhagic shock

Parameter	Class I	Class II	Class III	Class IV
Volume blood loss (%)	0–15	15–30	30–40	>40
Heart rate	Normal	Increased	Increased	Increased
Blood pressure	Normal	Normal	Decreased	Decreased
Pulse pressure	Normal	Decreased	Decreased	Decreased
Mentation	Normal	Anxious	Confused	Altered, lethargic
Respirations	Normal	Normal	Increased	Increased

Table 2.4 Sequential Organ Failure Assessment (SOFA) Score

Organ system	0	1	2	3	4
Pulmonary (P_aO_2/ FIO_2)	>400	301–400	201–300	101–200	≤100
Cardiovascular (hypotension/ vasopressors)	None	MAP <70 mmHg	Dopamine <5 or Dobutamine (any dose)[a]	Dopamine 5.1–15 or Epineprhine ≤0.1 or Norepinephrine ≤0.1[a]	Dopamine >15 or Epineprhine >0.1 or Norepinephrine >0.1[a]
Coagulation (PLTs × 10^3/mm^3)	≥150	<150	<100	<50	<20
Renal (Cr, mg/dL)	<1.2	1.2–1.9	2.0–3.4	3.5–4.9	≥5.0
Neurological (GCS)	15	13–14	10–12	6–9	<6
Hepatic (TB, mg/ dL)	<1.2	1.2–1.9	2.0–5.9	6.0–11.9	≥12.0

P_aO_2 arterial partial oxygen pressure, *FIO_2* fraction of inspired oxygen, *MAP* mean arterial pressure, *PLTs* platelets, *Cr* creatinine, *GCS* Glasgow coma scale, *TB* total bilirubin.
[a]Catecholamine doses in mg/kg/min for ≥1 h

Table 2.5 Hemodynamic changes in shock

Categories of shock	CO	SVR	CVP & PCWP	S_VO_2
Hypovolemic	↓	↑	↓	↓
Septic	↑	↓	↓	↑
Cardiogenic	↓	↑	↑	↓
Neurogenic	↓	↓	↓	↓
Obstructive	↓	↑	↑	↓

CO Cardiac output, *SVR* Systemic vascular resistance, *CVP* Central venous pressure, *PCWP* Pulmonary capillary wedge pressure, *SvO_2* venous oxygen saturation

underlying etiologies are classified as cardiomyopathic (e.g., myocardial infarction, congestive heart failure), arrhythmic (atrial and ventricular tachyarrhythmias or bradyarrhythmias), or mechanical (e.g., valvular dysfunction) [1, 25]. Obstructive shock is the manifestation of an extracardiac problem (e.g., pulmonary embolism, cardiac tamponade, or tension pneumothorax) resulting in reduced cardiac output [25]. Finally, neurogenic shock results from damage to the central nervous system, typically injury on the cervical or upper thoracic spinal cord. Disruption of the autonomic pathways resulting in diminished sympathetic tone is the hallmark of neurogenic shock. Patients may exhibit bradycardia, hypotension due to decreased systemic vascular resistance, and possible disruption in respiratory mechanics dependent upon the level of the injury [1, 25]. The aforementioned categories of shock are defined not only by their underlying etiology but also by the changes in various hemodynamic parameters as shown in Table 2.5.

With perfusion impaired due to hemorrhage, shock, or arterial occlusion, the ischemic cascade is set in motion and ultimately terminates with cell death via necrosis or apoptosis [24]. An inadequate supply of oxygen results in the depletion and decreased synthesis of ATP, due to an inability to proceed with oxidative phosphorylation and the electron transport chain. In the absence of ATP, cells turn to anaerobic metabolism resulting in the accumulation of lactic acid, and consequently cellular enzymatic activity is reduced within the acidic cell environment. Additionally, an inactive Na^+/K^+-ATPase channel results in retention of sodium and consequent cellular swelling, disruption of cellular membrane permeability, and an influx of calcium ions due to cellular depolarization. Increased levels of Ca^{2+} cause cell membrane and nuclear damage, alongside mitochondrial dysfunction resulting in tissue death via cell necrosis and/or apoptosis.

As previously mentioned, tissues undergo a period of reversible ischemic injury during which there is potential for recovery with restoration of blood flow; however, tissues remain susceptible to damage via reperfusion injury mediated by inflammation and oxidative damage [9, 24]. During the reperfusion period, cells undergo oxidative stress, resulting in the formation of reactive oxygen species (RoS) which cause disruption of cellular plasma membranes, decreased enzymatic activity, abnormal protein folding, and DNA mutations or breaks [28]. Reperfusion of tissues activates the inflammatory response by stimulating endothelial cells to release cytokines and recruit neutrophils; additionally, reperfusion inflammatory injury has the potential to affect tissues which initially were unaffected by the ischemic insult [27]. While all tissues suffering from ischemia are susceptible to reperfusion injury, frequently encountered is the development of compartment syndrome after restoration of blood flow in the setting of acute limb ischemia or traumatic vascular injuries. Such ischemia and reperfusion injury of the muscle can lead to rhabdomyolysis and can mandate further surgical and medical intervention, in the form of fasciotomies to relieve compartment pressures in addition to monitoring renal function for the development of rhabdomyolysis respectively [21].

Conclusion

Hemorrhage and thromboembolic disease are two potentially devastating conditions which can culminate in irreversible ischemic tissue injury. Although this review discussed the basic principles, various etiologies, diagnostic workup, treatment options, and examples of hemorrhagic versus thromboembolic disease, the fundamental concept is early recognition and appropriate management. What must not elude the reader is that while hemorrhage and thromboembolic disease are entities believed to be inherently antagonistic to one another, these processes typically affect patients with a continuously changing physiologic state and disrupted homeostatic mechanism; therefore, the individual or synergistic effects can ultimately prove to be fatal.

References

1. Kumar V, Abbas AK, Aster JC. Hemodynamic disorders, thromboembolic disease, and shock. In: Robbins and Cotran pathologic basis of disease. 9th ed. Philadelphia: Elsevier/Saunders; 2015. p. 113–35.

2. O'Keeffe T. Coagulopathy in the critically ill patient. In: Current surgical therapy. 13th ed. Philadelphia: Elsevier; 2020. p. 1457–66.
3. Stephen AH, Adams CA, Cioffi WG. Surgical critical care. In: Sabiston textbook of surgery. 20th ed. Philadelphia: Elsevier; 2017. p. 547–76.
4. Colwell C, Moreira ME, Grayzel J. Initial management of moderate to severe hemorrhage in the adult trauma patient. UpToDate. 2019. https://www.uptodate.com/contents/initial-management-of-moderate-to-severe-hemorrhage-in-the-adult-trauma-patient.
5. Peitzman AB, Rhodes M, Schwab CW, Yealy DM, Fabian TC. The trauma manual: trauma and acute care surgery. 3rd ed. Lippincott Williams & Wilkins; 2008.
6. Kumar V, Abbas AK, Aster JC. Red blood cell and bleeding disorders. In: Robbins and Cotran pathologic basis of disease. 9th ed. Philadelphia: Elsevier/Saunders; 2015. p. 629–67.
7. Amitrano L, Guardascione MA, Brancaccio V, Balzano A. Coagulation disorders in liver disease. Semin Liver Dis. 2002;22(1):83–96.
8. Ageno W, Gallus AS, Wittkowsky A, Crowther M, Hylek EM, Palareti G. Oral anticoagulant therapy: antithrombotic therapy and prevention of thrombosis, 9th ed: American College of Chest Physicians evidence-based clinical practice guidelines. Chest. 2012;141(2, Supplement):e44S–88S.
9. Rhee P, Joseph B. Shock, electrolytes, and fluid. In: Sabiston textbook of surgery. 20th ed. Philadelphia: Elsevier; 2017. p. 44–97.
10. Taylor JR, Cotton BA. Coagulation issues and the trauma patient. In: Current surgical therapy. 13th ed. Philadelphia: Elsevier; 2020. p. 1251–9.
11. Ker K, Kiriya J, Perel P, Edwards P, Shakur H, Roberts I. Avoidable mortality from giving tranexamic acid to bleeding trauma patients: an estimation based on WHO mortality data, a systematic literature review and data from the CRASH-2 trial. BMC Emerg Med. 2012;12(1):3.
12. Holcomb JB, Jenkins D, Rhee P, Johannigman J, Mahoney P, Mehta S, et al. Damage control resuscitation: directly addressing the early coagulopathy of trauma. J Trauma Acute Care Surg. 2007;62(2):307–10.
13. Hébert PC, Wells G, Blajchman MA, Marshall J, Martin C, Pagliarello G, et al. A multicenter, randomized, controlled clinical trial of transfusion requirements in critical care. N Engl J Med. 1999;340(6):409–17.
14. Holcomb JB, Tilley BC, Baraniuk S, Fox EE, Wade CE, Podbielski JM, et al. Transfusion of plasma, platelets, and red blood cells in a 1:1:1 vs a 1:1:2 ratio and mortality in patients with severe trauma: the PROPPR randomized clinical trial. JAMA. 2015;313(5):471–82.
15. Cardella JA, Amankwah KS. Venous thromboembolism: prevention, diagnosis, and treatment. In: Current surgical therapy. 13th ed. Philadelphia: Elsevier; 2020. p. 1072–82.
16. Caprini JA, Arcelus JI, Hasty JH, Tamhane AC, Fabrega F. Clinical assessment of venous thromboembolic risk in surgical patients. Semin Thromb Hemost. 1991;17(Suppl 3):304–12.
17. Gould MK, Garcia DA, Wren SM, Karanicolas PJ, Arcelus JI, Heit JA, et al. Prevention of VTE in nonorthopedic surgical patients. Chest. 2012;141(2 Suppl):e227S–77S.
18. Sarwar S, Narra S, Munir A. Phlegmasia cerulea dolens. Tex Heart Inst J. 2009;36(1):76–7.
19. Holscher CM, Reifsnyder T. Acute mesenteric ischemia. In: Current surgical therapy. 13th ed. Philadelphia: Elsevier; 2020. p. 1057–61.
20. Luís Foroni Casas A. Acute arterial embolism of the lower limb. In: Embolic diseases - evolving diagnostic and management approaches. IntechOpen; 2019.
21. Seegmiller CJ, Cogbill TH. Management of peripheral arterial thromboembolism. In: Current surgical therapy. 13th ed. Philadelphia: Elsevier; 2020. p. 1013–7.
22. Rutherford RB, Baker JD, Ernst C, Johnston KW, Porter JM, Ahn S, et al. Recommended standards for reports dealing with lower extremity ischemia: revised version. J Vasc Surg. 1997;26(3):517–38.
23. Lip GYH, Nieuwlaat R, Pisters R, Lane DA, Crijns HJGM. Refining clinical risk stratification for predicting stroke and thromboembolism in atrial fibrillation using a novel risk factor-based approach: the euro heart survey on atrial fibrillation. Chest. 2010;137(2):263–72.
24. Kumar V, Abbas AK, Aster JC. Cellular responses to stress and toxic insults: adaptation, injury, and death. In: Robbins and Cotran pathologic basis of disease. 9th ed. Philadelphia: Elsevier/Saunders; 2015. p. 31–68.

25. Gaieski DF, Mikkelsen ME, Parsons PE, Finlay G. Definition, classification, etiology, and pathophysiology of shock in adults. UpToDate. 2020. https://www.uptodate.com/contents/definition-classification-etiology-and-pathophysiology-of-shock-in-adults.
26. Henry S. ATLS 10th edition offers new insights into managing trauma patients. Bull Am Coll Surg. 2018. https://bulletin.facs.org/2018/06/atls-10th-edition-offers-new-insights-into-managing-trauma-patients/#Chapter_3_Shock.
27. Singer M, Deutschman CS, Seymour CW, Shankar-Hari M, Annane D, Bauer M, et al. The third international consensus definitions for sepsis and septic shock (Sepsis-3). JAMA. 2016;315(8):801–10.
28. Carden DL, Granger DN. Pathophysiology of ischaemia–reperfusion injury. J Pathol. 2000;190(3):255–66.

Principles of Vascular Imaging

3

Veronica Lenge de Rosen

Introduction

Imaging plays an increasingly important role in the assessment of postoperative vascular complications, especially as surgical and interventional techniques become more compound. A variety of modalities are available to evaluate and follow truncal and extremity vessels. Advances in imaging technology over the past two decades have greatly expanded the role of noninvasive cross-sectional imaging in the detection of postoperative complications. The American College of Radiology (ACR) has developed specific guidelines, referred to as ACR Appropriateness Criteria (AC) to assist referring physicians and other providers in making the most appropriate imaging or treatment decision for a specific clinical condition.

This review will mainly focus on providing information to healthcare professionals about the most commonly available imaging modalities with their advantages and disadvantages for assessment of postoperative vascular complications. Currently, radiograph, ultrasonography, computed tomography angiography (CTA), magnetic resonance imaging (MRI), and conventional angiography all have been used and compliment one to another by providing supplementary information.

Imaging Modalities and Protocols

CT Angiography (CTA)

Per ACR Appropriateness Criteria [1], CTA is the preferred imaging modality for the evaluation of truncal and extremity arteries due to its precise anatomic definition

V. L. de Rosen (✉)
Department of Radiology, Department of Internal Medicine, Baylor College of Medicine, Houston, TX, USA
e-mail: vvrosen@bcm.edu

R. Gilani, J. L. Mills Sr. (eds.), *Vascular Complications of Surgery and Intervention*, https://doi.org/10.1007/978-3-030-86713-3_3

and dynamic contrast visualization. However, it is important to keep in mind the trade-off between fineness of resolution determined by slice thickness and the allowable range to be imaged. An often employed solution is to initially obtain a less detailed examination over a large region of the body, followed by a more resolute scan when allowable focusing on the area of interest.

State-of-the-art technology and standardized protocols are crucial to obtain outstanding image quality to assess postoperative vascular complications. Protocols are often tailored to answer specific questions related to the type of surgery performed. For instance, electrocardiogram (ECG) gating can be critical in patients with type I aortic dissection for visualization of the aortic root as well as presence of post operative complications such as development of pseudoaneurysms (Fig. 3.1). The addition of ECG gating allows minimization of cardiac motion artifact, which is quite significant in the proximal aorta and aortic root.

Moreover, acquisition of multiple phases allows a better characterization of findings given the addition of a time variable. While arterial phase will suffice to assess large vessel hemorrhage, hematoma, dissection, thrombosis, surgical graft integrity, device migration, or presence of postoperative pseudoaneurysm, it may be inadequate for evaluation of contrast extravasation particularly low volume phenomenon. For example, the addition of pre-contrast and delayed phases is critical to evaluate endoleaks after endovascular aneurysm repair (Fig. 3.2). One benefit of the unenhanced phase is to differentiate extraluminal calcification or post-endoleak intervention material from extraluminal contrast seen on contrast-enhanced images. The main advantage of the delayed phase is to detect slow-flow endoleaks that may not be present on arterial phase. Therefore, standard protocol for endovascular repair evaluation is triphasic, including pre-contrast, arterial, and delayed phase (60–120 s after injection). An additional late phase (300 s after injection) can be obtained for higher detection of partial thrombosis in patients with repaired aortic dissection or to better visualize low-flow endoleaks.

CTA is also the preferred modality for assessment of aortic graft infection by demonstrating perigraft inflammation or erosion of adjacent structures, such as an aorto-esophageal fistula. These conditions are supported by pathognomonic imaging findings on CTA such as circumferential graft stranding, circumferential aortic thickening, air in proximity of the graft, loss of plain between the duodenum and

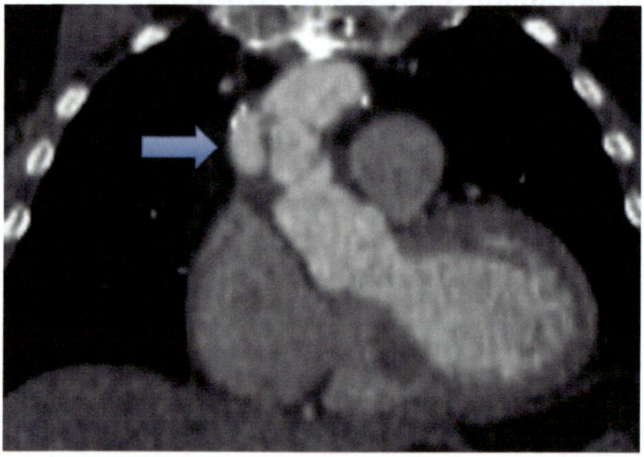

Fig. 3.1 Coronal CTA image demonstrates focal contrast outpouching at the distal graft anastomosis in a patient with prior type I aortic dissection repair consistent with postoperative pseudoaneurysm

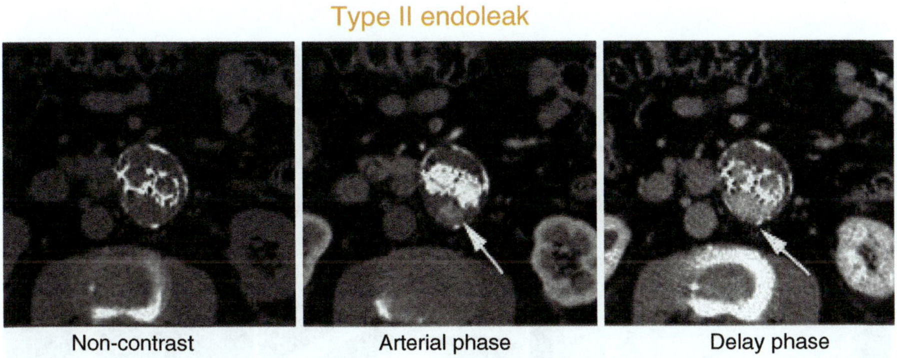

Fig. 3.2 Axial CTA images demonstrate contrast extravasation in the posterior aspect of the excluded aneurysm on arterial phase that increases on delay phase but not present on pre-contrast images consistent with type II endoleak

aorta, anastomotic disruption, and presence of fluid tracking along the length of the graft. Addition of 18F-fluorodeoxyglucose positron emission tomography (PET)/CT is increasing for determination of graft infection presence. This modality demonstrates strong sensitivity of detection when findings are analyzed to include maximum standardized uptake value (SUVmax), uptake pattern, and uptake distribution. However, its availability remains a significant barrier to utilization.

Post-processing techniques have become standard of care and provide more accurate measurements as well as detection of small lesions such as pseudoaneurysms. These techniques include multiplanar reformation, maximum intensity projection, curved planar reformation, and 3D volume rendering. CTA imaging 3D datasets should be reviewed on a workstation with multiplanar reformatting and measurement capabilities. Images should be manipulated such that reported aortic diameters are measured orthogonally to the aortic lumen, as measurements that are off-axis may significantly overestimate the true aortic diameter (Fig. 3.3a, b).

Disadvantages of CTA include potential nephrotoxicity and cumulative radiation dose, especially in younger patients who would require multiple exams along their lifetime. This issue partially has been ameliorated with the development of dual-energy acquisition, which offers the possibility of eliminating the unenhanced phase via the creation of a virtual noncontrast image set.

In patients with renal insufficiency, unenhanced CT can be an alternate exam that can be valuable for identification of aortic size, acute intramural hematoma (IMH), and aortic calcification. Moreover, in the immediate postoperative state, unenhanced CT can delineate complications related to acute aortic syndromes such as mediastinal or pericardial hemorrhage and rupture.

Magnetic Resonance Angiography (MRA)

Magnetic resonance imaging (MRI) of vessels can be performed with and without intravenous contrast and is a viable alternative for imaging a variety of conditions. Due to lack of ionizing radiation, it is an attractive alternative for surveillance of conventional

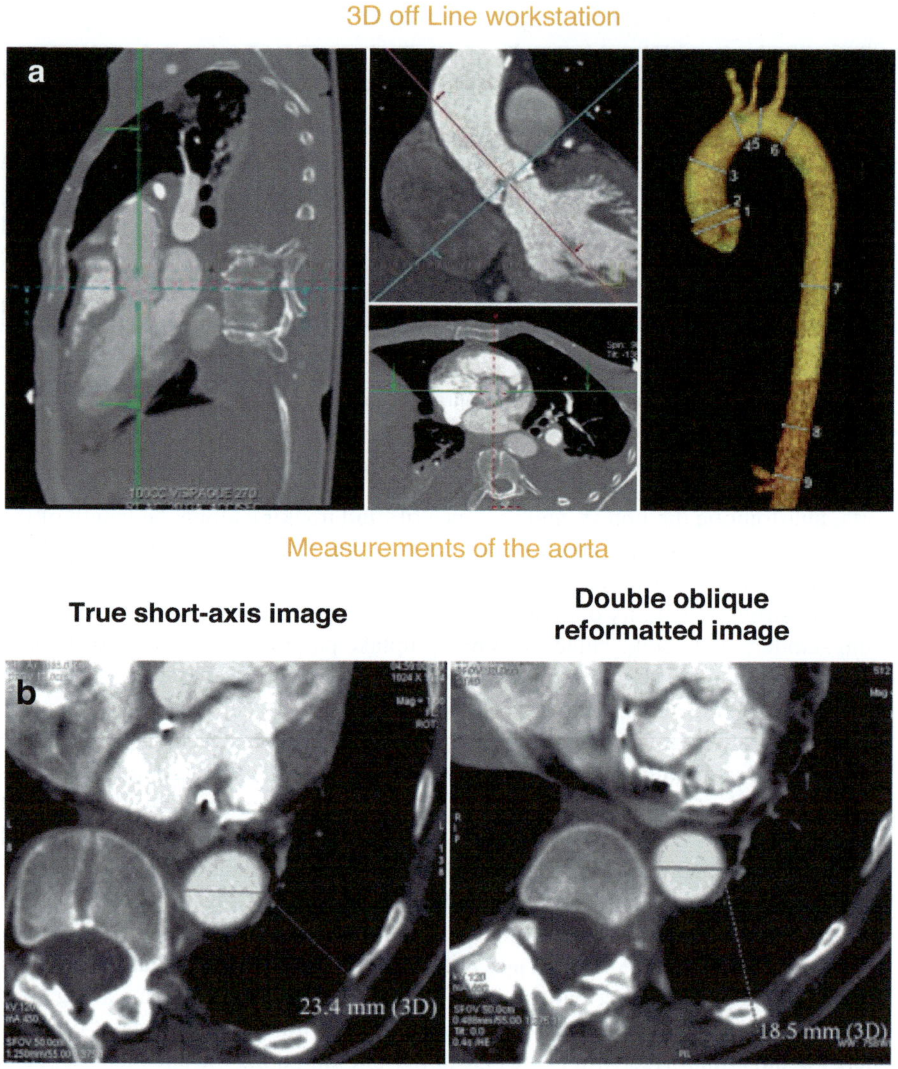

Fig. 3.3 (**a**) Multiplanar reformatting of the thoracic aorta in a 3D offline workstation. (**b**) Multiplanar reformatting of the thoracic aorta in a 3D offline workstation depicted a true short-axis diameter (right) which differs from the diameter obtained with a double oblique reformatted image (left)

surgical repair of the aorta in young patients that require multiple exams. However, in the evaluation of endovascular repairs, metallic stent grafts and other materials can obscure fine details that are often essential in postoperative assessment, resulting in inability to assess stent patency. In those cases, CTA is the preferred modality.

Most MRA protocols have been particularly helpful for evaluation of the lower extremity arteries providing both excellent soft-tissue differentiation and subtracted images demonstrating the vasculature in 2D and 3D representations similar to those provided during conventional angiography. In the current era, the accuracy of CTA and contrast-enhanced MRA (CEMRA) for the detection of hemodynamically significant peripheral artery disease (PAD) has become essentially equivalent, with an edge for CTA in the aortoiliac segment and for MRA in the infrageniculate distribution. Sjoerd et al. analyzed 12 CTA and 30 CEMRA studies and estimated a sensitivity and specificity of 96% (95% CI, 93–98%) and 95% (95% CI, 92–97%) for CTA, and 93% (95% CI, 91–95%) and 94% (95% CI, 93–96%) for CEMRA [2].

Furthermore, MRA is considered effective for lower extremity runoff and feet evaluation of diabetic patients because of its superior ability to detect flow in small, calcified vessels, and the capability to perform an unenhanced MR. Liu et al. found in a prospective study that unenhanced MR angiography with use of flow-sensitive dephasing (FSD)-prepared steady-state free precession (SSFP) sequence allows clear depiction of the foot arterial tree and accurate detection of significant arterial stenosis as compared to conventional contrast-enhanced MR angiography. The average sensitivity, specificity, positive predictive value, negative predictive value, and accuracy of the two readers for unenhanced MR angiography were 88%, 93%, 81%, 96%, and 92%, respectively [3].

Disadvantages of MRI embrace a more time-consuming study than CT, require more hands-on expertise, and necessitate a stable patient.

Other important issues with MRA imaging include poor spatial resolution, inability to detect wall calcification (especially problematic in patients with diabetes and chronic limb-threatening ischemia), and potential development of nephrogenic systemic fibrosis (NSF) in renal failure patients. NSF is a rare disorder that occurs in some individuals with reduced kidney function, who have been exposed to an intravenous contrast material that contains gadolinium. Currently, with the development of new gadolinium-based contrast agents, such as class II agents, the risk of NSF is low or nonexistent. As a result, and in alignment with the ACR Manual Contrast Media Version 2020 guidelines, no screening of any kind is necessary prior to single-dose administration of class II agents (such as Dotarem, Multihance, and Gadavist) as there is no documented risk of harm. Patients on dialysis do not need to alter their dialysis schedule and may be imaged before or after dialysis. Use of class I and III agents does still require pre-procedure renal function screening as they have been associated with NSF in patients with renal dysfunction.

Conventional Angiography

Catheter angiography has largely been replaced by cross-sectional imaging in the evaluation of patients with suspected truncal, head/neck, and proximal extremity arterial pathology. Angiography is still considered in symptomatic patients with coexistent malperfusion or suspected acute interventional complication to allow simultaneous evaluation and possible revascularization of the affected vascular bed. Also, angiography has gained popularity in the hybrid operating room, in which diagnostic and interventional angiography techniques are combined with open surgical repair.

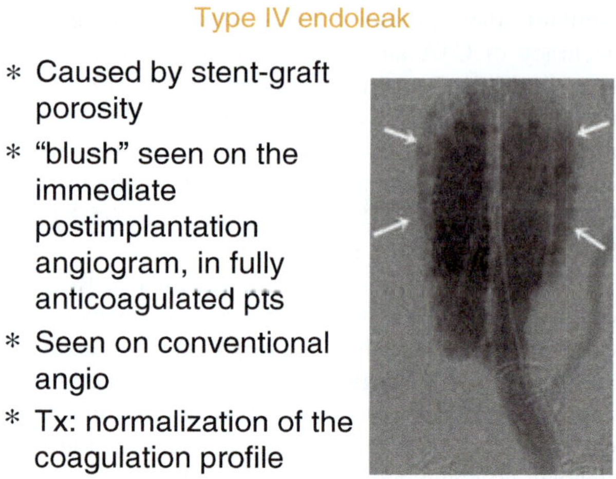

Fig. 3.4 Conventional angiography of the thoracic aorta depicted diffuse periaortic blush (arrows) post implantation of an endovascular stent graft consistent with type IV endoleak

In the postoperative follow-up, conventional angiography is useful for detection of occult leaks such as suspected type IV endoleak, which is not visualized by noninvasive imaging (Fig. 3.4) or nonlocalized gastrointestinal bleeding.

Noninvasive Hemodynamic Testing

Noninvasive testing (NIVT), both before and after intervention, has been used for decades as a first-line diagnostic tool to assess peripheral artery disease (PAD). It is widely available and provides a great deal of information at low cost. NIVT consists of one or more of the following components: the ABI, segmental pressure measurements (SPMs), pulse-volume recordings (PVRs), photoplethysmography (PPG), toe systolic pressure and toe-brachial index (TBI), and transcutaneous oxygen pressure measurement (TcPO2).

The ABI is defined as the ratio between the higher of the brachial artery pressures and the higher of the dorsalis pedis or posterior tibial artery pressures in each leg at the level of the ankle. A normal ABI value ranges between 0.9 and 1.31, a value less than 0.9 is suggestive of PAD, while values >1.3 indicate severe vessel disease, usually chronic. This technique may underestimate PAD by 30% when compared to CTA as demonstrated by Ro et al. [4]. The toe-brachial index (TBI) has been shown to provide a more accurate estimation of the presence of PAD in these subgroups, with a TBI <0.7 considered abnormal [6]. Toe pressures are preferred for hemodynamic assessment of patients with chronic limb-threatening ischemia, especially in people with diabetes.

SPMs compare systolic pressures at sequential levels in the extremities to evaluate for significant drops between one level and the next. A pressure drop of 20 mm Hg between adjacent measurements suggests one or more hemodynamically significant stenoses between them.

PVRs provide a qualitative measurement of limb perfusion. PVRs are created by inflating pneumoplethysmography cuffs to a specified pressure on each limb. Each cuff measures the miniscule change in the volume of the limb under the cuff with each pulse, creating a tracing of volume versus time. The resultant waveforms can be compared to determine segmental disease, providing insight into the quality of arterial blood flow at each station simultaneously.

PPG involves the detection of a transmitted infrared signal through each of the digits. The degree of transmitted signal varies depending on blood volume within the digit. PPG is useful for detection of disease below the knee as well as disease isolated to the forefoot and digits.

TcPO2 measurement allows the determination of the oxygen tension within the tissue. An improvement in the TcPO2 value postintervention compared with preintervention has been validated as an excellent marker of tissue reperfusion.

These tests may be limited by their availability in the office setting and patient resistance to avoiding smoking and caffeine before the test.

Ultrasonography

Duplex US (DUS) is an alternative modality for follow-up of abdominal aortic endovascular aneurysm repair with high specificity for detection of endoleaks and high accuracy for evaluation of aneurysm sac size. The addition of contrast material makes US an even more sensitive and specific test for characterization of endoleaks. Moreover, DUS has a more important role in assessing asymptomatic patients with previous infrainguinal endovascular therapy or bypass. By ACR Appropriateness Criteria, DUS is considered usually appropriate for surveillance in asymptomatic patients with previous infrainguinal endovascular therapy or bypass and can help to determine a baseline for future follow-up [5].

Echeverria et al. [7] assessed the utility of routine duplex surveillance in 379 infrainguinal reversed vein grafts performed at 2 independent teaching hospitals. Only 29% of grafts identified as failing (defined as duplex graft flow velocity (GFV) measurements less than 45 cm/sec) by duplex scan were associated with a reduction in ankle-brachial index of greater than 0.15. Secondary reconstructions were performed in 48 grafts based on detection of a reduced GFV measurement; all such reconstructions were patent after a mean follow-up of 5 months. The authors concluded that duplex surveillance is more reliable in identification of failing vein grafts than in determination of ankle-brachial index [6].

Its use in the chest is impractical given poor acoustic windows.

Radiograph

This procedure may be helpful for assessment of stent migration and stent integrity (fracture) following endovascular repair. However, it is unable to demonstrate other types of post-endograft or surgical graft complications. Radiographs cannot be used as a stand-alone method of follow-up.

Nuclear Medicine

Nuclear medicine scans are not the first choice for evaluation of postoperative vascular complications. However, recent research has shown that (99m)Tc-human serum albumin diethylenetriamine pentaacetic acid ((99m)Tc-HSAD) SPECT proved less sensitive than three-phase CT but depicted endoleaks with volumes 5.2 cm^3 or greater as perigraft radioisotope accumulation. Slow-filling endoleaks can be visualized with (99m)Tc-HSAD SPECT, which can be used to evaluate the efficacy of embolization [8].

Summary of Recommendations

A widespread variety of imaging modalities are available in current clinical practice. Vascular surgeons and referring providers need to be able to use combinations of these modalities at different stages of management.

Lifelong imaging follow-up is necessary in EVAR and TEVAR patients as endoleaks and other graft-related complications may develop at any time. The precise surveillance interval is still in debate and may be procedure and patient specific. CTA is the imaging modality of choice, given its sensitivity for the detection of endoleaks, changes in aortic/aneurysm diameter, and evaluation of false lumen thrombosis. Contrast-enhanced MRA is the preferred imaging modality in young patients requiring repetitive imaging follow-up. Unenhanced MRI is a more suitable modality for diabetic patients with renal dysfunction and peripheral arterial disease.

References

1. Expert Panels on Vascular Imaging and Interventional Radiology, Bonci G, Steigner ML, Hanley M, Braun AR, Desjardins B, Gaba RC, Gage KL, Matsumura JS, Roselli EE, Sella DM, Strax R, Verma N, Weiss CR, Dill KE. ACR appropriateness criteria. Thoracic aorta interventional planning and follow-up. J Am Coll Radiol. 2017;14:S570–83. Copyright 2017 American College of Radiology.
2. Jens S, Koelemay MJW, Reekers JA, Bipat S. Diagnostic performance of computed tomography angiography and contrast-enhanced magnetic resonance angiography in patients with critical limb ischaemia and intermittent claudication: systematic review and meta-analysis. Eur Radiol. 2013;23:3104–14.
3. Liu X, Fan Z, Zhang N, Yang Q, Feng F, Liu P, Zheng H, Li D. Unenhanced MR angiography of the foot: initial experience of using flow-sensitive dephasing–prepared steady-state free precession in patients with diabetes. Radiology. 2014;272:3. radiology.rsna.org.
4. Ro DH, Moon HJ, Kim JH, Lee KM, Kim SJ, Lee DY. Photoplethysmography and continuous-wave doppler ultrasound as a complementary test to ankle–brachial index in detection of stenotic peripheral arterial disease. Angiology. 2013;64(4):314–20.
5. Expert Panel on Vascular Imaging, Cooper K, Majdalany BS, Kalva SP, Chandra A, Collins JD, Francois CJ, Ganguli S, Gornik HL, Kendi AT, Khaja MS, Minocha J, Norton PT, Obara P, Reis SP, Sutphin PD, Rybicki FJ. ACR appropriateness criteria lower extremity arterial revascularization—post-therapy imaging. J Am Coll Radiol. 2018;15:S104–15. Copyright 2018 American College of Radiology.

6. Høyer C, Sandermann J, Petersen LJ. The toe-brachial index in the diagnosis of peripheral arterial disease. J Vasc Surg. 2013;58(1):231–8.
7. Echeverria AB, Branco BC, Goshima KR, Hughes JD, Mills JL Sr. Outcomes of endovascular management of acute thoracic aortic emergencies in an academic level 1 trauma center. Am J Surg. 2014;208(6):974–80; discussion 979–980.
8. Nakai M, Sato H, Sato M, Ikoma A, Sonomura T, Nishimura Y, Okamura Y. Utility of ^{99}mTc-human serum albumin diethylenetriamine pentaacetic acid SPECT for evaluating endoleak after endovascular abdominal aortic aneurysm repair. AJR Am J Roentgenol. 2015;204(1):189–96. https://doi.org/10.2214/AJR.13.12383.

Part II

Perioperative

Perioperative Venous Thromboembolism

4

Nawar Hudefi and Jayer Chung

Introduction

Venous thromboembolism (VTE) includes deep vein thrombosis (DVT) and pulmonary embolism (PE). VTE is a multifactorial disease process that refers to the formation of a blood clot in a deep vein. PE occurs when the clot then travels to the pulmonary arteries, thereby preventing effective gas exchange. All hospitalized patients are at risk for a VTE. There are measures to pharmacologically and mechanically prevent VTE while in hospital. Unfortunately, studies demonstrate that 50% of thromboembolic events are healthcare-related, occurring during or soon after a hospital stay. In fact, up to 20% of hospitalized patients will develop a VTE [1].

Risk Factors and Epidemiology of VTE

In a review of 1231 patients treated for VTE, 96% had one or more recognized risk factor [15]. Major surgery as a risk factor for VTE has been extensively studied, with trauma, hip or knee replacement, and spinal cord injury reported as strong risk factors among hospitalized patients [16]. One-third of VTE-associated deaths occur after surgical procedures. Additional risk factors demonstrating a moderate to low risk consist of chemotherapy, hormone replacement therapy, malignancy, and thrombophilia, with the likelihood of a VTE proportionally increasing with the number of risk factors present [16] (Table 4.1). The two most common genetic hypercoagulable disorders that predispose to VTE are factor V Leiden and prothrombin G20210A. A systematic review found that approximately 20% of patients

N. Hudefi · J. Chung (✉)
Division of Vascular Surgery and Endovascular Therapy, Michael E DeBakey Department of Surgery, Baylor College of Medicine, Houston, TX, USA
e-mail: Jayer.Chung@bcm.edu

R. Gilani, J. L. Mills Sr. (eds.), *Vascular Complications of Surgery and Intervention*, https://doi.org/10.1007/978-3-030-86713-3_4

Table 4.1 Risk factors for the development of venous thromboembolism

Strong risk factors (odds ratio >10)	Moderate risk factors (odds ratio 2–0)	Weak risk factors (odds ratio <2)
Fracture (hip or leg) Hip or knee replacement Major general surgery Major trauma Spinal cord injury	Arthroscopic knee surgery Central venous lines Chemotherapy Congestive heart or respiratory failure Hormone replacement therapy Malignancy Oral contraceptive therapy Paralytic stroke Pregnancy Previous thromboembolism Thrombophilia	Bed rest >3 days Immobility (long travel times) Age Laparoscopic surgery Obesity Varicose veins

experienced a first-ever VTE compared to 10% of patients with prothrombin G20210A [17]. Additional hematologic disorders associated with VTE include heparin-induced thrombocytopenia, disseminated intravascular coagulation (DIC), antiphospholipid antibody syndrome, and hemolytic uremic syndrome (HUS). First-time VTEs have a higher incidence in African-American populations when compared to Caucasians and Asian/Pacific Islanders [12]. A primary DVT occurs in the absence of known risk factors, and is also referred to as an "unprovoked" DVT. Conversely, secondary DVTs refer to thromboses in the presence of a recognized risk factor, and are referred to as "provoked" DVT.

VTE is a major health and financial burden on a national and global scale. The exact incidence of VTE is unknown as VTE remains underdiagnosed. However, approximately 900,000 people are estimated to develop a VTE in the United States. One-third of this population will experience recurrence within 10 years. VTE recurrence has been shown to be dependent on the original mode of presentation. This means that a patient who originally presented with a DVT is more likely to develop another DVT instead of a PE [11]. Research has shown that the risk of a developing a recurrent PE is three times greater in patients who initially presented with a PE [11].

Despite recent advancements in diagnosis, treatment, and prophylaxis of VTE over the last decade, the disease continues to be the third most common vascular pathology after myocardial infarction and stroke. VTE is responsible for approximately 250,000 hospitalizations per year [28]. PE is directly responsible for or associated with 100,000 deaths annually in the United States [28]. Mortality associated with PE is as high as 30% if untreated compared to an 8% mortality with appropriate treatment [27]. Acutely, up to 10% of patients will succumb to the PE and die suddenly, and two-thirds will die within 2 h of presentation [27]. After the acute event, 3-month mortality sits 17.5% [27]. To put it in perspective, more deaths annually can be owed to VTE than car crashes and breast cancer combined [27]. Thus, it is of utmost importance to recognize risk factors that lead to VTE and be familiar with initial diagnosis and treatment to further minimize morbidity and mortality.

Pathophysiology

Virchow's triad represents three discrete groups of risk factors that serve to describe the pathophysiology behind the formation of a thrombus: stasis of flow, a hypercoagulable state, and intravascular endothelial injury. Each of these factors in isolation may be responsible for VTE. However, it is the synergy between the three factors which can exponentially increase one's risk of VTE.

Damage to the wall of a vessel results in local alterations of blood flow and exposes endothelial cell and subendothelial proteins that promote the activation and circulation of coagulation pathways and enzymes. Such damage can occur from smoking, iatrogenic instrumentation, and trauma. Venous stasis occurs during times of immobility and trauma and in medical conditions such as arrhythmias, valvular heart disease, and congestive heart disease. Stasis increases the duration of contact between coagulation factors with each other and the endothelium, subsequently inducing endothelial damage and reducing fibrinolysis. Research has implicated smoking in various coagulation abnormalities mainly related to inflammation and increased fibrinogen. Fibrinogen is an acute phase reactant, and part of its contribution as a risk factor is by virtue of producing a vascular endothelial inflammatory state. It also plays an essential role in thrombus formation as fibrinogen is a thrombin substrate in the formation of fibrin [18]. Additional studies have demonstrated a rapid decline in fibrinogen concentration after the cessation of smoking. Fibrinogen levels are nearly equal in previous smokers and never smokers after 2 weeks of smoking cessation [19].

The delicate balance between clot formation and breakdown generally shifts toward thrombus generation in hereditary and acquired hypercoagulable conditions. It is important to note, however, that thrombophilias can be distinguished by associated risk for venous thrombus versus arterial thrombus versus both. Factor V Leiden and prothrombin G20210A, the most common inherited thrombophilias, have increased risk of venous thromboembolism with no consistent association with arterial thrombosis [20]. This pattern is also seen in protein C and S deficiencies and antithrombin deficiency. In contrast, antiphospholipid syndrome has a propensity for both venous and arterial thromboses, while homocysteinemia has been demonstrated to predispose patients to arterial thrombosis only [20]. Acquired hypercoagulable states seen in chemotherapy, cancer, pregnancy, oral contraceptives and hormone replacement therapy, and obesity further change coagulation pathways and create a thrombogenic state. There are few tests that qualitatively assess the ongoing clotting process in a patient. Conventional plasma tests such as prothrombin time, partial thromboplastin time, and INR are plasma-based studies that are inadequate in assessing coagulopathies. Thromboelastography (TEG) is a point-of-care test that evaluates the viscoelastic properties of whole blood, providing information about initial clot formation, fibrinolysis, and platelet aggregation. Studies have found that a collection of individual TEG parameters can be used as a marker for hypercoagulability and help identify patients at risk for VTE [32]. Subsequently, goal-directed therapies for intervention can be initiated and precision medicine practiced.

Deep Vein Thrombosis

Lower Extremity

The vast majority of DVTs are distal, occurring in the veins of the calf, while proximal DVTs, located in thigh veins, are less common. Up to half of all DVT patients are asymptomatic [25]. Symptomatic patients classically complain of a unilateral, dull ache in the leg, swelling, or erythema [24]. There may be significant swelling, cyanosis, and non-varicose, dilated superficial veins in patients with extensive iliofemoral DVT [24]. This classic presentation remains rare – less than 50% of cases [25]. Hence, physicians should remain vigilant in spite of the absence of the classic presentation, especially if other risk factors are present. With prompt recognition and anticoagulation therapy, some DVT may dissolve and recede within weeks to months, particularly those in the lower leg. Without appropriate anticoagulation, however, DVTs may extend and/or embolize.

Burdensome and lifestyle limiting sequelae include chronic venous insufficiency secondary to post-thrombotic syndrome. Post-thrombotic syndrome develops in up to 20–50% of patients within 7 years after the initial VTE [23]. While the pathophysiology is complex, most studies suggest that ambulatory venous hypertension is a result of outflow obstruction and/or valvular insufficiency. The sustained venous hypertension leads to structural and biochemical abnormalities that damage the vein walls and create a state of chronic inflammation, which results in pathologic skin and subcutaneous tissue effects. The most important risk factor for developing PTS is recurrent ipsilateral DVT, resulting in a sixfold increase in one study [29]. Additionally, DVT in multiple segments with iliac involvement increased the risk for developing PTS. Additional studies demonstrated that patients with popliteal vein abnormalities were also at an increased risk to develop PTS compared to those without popliteal vein involvement [29].

However, even with appropriate and timely treatment of DVT, the resulting inflammatory process can lead to permanent scarring and valvular dysfunction, ultimately leading to venous reflux and chronic venous hypertension [23]. The Villalta score diagnoses and stratifies the severity of post-thrombotic syndrome by assessing clinical signs and symptoms [22]. The higher the score, the greater the severity and disability [22]. The ATTRACT trial, a multicentered, randomized control trial, showed that the occurrence of moderate to severe post-thrombotic syndrome was greatly dependent on the location of the primary thrombosis. Patients had a greater risk of developing post-thrombotic syndrome after an iliofemoral DVT than following isolated femoropopliteal DVT [20]. Post-thrombotic syndrome can greatly reduce patient health-related quality of life and subjects patients to lifelong lower extremity pain, edema, venous ulceration, and lipodermatosclerosis [3] (Fig. 4.1).

A less frequent complication, seen in massive pelvic DVT, is the development of phlegmasia alba dolens and phlegmasia cerulea dolens, which occur when venous hypertension due to clot and edema obstructs arterial inflow, inducing tissue ischemia [2] (Fig. 4.2). Although this is not a common sequela, it is acutely life- and

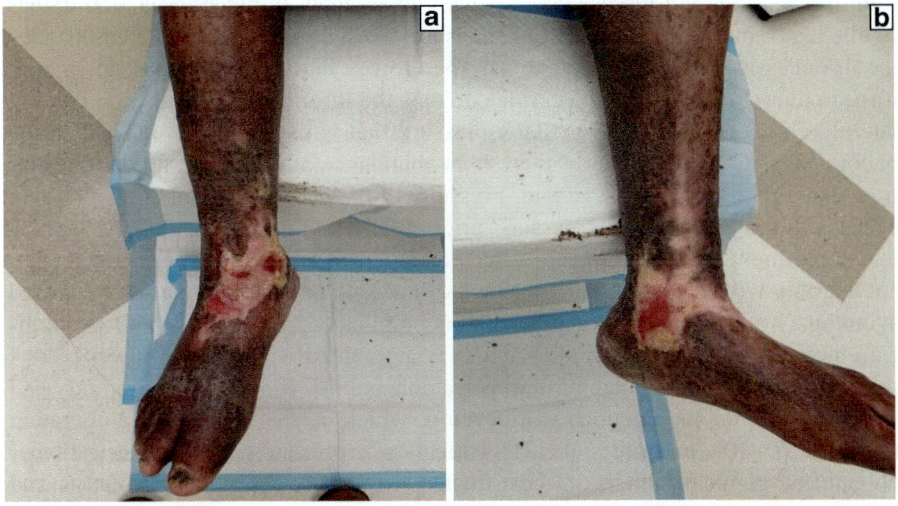

Fig. 4.1 Physical findings consistent with chronic venous insufficiency on the anterior (**a**) and medial aspect of the lower leg, ankle, and foot (**b**). Note the areas of hemosiderin deposition, resulting in hyperpigmentation, or rust-colored discoloration of the skin. Note also the medial location of both ulcers, which are in various stages of healing, typical for venous stasis ulceration

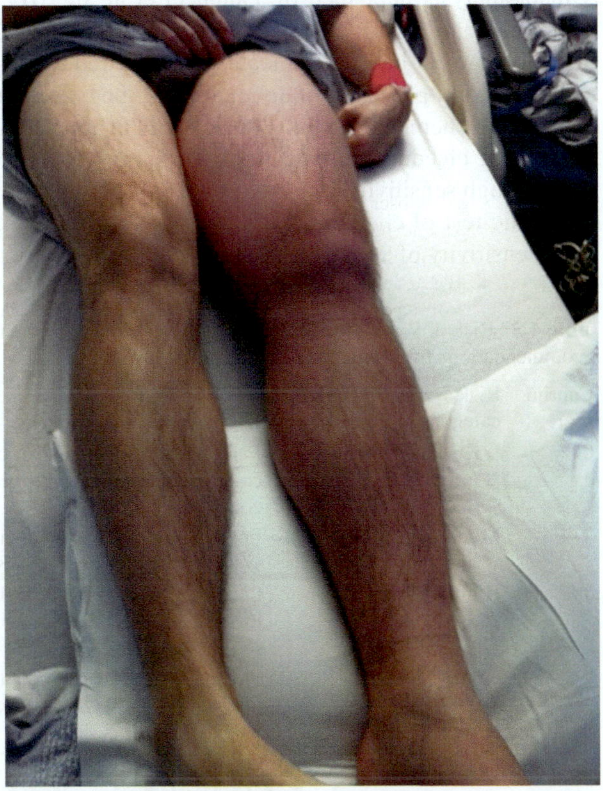

Fig. 4.2 Phlegmasia cerulea dolens of the left lower extremity

limb-threatening, and represents a surgical emergency. In phlegmasia alba dolens (white leg or milk leg), venous drainage is present but significantly decreased since the thrombosis spares collateral veins. Therefore, cyanosis will be absent. In contrast, in those with phlegmasia cerulea dolens, the thrombosis extends into the collateral veins, resulting in hydrostatic pressure that is exceedingly higher than the oncotic pressure. Consequently, there is an abundance of interstitial fluid sequestration that rapidly increases venous pressure [30]. When the interstitial pressure exceeds that of the capillary pressure, arterial ischemia ensues, potentially leading to compartment syndrome and so called venous gangrene. These patients will present not only with severe edema, pain, and cyanosis but also absent pulses, signs and symptoms not found in individuals with uncomplicated DVT. While both are surgical emergencies, phlegmasia alba dolens is associated with a much lower risk of major amputation than phlegmasia cerulea dolens [33]. If not treated promptly and aggressively, venous gangrene can develop, which carries a 20–50% amputation rate and a 20–40% mortality rate [21]. Patients who present with phlegmasia alba or phlegmasia cerulean dolens are best treated with therapeutic anticoagulation and thrombus removal [30].

The optimal approach to diagnosing DVT is a combination of risk stratification, laboratory testing, and, if appropriate, diagnostic imaging. One highly validated model that stratifies the risk for VTE and provides recommendations regarding prophylaxis during the hospital stay and upon discharge is the Caprini score (Table 4.2). A meta-analysis published by Pannucci et al. in 2017 demonstrated that patients with a higher Caprini score were more likely to develop a VTE and those with a Caprini score >7 had a significant VTE risk reduction in the perioperative period with chemoprophylaxis. Individualizing medicine by risk stratifying patients ensures that chemoprophylaxis is used only in appropriate surgical patients, thereby minimizing bleeding complications.

With high sensitivity and specificity, duplex ultrasound continues to be the initial diagnostic test of choice to diagnose DVT. One study reported duplex ultrasound had a sensitivity of 96% in a proximal DVT, sensitivity of 71% in a distal DVT, and

Table 4.2 Risk of venous thromboembolism as stratified by the Caprini score, with the attendant recommendations for adequate prophylaxis

Caprini score	Risk category	Risk percent	Recommended prophylaxis	Duration of prophylaxis
0–2	Low	Minimal	Early ambulation, pneumatic compression devices, +/− graduated compression stockings	During hospitalization
3–4	Moderate	0.7%	Pneumatic compression devices, +/− graduated compression stockings	During hospitalization
5–8	High	1.8–4%	Pneumatic compression devices *AND* low-dose heparin *OR* low molecular weight heparin	7–10 days
≥9	Highest	10.7%	Pneumatic compression devices *AND* low-dose heparin *OR* low molecular weight heparin	30 days

an overall specificity of 94% [34]. It is easily reproducible, noninvasive, painless, cost-effective, and safe to use during pregnancy. Even though it is thought to be less accurate in assessing veins below the knee, it is still a widely accepted technique.

In cases of iliofemoral DVT, the duplex ultrasound shows loss of respiratory variation at the common femoral vein [25]. Recognizing this finding is important since treatment of iliofemoral DVT differs compared to distal DVT due to higher risk of post-thrombotic syndrome. In the absence of flattened common femoral waveforms, one can safely assume that the proximal iliofemoral veins are patent (Fig. 4.3). Hence, an accurate negative duplex justifies withholding intervention (thrombolysis, balloon venoplasty, and/or stenting) for a suspected iliofemoral DVT. If a duplex is indeterminate, treatment administration can be decided based on other risk factors and laboratory testing. Duplex is limited in obese patients, those with marked edema, and areas not amenable to compression like the subclavian veins, iliac veins, and femoral vein at the adductor canal and is notoriously user-dependent.

Additional imaging includes contrast venography, computed tomographic venography, and magnetic resonance imaging. These modalities can be considered when DVT diagnosis remains uncertain after a duplex ultrasound or when the DVT in question is located in the pelvis or an upper extremity. CTV and MRV are useful diagnostic tools for overcoming anatomic limitations or diagnosing inferior vena caval thrombosis when other imaging is contraindicated or inadequate. It is important to highlight the fact that the most common etiology of a massive iliofemoral DVT arises from extrinsic compression, whether from compression of the left iliac vein between the right iliac artery and a vertebral body (May-Thurner syndrome), trauma, or, most commonly, compression via tumor [26]. In these scenarios, note that an MRV or CTV is necessary to diagnose and evaluate the mass effect. Overall, however, CTV and contrast venography are less preferred due to cost, invasiveness, and risk of renal dysfunction, and MRI is time-consuming and contraindicated in patients with certain hardware.

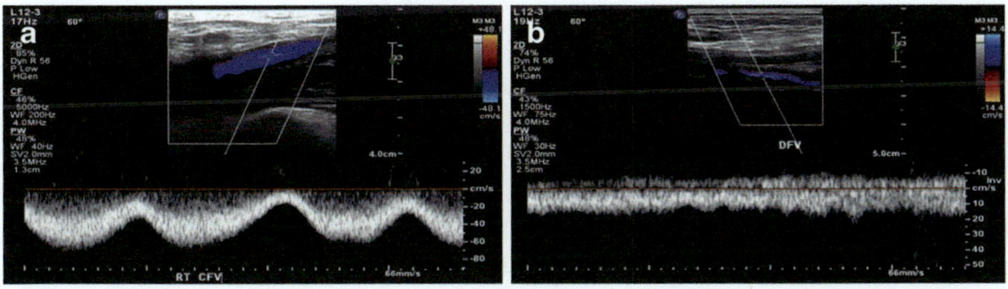

Fig. 4.3 Note the normal, respire-phasic waveforms with the gentle undulation with expiration and inspiration in (**a**). With proximal obstruction, the ability for changes in intra-abdominal pressure to influence the flow is obliterated, resulting in a non-phasic, flattened, or continuous Doppler venous waveform (**b**). (**a**) Normal phasic waveform in the common femoral vein that varies with respiration during the cardiac cycle. (**b**) Abnormal waveform in the common femoral vein. The absence of phasicity indicates an iliocaval venous obstruction. (Images courtesy of J. Chung)

Wells et al. created a scoring system based on risk factors and physical presentation that can be utilized to exclude the diagnosis of DVT without the need for a duplex ultrasound. A negative D-dimer in a patient combined with a low or intermediate Wells score has a negative predictive value of nearly 100%. However, use of the Wells score becomes more problematic when assessing patients categorized as high risk with a negative D-dimer. In these cases, it is recommended to proceed with duplex ultrasound. A resulting negative duplex is sufficient for ruling out a DVT, while a positive duplex warrants treatment with anticoagulation.

Upper Extremity

Thrombosis in upper extremity veins is far less common, accounting for 4% of all VTE cases. The most common locations of upper extremity DVT are the subclavian and axillary veins [3], though the jugular, brachiocephalic, distal brachial, ulnar, and radial veins are all possible sites. Although primary axillary and subclavian DVTs are rare, 10–15% cause PE.

Primary axillary/subclavian thrombosis is typically due to Paget-Schroetter syndrome (PSS), a venous form of thoracic outlet syndrome sometimes seen in young athletes or workers who use their arms repetitively. This occurs due to compression of the exiting vein in the thoracic outlet in the presence of anatomic abnormalities. Primary upper extremity DVT can also be a consequence of hypercoagulability. Secondary axillary/subclavian thromboses are more common, partly owing to the frequency of indwelling devices such as central venous catheters, pacemaker, or defibrillator leads [4]. Other risk factors include congestive heart failure and mediastinal tumors. As with lower extremity thrombosis, these clots may be occult or symptomatic. Suspicion for DVT should arise in patients presenting with unilateral upper extremity edema, pain, and cyanosis.

These veins can be difficult to directly visualize with duplex due to location and the shadowing of the clavicle. Nevertheless, duplex remains the dominant diagnostic test. If the duplex is indeterminate, CT or MRI can be used.

Pulmonary Embolism

A pulmonary embolism is a devastating and potentially fatal complication of DVT, occurring in up to 40% of patients with DVT and accounting for a majority of DVT-related deaths [13]. Clot from a DVT embolizes and travels into the pulmonary arteries, causing occlusion. These clots may range from small, sub-segmental emboli to massive emboli that lead to cardiogenic shock or cardiac arrest. Presentation is usually nonspecific; signs and symptoms include tachypnea, tachycardia, shortness of breath, dyspnea, pleuritic chest pain, and hemoptysis. Left untreated, PE carries a mortality rate of up to 25% [13]. The PIOPED II trial investigated the diagnostic accuracy of a CTA and indicated a 96% specificity in diagnosing a PE. Consequently, CTA became the modality of choice in assessing pulmonary vasculature [14].

V/Q scans and pulmonary arteriography have fallen out of favor due to inferior specificity and invasiveness, respectively.

Prophylaxis

VTE prophylaxis includes limiting venous stasis, reducing coagulability, or a combination of both. Mechanical prevention with graduated compression stockings or sequential compression devices (SCDs) compresses the leg compartments, resulting in an increase in venous return and fibrinolytic activity. Employing mechanical prophylaxis reduces the risk for DVT in surgical patients by two-thirds when used alone and by an additional 50% when used in conjunction with drug prophylaxis [6]. A Cochrane review found that monotherapy with graduated compression stockings reduced the risk of a DVT from 27% to 13% and, if added to any other prophylactic measure, further reduced the risk of a DVT from 15% to 2% [5]. In most hospital settings, utilization of SCDs is prevalently preferred over static graduation compression stockings. A meta-analysis demonstrated that sequential compression devices decrease the relative risk of DVT by 62% compared to placebo and 47% compared to graduated compression stockings [7].

In addition to sequential compression devices, other means of counteracting venous stasis have been investigated, such as physical exercises. One study aimed to identify forceful foot exercises that engaged the calf muscle pump, thereby increasing venous return [31]. Six exercises were performed, and peak systolic velocity was measured via Doppler ultrasound and recorded. While all exercises resulted in a marked increase in peak systolic velocity, the highest was achieved by forceful dorsiflexion with toe extension followed by plantar flexion with 250 Newtons and forceful flexion of all toes [31]. These simple maneuvers can be taught to patients prior to long periods of immobilization or during hospital admission stays.

The value of anticoagulation in the prevention of DVT has long been established. Studies have shown that unfractionated heparin (UFH) and low molecular weight heparin (LMWH) each reduce the risk of DVT and PE by approximately 60%. Notably, LMWH carries a lower risk of major bleeding compared to UFH due to its decreased ability to bind and inhibit thrombin [8]. Although the risk of complications from prophylactic levels of anticoagulation remains low, platelet counts should be closely monitored in any patient receiving heparin for the development of heparin-induced thrombocytopenia (HIT). This is a dose-independent reaction that should be suspected when platelet counts fall below 100,000 or where there ≥50% drop in platelet count occurs following the administration of heparin. When suspected, heparin should be immediately stopped and an alternate form of anticoagulation initiated. It is important to note, however, there are two types of HIT. Type I HIT is a nonimmune-mediated reaction resulting from platelet aggregation that is more common than type II and is of mild consequence. It can be seen as soon as after 1 day of therapy, and the platelet counts will spontaneously normalize even if heparin is continued [35]. Type II HIT is an immune-, antibody-mediated reaction and will therefore usually occur 5–14 days after receiving heparin [35]. The resulting hypercoagulable state can lead to life-threatening complications. As such, calculating the "4 T score" is the first step in diagnosing type II HIT. A score of 0–3 points indicates that HIT is unlikely and heparin therapy may precede as the other causes of thrombocytopenia are explored. A score of 4–5 corresponds to an intermediate probability, while a score of 6–8 is a high probability of HIT [35]. A score of 4+ warrants immediate discontinuation of all forms of heparin with the initiation of a direct thrombin inhibitor for further anticoagulation.

Treatment

Anticoagulation is the mainstay of treatment for DVT and should be initiated promptly when there is high suspicion for a DVT, regardless if there is a delay in diagnosis. Patients will be placed on an anticoagulation regimen for at least 3–6 months, depending on the absence or presence of propagating factors. Traditionally, treatment of a DVT began with the administration of heparin and then bridged to warfarin after 2–3 doses which typically places the INR between 2.5–3.0. Although heparin does not have thrombolytic activity, it is effective in preventing the propagation of the thrombus. It is relatively safe, is easy to administer, has a quick onset of action, has a relatively short half-life, and can be monitored.

Warfarin creates a hypercoagulable state in the first several days of its administration due to its inhibition of anticoagulant proteins C and S. Therefore, unopposed warfarin will exacerbate thrombus extension and can lead to warfarin-induced skin necrosis, a rare complication occurring in 1:10,000 [34]. For these reasons, warfarin therapy is always initiated in conjunction with parenteral anticoagulation until there is effective reduction of coagulation factors, which usually requires several days because of the varying half-lives of the vitamin-K dependent factors. Because of warfarin's narrow therapeutic window and drug and dietary interactions, patients will also require ongoing monitoring of their INR, aiming for an INR range between 2.0 and 3.0.

Novel oral anticoagulants (NOACs) such as direct-acting oral anticoagulants (apixaban, rivaroxaban, edoxaban) and direct factor IIa inhibitors (dabigatran) have recently been introduced as options for long-term anticoagulation. Both classes have been shown to be non-inferior to LMWH and warfarin. Instead of being bridged to warfarin, patients can now be transitioned to a DOAC/NOAC and sent home. The lack of requirement for routine laboratory monitoring is an added benefit of DOACs.

Anticoagulants alone are sufficient to prevent thrombus extension and recurrence in most DVTs. However, in cases of iliofemoral DVT or severe obstruction (Fig. 4.4), as seen in phlegmasia, where edema threatens limb viability, there is a marked increase in long-term morbidity. Studies show 95% of patients with iliofemoral DVT have valvular dysfunction 5 years after the initial DVT and 30% developed venous ulceration or claudication [9]. Therefore, in these patients intervention should be strongly considered. Suction thrombectomy and rheolytic thrombectomy

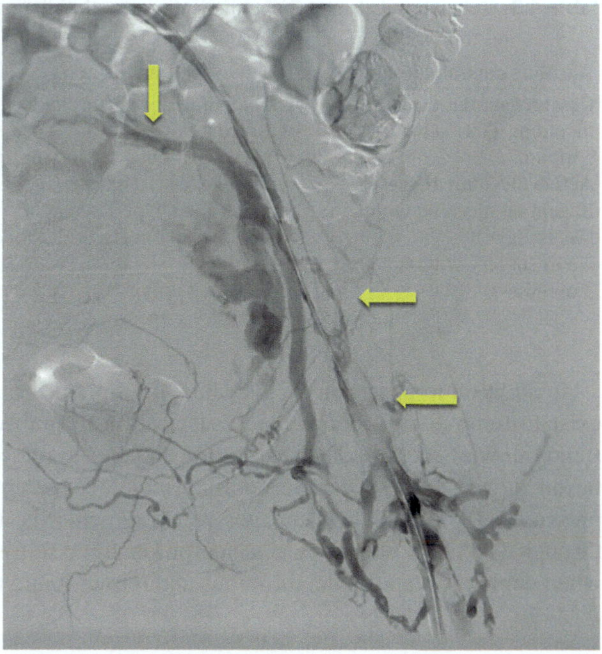

Fig. 4.4 Venogram of an extensive iliofemoral vein deep venous thrombosis. The areas free of thrombus show contrast partially filling the lumen of the vein segment. Areas of flow defects, as seen in the common femoral vein, and the external iliac vein, show where the acute thrombus is present (yellow arrows)

are two procedures designed to retrieve clots via catheter aspiration. The primary purpose of the ATTRACT trial was to investigate the risk of post-thrombotic syndrome development after treatment of DVT with either pharmacomechanical thrombolysis followed by anticoagulation or oral anticoagulation only [20]. Of the patients in the treatment arm who underwent catheter-directed thrombolysis, 46.7% went on to develop post-thrombotic syndrome, while 48.2% of patients who received anticoagulation alone went on to develop post-thrombotic syndrome [20]. The study concluded that there was no difference in prevalence of post-thrombotic syndrome between the two treatment arms ($p = 0.56$). However, the arm receiving pharmacomechanical thrombolysis had less moderate/severe post-thrombotic syndrome compared to the arm receiving thrombolysis alone ($p = 0.04$).

Thrombolysis using agents such as urokinase, streptokinase, and tissue plasminogen activator is commonly delivered through a catheter instead of systemically. This catheter-directed thrombolysis (CDT) is a minimally invasive endovascular approach that has become increasingly popular over the past decade. The 2011 CaVent trial revealed that long-term occurrence of post-thrombotic syndrome is reduced in patients who receive CDT compared to those who received traditional treatment with anticoagulation and compression stockings. However, CDT was associated with increased risk of bleeding [10] (Table 4.3).

While studies favor the addition of CDT, especially for iliofemoral DVT, it is important to be aware that not all patients are suitable candidates for this approach. Absolute contraindications to CDT include active internal bleeding and recent stroke [36]. Relative contraindications involve recent eye surgery, major surgery, or trauma [36].

Table 4.3 Relative and absolute contraindications for the administration of thrombolytic therapy

Absolute contraindications	Relative contraindications	Minor contraindications
Cerebrovascular events, including TIA, in the last 3 months Active bleeding diathesis Recent GI bleeding within the last 10 days Neurosurgery within the last 3 months	Cardiopulmonary resuscitation within the last 10 days Major nonvascular surgery or trauma within the last 10 days Uncontrolled hypertension of systolic >180 mmHg or diastolic >100 mmHg Intracranial tumor Recent eye surgery	Hepatic failure Bacterial endocarditis Pregnancy Diabetic hemorrhagic retinopathy

In addition to pharmacologic agents, multiple percutaneous mechanical devices exist to remove clot. Percutaneous aspiration thrombectomy devices rely upon a steady flow of suction via an aspiration catheter to remove the clot. Rheolytic aspiration devices utilize the Bernoulli principle by creating a vacuum with high-pressure hypotube, which engages and fragments the thrombus before aspiration through a catheter. Other devices incorporate three self-expanding nitinol disks that, when deployed, capture the thrombus and retract it into the aspiration catheter [37].

Future Investigation

Clinical investigation is ongoing in the areas of pharmacologic and mechanical prophylaxis, venous stenting, and prosthetic venous valves. Additionally, the quest to determine the optimal duration of anticoagulation after discharge using the safest and most efficacious medication is a top priority.

With the wider adoption of the direct oral anticoagulants, the management of VTE in the acute and long-term setting has been simplified. Direct thrombin (dabigatran) and factor Xa inhibitors (apixaban, rivaroxaban, and edoxaban) are first-line oral anticoagulants in nonpregnant patients without renal insufficiency or active cancer [37]. Unlike warfarin, routine lab testing and dose adjustments are not required for these medications. In nonpregnant patients with renal dysfunction, warfarin is the medication of choice for long-term anticoagulation [37]. However, warfarin does require bridging with heparin as it does not reach its full therapeutic effect until 5–7 days after beginning therapy. Premature discontinuation of heparin prior to warfarin reaching a full therapeutic effect can result in insufficient protection against DVT [37]. In patients without renal insufficiency who are unable to tolerate oral medications, low molecular weight heparin can be used, as it is as effective as warfarin in the prevention of VTE [39].

When assessing duration of anticoagulation, it is of utmost importance to individualize therapy based on risk factors and bleeding risks. In general, current guidelines recommend a minimum of 3 months of anticoagulation in patients with a first episode of VTE [37]. In patients with transient risk factors that are no longer present, isolated distal DVT, or if the bleeding risk is high, extending anticoagulation for longer than 3 months is not recommended [37]. The populations that are likely to benefit from indefinite anticoagulation include those who experience an unprovoked proximal DVT or PE and recurrent unprovoked VTE, patients with active cancer, and those with antiphospholipid antibody syndrome.

Advances in prophylactic strategies have led to the development of game-based exercises that augment blood flow in the deep venous system. A pilot study demonstrated that a series of foot exercises increases the average volume flow volume, flow velocity, and peak systolic velocity in the femoral vein by approximately 50% [38]. In doing so, patients can help mitigate the risk of clot formation.

In recent years, the role of venous stenting in acute and chronic venous insufficiency has received increased attention as treatment in patients with proximal venous disease, especially those with compressive pathologies, such as May-Thurner syndrome or pelvic tumors. One of the first large studies to look at stenting in chronic venous disease found an overall improvement in pain and swelling and healing of half of venous ulcers after venoplasty and stenting, suggesting a role for stenting in chronic venous disease [40]. Stenting has also attracted attention in the setting of acute venous disease for the alleviation of symptoms. Research has been focused on assessing the efficacy of invasive management versus anticoagulation alone. Park et al. conducted a study looking at venous stent placement following CDT. A venogram was used to evaluate the degree of stenosis after completion of CDT, and in patients that continued to have severe stenosis or those with May-Thurner syndrome, a stent was placed. At 5 years, those that received a stent had a venous patency rate of 77.8% compared to 42.1% in non-stented patients [41]. Additionally, DVT recurrence was markedly increased in the non-stented arm [41]. Regardless, stenting in acute DVT warrants further investigation as there is a paucity of studies examining the long-term efficacy of this intervention. (Insert venogram pictures here.)

Currently there are no FDA-approved thrombolytics approved for the treatment of DVT. However, alteplase, urokinase, and streptokinase have been well-studied and are FDA-approved for the treatment of PE [42]. Utilization of newer thrombolytics, such as tenecteplase, for DVT has been reported in small case studies. Development of agents that are increasingly specific and effective at dissolving clot continues to be one such area of future investigation [42].

In the last several decades, there has been experimental work regarding prosthetic and autogenous valve replacement in the treatment of chronic venous insufficiency. One study showed autogenous valve transplants to be patent and competent for up to 3 months, and while these short-term results appeared to be promising, long-term results remain disappointing [42]. Percutaneous prosthetic or autogenous venous valves may prove to be a minimally invasive treatment, but further studies are required to document their success.

Summary

Venous thromboembolism (VTE) continues to be a significant source of inhospital morbidity, complicating up to 20% of hospital admissions. The most recent epidemiologic data shows that approximately 900,000 patients suffer VTE per year in the United States, and is responsible for approximately 100,000 deaths. This makes VTE the third most lethal cardiovascular disease in America. Virchow's triad, comprised of stasis, hypercoagulability, and endothelial cell damage, underpins the risk factors for the development of VTE. The Caprini score has been validated to help practitioners risk stratify patients for the potential to develop VTE, and hence their need for prophylactic measures. Most VTE occurs in the lower extremity and pelvic veins, though a significant minority may develop in the upper extremities. Duplex ultrasound, D-dimer, and application of Wells criteria remain the mainstays of the diagnosis of deep vein thrombosis (DVT). Identification of pulmonary embolus hinges mostly upon computed tomographic angiography. Physicians continue to rely upon systemic anticoagulation to manage DVT. Novel oral anticoagulants (NOACs) have been rapidly supplanting more traditional means of anticoagulation with similar efficacy. Thrombolysis and other devices to remove thrombus are reserved for more extensive thrombus burdens and in the setting of phlegmasia cerulean dolens and massive PE. Future investigations abound in the areas of pharmacologic and mechanical prophylaxis, venous stenting, and prosthetic valves.

References

1. Dobromirski M, Cohen AT. How I manage venous thromboembolism risk in hospitalized medical patients. Blood. 2012;120(8):1562–9. https://doi.org/10.1182/blood-2012-03-378901.
2. Cohen AT, et al. Venous thromboembolism risk and prophylaxis in the acute hospital care setting (ENDORSE Study): a multinational cross-sectional study. Lancet. 2008; 371(9610):387–94. https://doi.org/10.1016/s0140-6736(08)60202-0.
3. Muñoz FJ, et al. Clinical outcome of patients with upper-extremity deep vein thrombosis. Chest. 2008;133(1):143–8. https://doi.org/10.1378/chest.07-1432.
4. Douketis JD, et al. Deep venous thrombosis (DVT) – cardiovascular disorders. Merck Manuals Professional Edition. Merck Manuals; 2021.
5. Kahn SR. The post-thrombotic syndrome. Hematology. 2016;2016(1):413–8. https://doi.org/10.1182/asheducation-2016.1.413.
6. Prandoni P, et al. Below-knee elastic compression stockings to prevent the post-thrombotic syndrome: a randomized, controlled trial. J Vasc Surg. 2005;41(1):177. https://doi.org/10.1016/j.jvs.2004.10.021.
7. Amaragiri, Sachiendra V, and Timothy Lees. "Elastic compression stockings for prevention of deep vein thrombosis." Cochrane Database Syst Rev, 2000 (3):CD001484, doi:https://doi.org/10.1002/14651858.cd001484.
8. Roderick P, et al. Towards evidence-based guidelines for the prevention of venous thromboembolism: systematic reviews of mechanical methods, oral anticoagulation, dextran and regional anaesthesia as thromboprophylaxis. Health Technol Assess. 2005;9(49):iii–iv, ix–x, 1–78. https://doi.org/10.3310/hta9490.
9. Vanek VW. Meta-analysis of effectiveness of intermittent pneumatic compression devices with a comparison of thigh-high to knee-high sleeves. Am Surg. 1998;64(11):1050–8. https://www.crd.york.ac.uk/CRDWeb/ShowRecord.asp?AccessionNumber=11998001884&AccessionNumber=11998001884. Accessed 6 Oct 2019.
10. Laporte-Simitsidis S, et al. Prevention of venous thromboembolism in internal medicine with unfractionated or low-molecular-weight heparins: a meta-analysis of randomised clinical trials. Thromb Haemost. 2000;83(01):14–9. https://doi.org/10.1055/s-0037-1613749.
11. Watson L, et al. Thrombolysis for acute deep vein thrombosis. Cochrane Database Syst Rev. 2016;11(11):CD002783. https://doi.org/10.1002/14651858.cd002783.pub4.

12. Vedantham S, et al. Quality improvement guidelines for the treatment of lower-extremity deep vein thrombosis with use of endovascular thrombus removal. J Vasc Interv Radiol. 2014;25(9):1317–25. https://doi.org/10.1016/j.jvir.2014.04.019.
13. White RH. The epidemiology of venous thromboembolism. Circulation. 2003;107(23 Suppl 1):I4–8. https://doi.org/10.1161/01.cir.0000078468.11849.66.
14. Moheimani F, Jackson DE. Venous thromboembolism: classification, risk factors, diagnosis, and management. ISRN Hematol. 2011;2011:1–7. https://doi.org/10.5402/2011/124610.
15. Anderson FA, Wheeler HB. Physician practices in the management of venous thromboembolism: a community-wide survey. J Vasc Surg. 1992;16(5):707–14. https://doi.org/10.1016/0741-5214(92)90225-w.
16. Anderson FA. Risk factors for venous thromboembolism. Circulation. 2003;107(23 Suppl 1):I9–16. https://doi.org/10.1161/01.cir.0000078469.07362.e6.
17. Ho WK, et al. Risk of recurrent venous thromboembolism in patients with common thrombophilia. Arch Intern Med. 2006;166(7):729. https://doi.org/10.1001/archinte.166.7.729.
18. Tapson VF. The role of smoking in coagulation and thromboembolism in chronic obstructive pulmonary disease. Proc Am Thorac Soc. 2005;2(1):71–7. https://doi.org/10.1513/pats.200407-038ms.
19. Feher MD, et al. Acute changes in atherogenic and thrombogenic factors with cessation of smoking. J R Soc Med. 1990;83(3):146–8. https://doi.org/10.1177/014107689008300306.
20. Comerota AJ, et al. Endovascular thrombus removal for acute iliofemoral deep vein thrombosis. Circulation. 2019;139(9):1162–73. https://doi.org/10.1161/circulationaha.118.037425.
21. Doleman B, et al. Phlegmasia caerulea dolens secondary to pelvic plasmacytoma and left femoral deep vein thrombosis. Int J Surg Case Rep. 2013;4(10):825–7. https://doi.org/10.1016/j.ijscr.2013.07.010.
22. Kahn SR, et al. Determinants and time course of the postthrombotic syndrome after acute deep venous thrombosis. J Vasc Surg. 2009;49(5):1358. https://doi.org/10.1016/j.jvs.2009.03.021.
23. Farrell JJ, et al. Incidence and interventions for post-thrombotic syndrome. Cardiovasc Diagn Ther. 2016;6(6):623–31. https://doi.org/10.21037/cdt.2016.11.22.
24. Kearon C. Natural history of venous thromboembolism. Circulation. 2003;107(23 Suppl 1):I22–30. https://doi.org/10.1161/01.cir.0000078464.82671.78.
25. Min S-K, et al. Diagnosis and treatment of lower extremity deep vein thrombosis: Korean practice guidelines. Vasc Specialist Int. 2016;32(3):77–104. https://doi.org/10.5758/vsi.2016.32.3.77.
26. Casey ET, et al. Treatment of acute iliofemoral deep vein thrombosis. J Vasc Surg. 2012;55(5):1463–73. https://doi.org/10.1016/j.jvs.2011.12.082.
27. Bělohlávek J, et al. Pulmonary embolism, part I: epidemiology, risk factors and risk stratification, pathophysiology, clinical presentation, diagnosis and nonthrombotic pulmonary embolism. Exp Clin Cardiol. 2013;18(2):129–38.
28. Horlander KT, et al. Pulmonary embolism mortality in the United States, 1979–1998. Arch Intern Med. 2003;163(14):1711. https://doi.org/10.1001/archinte.163.14.1711.
29. Kahn SR, Ginsberg JS. Relationship between deep venous thrombosis and the postthrombotic syndrome. Arch Intern Med. 2004;164(1):17. https://doi.org/10.1001/archinte.164.1.17.
30. Mumoli N, et al. Phlegmasia cerulea dolens. Circulation. 2012;125(8):1056–7. https://doi.org/10.1161/circulationaha.111.051912.
31. Kropp AT, et al. The efficacy of forceful ankle and toe exercises to increase venous return: a comprehensive doppler ultrasound study. Phlebology. 2017;33(5):330–7. https://doi.org/10.1177/0268355517706042.
32. Bose E, Hravnak M. Thromboelastography: a practice summary for nurse practitioners treating hemorrhage. J Nurse Pract. 2015;11(7):702–9. https://doi.org/10.1016/j.nurpra.2015.05.006.
33. Chaochankit W, Akaraborworn O. Phlegmasia cerulea dolens with compartment syndrome. Ann Vasc Dis. 2018;11(3):355–7. https://doi.org/10.3400/avd.cr.18-00030.
34. Goodacre S, et al. Systematic review and meta-analysis of the diagnostic accuracy of ultrasonography for deep vein thrombosis. BMC Med Imaging. 2005;5(1):6. https://doi.org/10.1186/1471-2342-5-6.

35. Nicolas D, Nicolas S, Reed M. Heparin induced thrombocytopenia (HIT) [updated 2020 Feb 14]. In: StatPearls [internet]. Treasure Island (FL): StatPearls Publishing; 2020.
36. Morrison H. Catheter-directed thrombolysis for acute limb ischemia. Semin Interv Radiol. 2006;23(3):258–69. https://doi.org/10.1055/s-2006-948765.
37. Kearon C, et al. Antithrombotic therapy for VTE disease. Chest. 2012;141(2):E419S–96S. https://doi.org/10.1378/chest.11-2301.
38. Chung J, et al. Pilot study evaluating the efficacy of exergaming for the prevention of deep venous thrombosis. J Vasc Surg. 2017;66(3):e55–6. https://doi.org/10.1016/j.jvs.2017.05.071.
39. Van Der Heijden JF, et al. Vitamin K antagonists or low-molecular-weight heparin for the long term treatment of symptomatic venous thromboembolism. Cochrane Database Syst Rev. 2001;4:CD002001. https://doi.org/10.1002/14651858.cd002001.
40. Neglén P, et al. Endovascular surgery in the treatment of chronic primary and post-thrombotic iliac vein obstruction. Eur J Vasc Endovasc Surg. 2000;20(6):560–71. https://doi.org/10.1053/ejvs.2000.1251.
41. Srinivas BC, et al. Outcome of venous stenting following catheter directed thrombolysis for acute proximal lower limb venous thrombosis: a prospective study with venous doppler follow-up at 1-year. Cardiovasc Interv Ther. 2015;30(4):320–6. https://doi.org/10.1007/s12928-015-0317-5.
42. Vedantham S, et al. Guidance for the use of thrombolytic therapy for the treatment of venous thromboembolism. J Thromb Thrombolysis. 2016;41(1):68–80. https://doi.org/10.1007/s11239-015-1318-z.

Postoperative Spinal Cord Ischemia and Stroke

5

Xin Peng, Bruce L. Tjaden, and Kristofer M. Charlton-Ouw

Abbreviations

CAS	Carotid artery stenting
CEA	Carotid endarterectomy
CI	Cardiac index
CSF	Cerebrospinal fluid
CT	Computed tomography
EEG	Electroencephalography
EPD	Embolic protection device
ICA	Internal carotid artery
MEP	Motor evoked potential
NIRS	Near-infrared spectroscopy
SCI	Spinal cord ischemia
SSEP	Somatosensory evoked potential
TCD	Transcranial Doppler
TEVAR	Thoracic endovascular aortic repair
TPA	Tissue plasminogen activator

X. Peng
Division of Vascular Diseases and Surgery, Wexner Medical Center, The Ohio State University, Columbus, OH, USA

B. L. Tjaden
Division of Vascular and Endovascular Surgery, Cooper University Health Care, Camden, NJ, USA

K. M. Charlton-Ouw (✉)
HCA Gulf Coast Division, Vascular Surgery, Gulf Coast Vascular, HCA Houston Healthcare, Departments of Clinical and Biomedical Sciences, University of Houston College of Medicine, Houston, TX, USA
e-mail: kmcharlt@central.uh.edu

R. Gilani, J. L. Mills Sr. (eds.), *Vascular Complications of Surgery and Intervention*, https://doi.org/10.1007/978-3-030-86713-3_5

Introduction

Spinal cord ischemia (SCI) and stroke in the postoperative setting are potentially devastating complications that greatly affect patients' quality of life. It is crucial to identify patients at elevated risk for these complications and to diagnose them in a timely fashion. Having clear protocols to manage these complications is critical. In this chapter, we discuss the management strategies for both postoperative SCI and stroke.

Spinal Cord Ischemia

SCI is a feared risk; it occurs during and after operations involving the thoracoabdominal aorta but can also develop after aortic arch and infrarenal aortic repair. The rates of this complication are reported to be 3–10% among open thoracoabdominal aortic surgery [1] and 0.2–0.6% in infrarenal aortic surgery [2–4]. Risk factors for SCI include renal insufficiency, extent of aortic repair, use of surgical SCI mitigation adjuncts, previous aortic repair, and any postoperative hypotension (Table 5.1). Despite the decreased overall morbidity and mortality associated with endovascular aortic surgery, the rate of SCI has not changed greatly with this approach [5–7].

Immediate SCI is defined as that which occurs during the procedure, and is noted immediately upon patient arousal after anesthesia, regardless of severity. We define delayed SCI as occurring anytime after intervention in a patient previously noted to be neurologically intact after aortic surgery and after exclusion of stroke. For both immediate and delayed SCI, we categorize the severity using the modified Tarlov scale [8, 9] (Table 5.2). Recovery of function after immediate paraplegia is generally poor.

The pathophysiology leading to spinal ischemia is complex. In open thoracic aortic surgery, it is attributable to aortic cross-clamping, steal syndrome leading to back-bleeding into an open excluded aortic segment, insufficient reperfusion, spinal cord edema, and subsequent elevated intrathecal pressure [10–13]. Minimizing aortic cross-clamp time is also important, although due to the wide variation of collateral network supplying the spinal cord, there is no known absolute maximum time a patient may be able to tolerate aortic cross-clamping [11]. In endovascular surgery involving the thoracic aorta, pathogenesis of SCI is believed to be inadequate perfusion by the collateral network supplying the spinal cord after endograft coverage, and thromboembolic events involving the segmental spinal arteries [6]. Spinal ischemia from infrarenal aortic surgery is thought to result from atheroembolic events to the conus medullaris [4].

Intraoperative Prevention

Table 5.3 lists the SCI mitigation techniques for open and endovascular surgery. The choice depends on surgeon preference, local expertise, and previous experiences. Surgical adjuncts for spinal cord protection in open surgery include "permissive" hypothermia, sequential clamping technique, distal aortic perfusion, selective

Table 5.1 Risk factors for spinal cord ischemia in open and endovascular aortic surgery

Patient characteristic
Older age
Renal insufficiency
Peripheral arterial disease
Disease characteristic
Extent II or III thoracoabdominal aortic aneurysm
DeBakey type I aortic dissection
DeBakey type III aortic dissection
Prior intervention
Previous open aortic surgery
Previous endovascular aortic repair
Anatomic consideration
Endograft coverage >20 cm of thoracic aorta
Endograft coverage >4 cm of the aorta proximal to celiac trunk
Endograft coverage T8–L2
Bilateral hypogastric artery occlusion
Left subclavian artery occlusion
Perioperative factor
Hypotension
Pressor requirement
Transfusion requirement
Not using mitigation techniques
Refer to Table 5.3

Table 5.2 Modified Tarlov scale was used to categorize the severity of SCI

Modified Tarlov scale		
Grade	Motor function	Deficits
0	No lower extremity movement	Paraplegia
1	Lower extremity motion without gravity	Paraplegia
2	Lower extremity motion against gravity	Paraplegia
3	Able to stand without assistance	Paraparesis
4	Able to walk with assistance	Paraparesis
5	Able to perform all activity	Normal

reimplantation of intercostal arteries, and prophylactic lumbar cerebrospinal fluid (CSF) drainage [11, 14]. Intraoperative neurophysiologic monitoring, including electroencephalography, somatosensory evoked potential (SSEP), and motor evoked potential (MEP) are tools that assist in intraoperative decision-making with regard to resuscitative efforts, addition of vasoactive agents, lumbar drainage, and decision to reimplant intercostal arteries [15, 16]. Intraoperative loss of lower extremity evoked potentials can help guide therapy which might include CSF drainage via the lumbar drain, transfusion to hemoglobin above 10 mg/dL, driving the systolic blood pressure above 140 mmHg, and expeditious reimplantation of the intercostal arteries.

For those undergoing endovascular repair, preemptive CSF drainage is recommended in high-risk patients, such as those who have had previous aortic surgery,

Table 5.3 Techniques to mitigate SCI in open and endovascular surgery

Open
Permissive hypothermia
Sequential clamping
Distal aortic perfusion
Reimplantation of intercostal arteries
Prophylactic lumbar drain placement
Endovascular
Preemptive spinal artery embolization
Prophylactic lumbar drain placement

bilateral hypogastric artery occlusion, left subclavian occlusion without revascularization, or aortic coverage of T8 to L2 vertebral bodies, as this segment is thought to be the origin of the artery of Adamkiewicz [6, 17]. Preemptive embolization of spinal arteries and placement of perfusion branches to trigger the growth of more collaterals (essentially, ischemic preconditioning) prior to thoracic endovascular aortic repair (TEVAR) have also been described [17].

Postoperative Management

Postoperative patients are evaluated frequently for neurologic changes in an intensive care unit setting. As soon as the patient fully emerges from anesthesia, a baseline neurological exam is obtained.

SCI Treatment Protocol

Immediate evidence of SCI postoperatively, or the intraoperative loss of evoked potentials without recovery, should prompt initiation of a SCI treatment protocol (Fig. 5.1). Patients are kept flat and at bedrest, with goal spinal pressure of less than 5 mmHg, checked on an hourly basis with subsequent unlimited drainage until the goal is met. Patients' oxygen saturation is optimized, hemoglobin kept above 10 mg/dl, and cardiac index (CI) kept above 2.5 L/min/BSA through use of resuscitation and vasoactive agents. Systolic blood pressure goal is above 140 mmHg, with the goal of systolic blood pressure and CSF pressure gradient of >130 mmHg. Renal replacement therapy is avoided as much as possible to maintain a stable blood pressure that does not range more than 15 mmHg. In general, this protocol is implemented for at least 7 days before clamping of the lumbar drain is considered.

Modified SCI Prevention Protocol

Patients who have awakened from anesthesia and are found to be neurologically intact are closely monitored in the intensive care unit (Fig. 5.2). Delayed paresis and

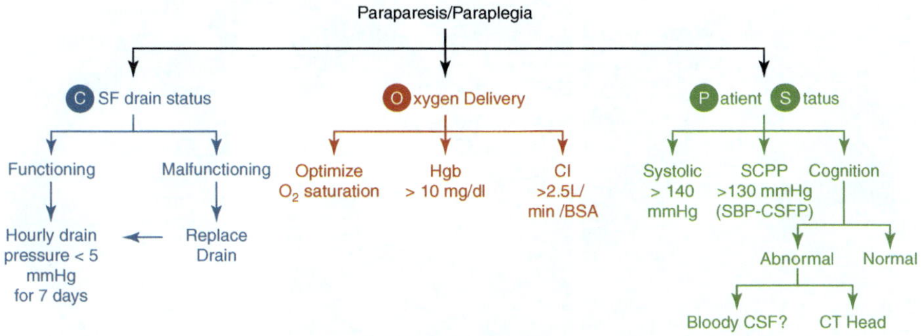

Fig. 5.1 SCI treatment protocol involves CSF drainage, maximization of oxygen delivery, and permissive hypertension

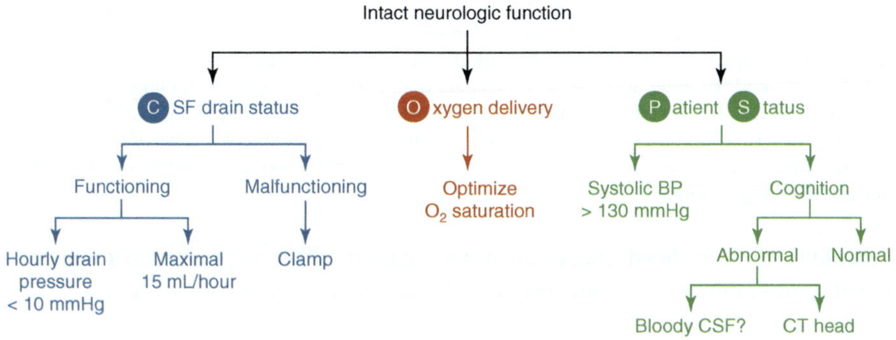

Fig. 5.2 SCI prevention protocol involves less aggressive CSF drainage and a lower systolic blood pressure goal

paralysis are most commonly reported an average of 1.8 days postoperatively, although delayed SCI has been seen 2 weeks after surgery and later. Therefore, for the first 24–48 h after surgery, an SCI prevention protocol is implemented. Spinal pressure is checked via the lumbar drain on an hourly basis, with goal pressure of less than 10 mmHg. If higher than 10 mmHg, CSF is drained up to a maximum of 15 mL per hour. Systolic blood pressure is maintained at above 130 mmHg, once again, taking care to avoid fluctuations of greater than 15 mmHg. On the second day, the lumbar drain is clamped. After endovascular surgery, the drain may be removed later on the second day if the patient remains neurologically intact. After open surgery, the drain may be removed on the third day. If the patient develops paresis or paralysis, then the formal SCI treatment protocol is initiated. Delayed SCI occurring after lumbar drain removal prompts urgent replacement of a new lumbar drain, and reinitiation of the formal SCI treatment protocol.

If there is any blood in the CSF fluid, the lumbar drain is immediately clamped and any coagulopathy corrected. Decision for definitive removal of the lumbar drain depends upon whether the patient remains neurologically intact. Any focal

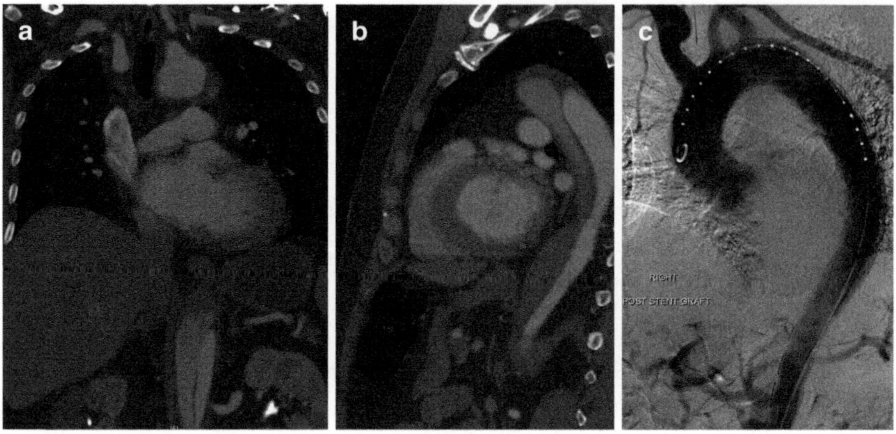

Fig. 5.3 (**a** and **b**): Coronal and sagittal views of CT angiography of a 56-year-old male who presented to our institution with an acute symptomatic DeBakey IIIb dissection complicated by right kidney malperfusion and acute renal failure. (**c**): completion angiography following an emergent thoracic endovascular aortic repair. This patient underwent placement of a lumbar drain prior to the procedure, which had to be clamped due to bloody CSF. He developed paraplegia on postoperative day 1, prompting lumbar drain replacement. He was initiated on 7 days of SCI treatment protocol and regained all neurologic function of the bilateral lower extremities. He was subsequently discharged home

neurologic deficits, headache, or altered mentation will prompt an immediate computed tomography (CT) of the head to rule out intracranial hemorrhage.

Recovery

Patients who have recovered successfully with modified SCI prevention protocol will generally not require other adjuncts to maintain spinal cord perfusion. Those who have required the formal SCI treatment protocol are generally successfully weaned off the multimodal management strategy (Fig. 5.3). Rarely, patients will require long-term permissive hypertension for the purpose of maintaining adequate spinal cord perfusion pressures.

Stroke

Postoperative strokes can be classified based on the timeframes in which they occur: intraoperative (apparent upon emergence from anesthesia) or postoperative (occurring after a period of normalcy postoperatively) [18]. Postoperative strokes may occur anywhere from hours to days after surgery [19]. Studies performed on perioperative strokes associated with carotid endarterectomy (CEA) indicate numerous different mechanisms for stroke, including embolic and thrombotic events, hemodynamic alterations leading to cerebral hypoperfusion, and hemorrhage [20]. The most frequent causes are arterial thrombosis and embolization as a result of technical errors, including intimal disruption during placement of an intraluminal shunt, intimal flaps following endarterectomy, and residual intraluminal thrombi [21]. Clinically significant cerebral ischemia can develop and be sustained during clamping of the carotid artery. This mechanism may account for up to one-third of perioperative strokes in carotid surgery [22, 23]. Sustained bradycardia and hypotension intraoperatively and postoperatively can lead to global cerebral ischemia. Intracerebral hemorrhage can occur as a sequela of carotid surgery, though the incidence of this is reported to be low at 0.6% [24]. In total, the incidence of stroke associated with CEA ranges from 2% to 3%, and with carotid artery stenting (CAS) from 5% to 8% [25]. The strongest risk factor for perioperative stroke is a history of preoperative stroke [26, 27]. Completion angiography has not proven to reduce the risk of stroke or death, and, therefore, no standardized recommendations exist [28].

The incidence and etiology of stroke associated with thoracic aortic surgery have not been studied as extensively as other complications, such as death, bleeding, and paraplegia. Available studies cite a 6.9% postoperative stroke risk in operations involving the ascending aorta and 8.1% in the descending aorta. Similar to carotid procedures, most strokes are embolic in nature, followed by ischemic and hemorrhagic. Risk factors include emergency aortic surgery, surgery in the descending aorta, higher transfusion need for fresh frozen plasma, and history of diabetes mellitus [29]. In urgent, nonelective settings, neurologic complications may occur in up to 10–13% of cases [30].

The risk of stroke in patients undergoing abdominal aortic surgeries has been reported to be between 0.2% and 3.1%, while lower extremity procedures carry a stroke risk between 0.5% and 2% [31]. Risk factors for stroke in these situations included history of stroke and degree of critical illness.

Cerebral Protection Strategies

Various approaches have been undertaken to provide cerebral protection. The strategy employed is dependent upon the nature of the procedure.

During CEA, minimal manipulation of the diseased carotid bulb and early clamping of the internal carotid artery (ICA) will minimize distal embolic events [32]. Another benefit of this approach is that it can provide an early indication of whether shunting will be necessary.

Patients unable to tolerate the interruption of cerebral blood flow during carotid clamping may benefit from shunt placement. Some surgeons prefer to routinely shunt. The benefits of this approach include familiarity with the act of shunt insertion and the fact that it simplifies the operation and reduces the potential for intraoperative "surprises." There is reasonable evidence to support routine or selective shunting, but never has shunting been shown to be an inferior approach nor has it been associated with a substantially higher stroke rate [22]. Early literature recommended routine use, but later studies demonstrated that shunts themselves carry risks of complications [33]. Disadvantages for use include arterial dissection, air embolism, shunt thrombosis, dislodgement, increased time for insertion and removal, need for longer arteriotomy, and worse visualization of the endpoint [22, 34]. Therefore, the risks and benefits of shunting must be carefully considered. Various methods have been described to monitor cerebral function intraoperatively to determine need for shunting, such as electroencephalography (EEG) and transcranial Doppler (TCD). CEA can also be performed under local or regional anesthesia and neurologic status monitored to determine the need for a shunt. These techniques will be further discussed in the next section.

With respect to CAS (carotid artery stenting), several types of embolic protection devices (EPDs) are available, including distal filters, distal occlusion balloons, proximal occlusion balloons, and flow reversal systems [35, 36]. Studies comparing CEA with CAS and distal EPD in high-risk lesions have demonstrated noninferiority of CAS when comparing a composite 1-year end-point events of death, stroke, and myocardial infarction [37, 38]. High procedural success has been reported using distal filters and occlusive balloons, with a low rate of complications. These complications included ICA dissection secondary to device-induced injury, "trapped" guidewires, and transient arterial spasm [39]. The major limitation of distal EPDs is that they require crossing the stenosis with a wire and filter before initiation of protection, risking disturbance of the plaque and embolic events. This mechanism may contribute to 15% of clinical strokes [35, 40]. Distal occlusive balloons cause complete flow cessation, which may be intolerable for some patients. While filters avoid this and preserve some antegrade flow, this very characteristic renders them less effective than the balloon in capturing microemboli smaller than 100–150 micrometers in size [35]. Even miniscule particles of less than 10 micrometers that do not contribute to clinically significant strokes have been associated with cognitive deterioration. As such, the true incidence of long-term complications secondary to distal EPD may be underestimated [35].

Proximal EPDs that have been studied include both an occlusive balloon device and a flow reversal system. Again, balloons have the potential disadvantage of totally interrupting cerebral flow [36]. On the other hand, proximal control with flow reversal is believed to be favorable as it eliminates distal embolic events to the brain and allows the operator to avoid the aortic arch and supra-aortic vessels via direct transcervical common carotid artery access [41]. Furthermore, retrograde flow may theoretically reduce "stagnation" of flow by allowing for continued runoff through the carotid artery of interest and facilitating additional flow through the circle of Willis. Investigation of reversal of flow technique thus far has proven to be promising, as long as the anatomy of the patient permits its use [42].

Cerebral perfusion and hypothermia are established cerebral protection modalities in open aortic surgery [43]. Hypothermia exerts a protective effect by reducing the metabolic rate and, therefore, the consumption of oxygen, preserving phosphate-based energy storage units, and decreasing neurotransmitter release [44]. The optimal goal temperature of hypothermia is not strictly established. At its early inception, deep or profound hypothermia was utilized [29, 45]. However, profound hypothermia is associated with coagulopathy, dysfunction of the cerebral microvasculature, neuronal injury, and systemic inflammatory response syndrome [29, 46]. Moderate hypothermia with adjunctive cerebral perfusion in arch pathology has been studied as an alternative and found to be equally protective, although there remains a wide variation in practice [29, 44, 46, 47]. Use of cerebral perfusion leads to decreased stroke rate, and use of retrograde or antegrade modalities depends on the severity and location of aortic atherosclerotic disease [45, 48–50].

Intraoperative Monitoring Strategies

Cerebral protection strategies can only be adequately and optimally utilized in the setting of appropriate intraoperative monitoring. There are various means by which brain perfusion can be evaluated.

In many centers, CEA is performed in awake patients [22, 23]. This provides the most immediate and clinically relevant measure of cerebral perfusion [51–53]. Compared with concomitantly performed EEG and stump pressure measurements, awake CEA has been demonstrated to be the most sensitive and specific test to determine the need for shunting [52, 54, 55].

Carotid artery stump pressure measurement is a simple, inexpensive test of cerebral perfusion during proximal clamping which can be performed as an adjunct or independently. A stump pressure of >45 mmHg reliably predicts adequate cerebral perfusion [56]. Other authors have used a cutoff of 50 mmHg [57].

EEG measures electrical activities produced by the brain via electrodes placed on the scalp. Reliability of EEG is inconsistent. It may be both oversensitive and, at the same time, fail to detect all patients who would require shunting [52, 54, 58]. Cerebral ischemia deep in the basal ganglia or the white matter may not be captured—in these patients, EEG may only be diagnostic in 34% of cases [58]. If an abnormality is picked up on EEG, however, it correlates with a statistically significant increase in intraoperative stroke [59, 60].

TCD involves the insonation of the middle cerebral artery through the temporal window. It is a reliable modality to evaluate real-time hemodynamic abnormalities, including flow, thrombosis, and embolism, by measuring the velocity and evaluating the waveforms of the middle cerebral artery [61]. However, as anesthesia interferes with resistance of the intracranial arteries and, thus, cerebral blood flow, an absolute velocity may not suffice to determine the need for shunting. Rather, comparing the pre-clamp to post-clamp velocity may be the best guide in decision-making. A post-clamp velocity which decreases by more than two-thirds of the pre-clamp velocity indicates the need for a shunt [55]. The other advantage of TCD is its sensitivity in detecting microemboli, thus providing real-time information to guide the operator to adapt and finesse surgical technique [62]. While it is important to note that the exact number, size, composition, and, therefore, impact of the microemboli are incompletely understood, more than 10 embolic signals have been correlated with new ischemic lesions on postop magnetic resonance imaging [62].

Near-infrared spectroscopy (NIRS) is another noninvasive technique which monitors cerebral perfusion by way of cerebral hemoglobin oxygen desaturation. Its reliability is controversial, and the critical regional oxygen saturation threshold at which neurologic symptoms develop has not been determined [63–68]. Rather, a decrease in oxygen saturation of less than 20% from baseline is thought to reliably predict adequate cerebral perfusion with high specificity. However, a decrease of more than 20% does not necessarily correlate with poor perfusion, and sensitivity is quite low [63, 69].

SSEP involves measurement of electrical activity response at the skin. Studies have also shown conflicting results over its reliability as a stand-alone modality [70–72]. It has high specificity but low sensitivity to detect neurologic events—and patients with postoperative strokes are 14-fold more likely to have had SSEP changes [73].

Numerous studies have demonstrated that these cerebral monitoring strategies used in conjunction help to provide the most accurate real-time information about cerebral perfusion and embolic events. The combined use of these modalities may assist in intraoperative decision-making with the goal of minimizing neurologic events.

Intraoperative Stroke

An intraoperative stroke after carotid surgery is first diagnosed in the operating room upon emergence from anesthesia. The presence of neurologic deficits should prompt immediate re-exploration to examine the ICA. It is checked for flow using a Doppler, followed by Duplex ultrasonography or on-table angiography if flow is detected.

Abnormal or absent flow through the ICA must be re-explored by opening the endarterectomy. If thrombosis is encountered, careful thromboembolectomy is performed. The underlying cause must be identified, however, and careful inspection of the endarterectomy bed or the intimal ledge must be undertaken to rule out and repair the causative technical defect. Distal clamping of the ICA is not recommended. If a shunt is to be replaced, this must be performed with the utmost care so as to not injure the distal endpoint. In rare occasions, resection and interposition of the ICA may need to be performed with a graft.

If there is no abnormality upon re-exploration, then an embolic or ischemic event must be considered. At this juncture, angiography should be obtained to include the intracranial vessels. Intracranial pathology should prompt immediate consideration of intra-arterial thrombolysis by direct administration of tissue plasminogen activator (TPA) into the ICA and mandatory emergent consultation with neuroradiology interventionalists for consideration of microcatheter embolectomy, and/or mechanical or directed chemical thrombolysis. Patients with intraoperative stroke following carotid artery stenting should undergo immediate investigation with angiography to evaluate stent and intracranial vessel patency, and identification of intracranial thromboemboli should again lead to consideration of TPA and emergent neuroradiological interventional consultation.

Postoperative Stroke

Patients who awaken neurologically intact but then develop new deficits in the recovery area or later should be immediately evaluated with a Duplex ultrasound. Evidence of acute thrombosis, abnormalities within the lumen, or abnormalities in flow should prompt immediate return to the operating room for re-exploration. If the Duplex demonstrates no abnormalities in the neck, CT of the head must be immediately undertaken. If diagnostic imaging detects intracerebral hemorrhage, an immediate neurosurgical consultation must be sought, and decisions regarding antiplatelet reversal, blood pressure management, and additional interventions must be made.

If the head CT is negative, the possibility of intracranial thromboemboli must be entertained and should prompt emergent neuroradiological interventional consultation and performance of cerebrovascular angiography. Presence of cerebrovascular emboli should prompt intracerebral endovascular intervention, including mechanical thrombectomy and catheter-directed thrombolysis. Prompt intervention, within 1–2 h, has resulted in success [25, 74].

In patients who have undergone noncarotid vascular surgery, strokes are typically diagnosed postoperatively. In those who have undergone abdominal aortic and extremity interventions, the timing of stroke is most commonly in the first postoperative week [31]. Following thoracic aortic surgery, patients routinely remain intubated as they leave the operating room, and, therefore, the exact timing of postoperative stroke may be difficult to discern. As such, intraoperative stroke sustained from manipulation of the aortic arch and subsequent embolic strokes may be underreported and undertreated. Upon diagnosis of stroke, however, the patient must undergo immediate CT imaging of the head, followed by angiography, if necessary.

Finally, patients who have diagnosed cerebrovascular atherosclerotic pathology should be initiated on maximum medical therapy if they are not already on these medications. Diagnosis of asymptomatic cerebrovascular disease should be viewed as opportunities to intervene and reduce long-term stroke risks. Statins, angiotensin-converting enzyme inhibitors, beta-blockers, and antiplatelet agents should be considered, if appropriate.

Conclusion

Spinal cord ischemia and stroke are dreaded postoperative complications. With timely identification, prompt evaluation, and appropriate management, there is a chance to avert long-term consequences.

Disclosures Dr. Charlton-Ouw is a consultant for WL Gore & Associates and Medtronic. The other authors have no disclosures and no outside funding was used for this report.

References

1. Tanaka A, Safi HJ, Estrera AL. Current strategies of spinal cord protection during thoracoabdominal aortic surgery. Gen Thorac Cardiovasc Surg. 2018;66(6):307–14.
2. Rosenthal D, Chaikof EL, Williams GM, Gregory RT, Safi HJ, Gross GM, et al. Spinal cord ischemia after abdominal aortic operation: is it preventable? J Vasc Surg. 1999;30(3):391–9.
3. Berg P, Kaufmann D, Van Marrewijk CJ, Buth J. Spinal cord ischaemia after stent-graft treatment for infra-renal abdominal aortic aneurysms. Analysis of the Eurostar database. Eur J Vasc Endovasc Surg. 2001;22(4):342–7.
4. Maldonado TS, Rockman CB, Riles E, Douglas D, Adelman MA, Jacobowitz GR, et al. Ischemic complications after endovascular abdominal aortic aneurysm repair. J Vasc Surg. 2004 Oct;40(4):703–10.
5. Wong CS, Healy D, Canning C, Coffey JC, Boyle JR, Walsh SR. A systematic review of spinal cord injury and cerebrospinal fluid drainage after thoracic aortic endografting. J Vasc Surg. 2012;56(5):1438–47.
6. Awad H, Ehab Ramadan M, El Sayed HF, Tolpin DA, Tili E, Collard CD, et al. Spinal cord injury after thoracic endovascular aortic aneurysm repair. Can J Anaesth. 2017;64(12):1218–35.
7. Chiesa R, Melissano G, Marrocco-Trischitta MM, Civilini E, Setacci F. Spinal cord ischemia after elective stent-graft repair of the thoracic aorta. J Vasc Surg. 2005;42(1):11–7.
8. Izumi S, Okada K, Hasegawa T, Omura A, Munakata H, Matsumori M, et al. Augmentation of systemic blood pressure during spinal cord ischemia to prevent postoperative paraplegia after aortic surgery in a rabbit model. J Thorac Cardiovasc Surg. 2010;139(5):1261–8.
9. Maeda T, Yoshitani K, Sato S, Matsuda H, Inatomi Y, Tomita Y, et al. Spinal cord ischemia after endovascular aortic repair versus open surgical repair for descending thoracic and thoracoabdominal aortic aneurism. J Anesth. 2012;26(6):805–11.
10. Grabitz K, Sandmann W, Stuhmeier K, Mainzer B, Godehardt E, Ohle B, et al. The risk of ischemic spinal cord injury in patients undergoing graft replacement for thoracoabdominal aortic aneurysms. J Vasc Surg. 1996;23(2):230–40.
11. Griepp RB, Griepp EB. Spinal cord perfusion and protection during descending thoracic and thoracoabdominal aortic surgery: the collateral network concept. Ann Thorac Surg. 2007;83(2):S865–9.
12. Christiansson L, Ulus AT, Hellbergg A, Bergqvist D, Wiklund L, Karacagil S. Aspects of the spinal cord circulation as assessed by intrathecal oxygen tension monitoring during various arterial interruptions in the pig. J Thorac Cardiovasc Surg. 2001;121(4):762–72.
13. D'oria M, Chiarandini S, Pipitone M, Calvagna C, Ziani B. Coverage of visible intercostal and lumbar segmental arteries can predict the volume of cerebrospinal fluid drainage in elective endovascular repair of descending thoracic and thoracoabdominal aortic disease: a pilot study. Eur J Cardiothorac Surg. 2019;55(4):646–52.
14. Wynn M, Acher C, Marks E, Acher CW. The effect of intercostal artery reimplantation on spinal cord injury in thoracoabdominal aortic aneurysm surgery. J Vasc Surg. 2016;64(2):289–96.
15. Gombert A, Grommes J, Hilkman D, Kotelis D, Mess WH, Jacobs MJ. Recovery of lost motor evoked potentials in open thoracoabdominal aortic aneurysm repair using intercostal artery bypass. J Vasc Surg Cases Innov Tech. 2018;4(1):54–7.
16. Jacobs MJ, Mess W, Mochtar B, Nijenhuis RJ, Statius Van Eps RG, Schurink GWH. The value of motor evoked potentials in reducing paraplegia during thoracoabdominal aneurysm repair. J Vasc Surg. 2006;43(2):239–46.
17. Dias-Neto M, Reis PV, Rolim D, Ramos JF, Teixeira JF, Rgio SS. Strategies to prevent TEVAR-related spinal cord ischemia. Vascular. 2017;25(3):307–15.
18. Lennard N, Smith J, Dumville J, Abbott R, Evans DH, London NJM, et al. Prevention of postoperative thrombotic stroke after carotid endarterectomy: the role of transcranial Doppler ultrasound. J Vasc Surg. 1997;26(4):579–84.
19. Kwaan JH, Connolly JE, Sharefkin JB. Successful management of early stroke after carotid endarterectomy. Ann Surg. 1979;190(5):676–8.

20. Ellis M. Transcranial Doppler: preventing stroke during carotid endarterectomy. Ann R Coll Surg Engl. 1998;80(6):377–87.
21. Jacobowitz GR, Rockman CB, Lamparello PJ, Adelman MA, Schanzer A, Woo D, et al. Causes of perioperative stroke after carotid endarterectomy: special considerations in symptomatic patients. Ann Vasc Surg. 2001;15(1):19–24.
22. Schneider JR, Droste JS, Schindler N, Golan JF, Bernstein LP, Rosenberg RS. Carotid endarterectomy with routine electroencephalography and selective shunting: influence of contralateral internal carotid artery occlusion and utility in prevention of perioperative strokes. J Vasc Surg. 2002;35(6):1114–22.
23. Imparato AM, Ramirez A, Riles T, Mintzer R. Cerebral protection in carotid surgery. Arch Surg. 1982;117(8):1073–8.
24. Piepgras DG, Morgan MK, Sundt TM, Yanagihara T, Mussman LM. Intracerebral hemorrhage after carotid endarterectomy. J Neurosurg. 1988;68(4):532–6.
25. Wholey MH, Wholey MH, Tan WA, Toursarkissian B, Bailey S, Eles G, et al. Management of neurological complications of carotid artery stenting. J Endovasc Ther. 2001;8(4):341–53.
26. Halm EA, Tuhrim S, Wang JJ, Rockman C, Riles TS, Chassin MR. Risk factors for perioperative death and stroke after carotid endarterectomy: results of the New York carotid artery surgery study. Stroke. 2009;40(1):221–9.
27. Li Y, Walicki D, Mathiesen C, Jenny D, Li Q, Isayev Y, et al. Strokes after cardiac surgery and relationship to carotid stenosis. Arch Neurol. 2009;66(9):1091–6.
28. Wallaert JB, Goodney PP, Vignati JJ, Stone DH, Nolan BW, Bertges DJ, et al. Completion imaging after carotid endarterectomy in the Vascular Study Group of New England. J Vasc Surg. 2011;54(2):376–85, 385.e1–3.
29. Goldstein LJ, Davies RR, Rizzo JA, Davila JJ, Cooperberg MR, Shaw RK, et al. Stroke in surgery of the thoracic aorta: incidence, impact, etiology, and prevention. J Thorac Cardiovasc Surg. 2001;122(5):935–45.
30. Englum BR, He X, Gulack BC, Ganapathi AM, Mathew JP, Brennan JM, et al. Hypothermia and cerebral protection strategies in aortic arch surgery: a comparative effectiveness analysis from the STS adult cardiac surgery database. Eur J Cardiothorac Surg. 2017;52(3):492–8.
31. Axelrod DA, Stanley JC, Upchurch GR, Khuri S, Daley J, Henderson W, et al. Risk for stroke after elective noncarotid vascular surgery. J Vasc Surg. 2004;39(1):67–72.
32. Pratesi C, Dorigo W, Innocenti AA, Azas L, Barbanti E, Lombardi R, et al. Reducing the risk of intraoperative neurological complications during carotid endarterectomy with early distal control of the internal carotid artery. Eur J Vasc Endovasc Surg. 2004;28(6):670–3.
33. Bandyk DF, Thiele BL. Safe intraluminal shunting during carotid endarterectomy. Surgery. 1983;93(2):260–3.
34. Jamil M, Usman R, Ghaffar S. Advantages of selective use of intraluminal shunt in carotid endarterectomy: a study of 122 cases. Ann Vasc Dis. 2016;9(4):285–8.
35. Mousa AY, Campbell JE, Aburahma AF, Bates MC. Current update of cerebral embolic protection devices. J Vasc Surg. 2012;56(5):1429–37.
36. Ohki T, Parodi J, Veith FJ, Bates M, Bade M, Chang D, et al. Efficacy of a proximal occlusion catheter with reversal of flow in the prevention of embolic events during carotid artery stenting: an experimental analysis. J Vasc Surg. 2001;33(3):504–9.
37. Gray WA, Hopkins LN, Yadav S, Davis T, Wholey M, Atkinson R, et al. Protected carotid stenting in high-surgical-risk patients: the ARCHeR results. J Vasc Surg. 2006;44(2):258–68.
38. Matsumura JS, Gray W, Chaturvedi S, Gao X, Cheng J, Verta P. CAPTURE 2 risk-adjusted stroke outcome benchmarks for carotid artery stenting with distal embolic protection. J Vasc Surg. 2010;52(3):576–83, 583.e1-583.e2.
39. Cremonesi A, Manetti R, Setacci F, Setacci C, Castriota F. Protected carotid stenting clinical advantages and complications of embolic protection devices in 442 consecutive patients. Stroke. 2003;34(8):1936–41.
40. Coggia M, Goeau-Brissonniere O, Duval JL, Leschi JP, Letort M, Nagel MD. Embolic risk of the different stages of carotid bifurcation balloon angioplasty: an experimental study. J Vasc Surg. 2000;31(3):550–7.

41. Alvarez B, Matas M, Ribo M, Maeso J, Yugueros X, Alvarez-Sabin J. Transcervical carotid stenting with flow reversal is a safe technique for high-risk patients older than 70 years. J Vasc Surg. 2012;55(4):978–84.
42. Pinter L, Ribo M, Loh C, Lane B, Roberts T, Chou TM, et al. Safety and feasibility of a novel transcervical access neuroprotection system for carotid artery stenting in the PROOF study. J Vasc Surg. 2011;54(5):1317–23.
43. Pacini D, Leone A, Di Marco L, Marsilli D, Sobaih F, Turci S, et al. Antegrade selective cerebral perfusion in thoracic aorta surgery: safety of moderate hypothermia. Eur J Cardiothorac Surg. 2007;31(4):618–22.
44. Weiss AJ, Pawale A, Griepp RB, Di Luozzo G. Deep versus mild hypothermia during thoracoabdominal aortic surgery. Ann Cardiothorac Surg. 2012;1(3):329–33.
45. Griepp RB. Cerebral protection during aortic arch surgery. J Thorac Cardiovasc Surg. 2001;121(3):425–7.
46. Tian DH, Wan B, Bannon PG, Misfeld M, LeMaire SA, Kazui T, et al. A meta-analysis of deep hypothermic circulatory arrest versus moderate hypothermic circulatory arrest with selective antegrade cerebral perfusion. Ann Cardiothorac Surg. 2013;2(2):148–58.
47. Kamiya H, Hagl C, Kropivnitskaya I, Böthig D, Kallenbach K, Khaladj N, et al. The safety of moderate hypothermic lower body circulatory arrest with selective cerebral perfusion: a propensity score analysis. J Thorac Cardiovasc Surg. 2007;133(2):501–9.
48. Ueda Y, Miki S, Kusuhara K, Okita Y, Tahata T, Yamanaka K. Surgical treatment of aneurysm or dissection involving the ascending aorta and aortic arch, utilizing circulatory arrest and retrograde cerebral perfusion. J Cardiovasc Surg. 1990;31(5):553–8.
49. Coselli JS. Retrograde cerebral perfusion is an effective means of neural support during deep hypothermic circulatory arrest. Ann Thorac Surg. 1997;64(3):908–12.
50. Crittenden MD, Roberts CS, Rosa L, Vatsia SK, Katz D, Clark RE, et al. Brain protection during circulatory arrest. Ann Thorac Surg. 1991;51(6):942–7.
51. Peitzman AB, Webster MW, Loubeau J-M, Grundy BL, Bahnson HT. Carotid endarterectomy under regional (conductive) anesthesia. Ann Surg. 1982;196(1):59–64.
52. Evans WE, Hayes JP, Waltke EA, Vermilion BD. Optimal cerebral monitoring during carotid endarterectomy: neurologic response under local anesthesia. J Vasc Surg. 1985;2(6):775–7.
53. Benjamin ME, Silva MB, Watt C, McCaffrey MT, Burford-Foggs A, Flinn WR. Awake patient monitoring to determine the need for shunting during carotid endarterectomy. Surgery. 1993;114(4):673–9; discussion 679-81.
54. Hans SS, Jareunpoon O. Prospective evaluation of electroencephalography, carotid artery stump pressure, and neurologic changes during 314 consecutive carotid endarterectomies performed in awake patients. J Vasc Surg. 2007;45(3):511–5.
55. Giannoni MF, Sbarigia E, Panico MA, Speziale F, Antonini M, Maraglino C, et al. Intraoperative transcranial Doppler sonography monitoring during carotid surgery under locoregional anaesthesia. Eur J Vasc Endovasc Surg. 1996;12(4):407–11.
56. Jacob T, Hingorani A, Ascher E. Carotid artery stump pressure (CASP) in 1135 consecutive endarterectomies under general anesthesia: an old method that survived the test of times. J Cardiovasc Surg. 2007;48(6):677–81.
57. Tyagi SC, Dougherty MJ, Fukuhara S, Troutman DA, Pineda DM, Zheng H, et al. Low carotid stump pressure as a predictor for ischemic symptoms and as a marker for compromised cerebral reserve in octogenarians undergoing carotid endarterectomy. J Vasc Surg. 2018;68(2):445–50.
58. Green RM, Messick WJ, Ricotta JJ, Charlton MH, Satran R, Mcbride MM, et al. Benefits, shortcomings, and costs of EEG monitoring. Ann Surg. 1985;201(6):785–92.
59. Pinkerton JA. EEG as a criterion for shunt need in carotid endarterectomy. Ann Vasc Surg. 2002;16(6):756–61.
60. Plestis KA, Loubser P, Mizrahi EM, Kantis G, Jiang ZD, Howell JF. Continuous electroencephalographic monitoring and selective shunting reduces neurologic morbidity rates in carotid endarterectomy. J Vasc Surg. 1997;25(4):620–8.
61. Ackerstaff RGA, Jansen C, Moll FL, Vermeulen FEE, Hamerlijnck RPHM, Mauser HW. The significance of microemboli detection by means of transcranial Doppler ultrasonography monitoring in carotid endarterectomy. J Vasc Surg. 1995;21(6):963–9.

62. Jansen C, Vriens EM, Eikelboom BC, Vermeulen FEE, Van Gijn J, Ackerstaff RGA. Carotid endarterectomy with transcranial Doppler and electroencephalographic monitoring a prospective study in 130 operations. Stroke. 1993;24(5):665–9.
63. Samra SK, Dy EA, Welch K, Dorje P, Zelenock GB, Stanley JC. Evaluation of a cerebral oximeter as a monitor of cerebral ischemia during carotid endarterectomy. Anesthesiology. 2000;93(4):964–70.
64. Williams IM, Picton A, Farrell A, Mead GE, Mortimer AJ, McCollum CN. Light-reflective cerebral oximetry and jugular bulb venous oxygen saturation during carotid endarterectomy. Br J Surg. 1994;81(9):1291–5.
65. Cho H, Nemoto EM, Yonas H, Balzer J, Sclabassi RJ. Cerebral monitoring by means of oximetry and somatosensory evoked potentials during carotid endarterectomy. J Neurosurg. 1998;89(4):533–8.
66. Duffy CM, Manninen PH, Chan A, Kearns CF. Comparison of cerebral oximeter and evoked potential monitoring in carotid endarterectomy. Can J Anaesth. 1997;44(10):1077–81.
67. Beese U, Langer H, Lang W, Dinkel M. Comparison of near-infrared spectroscopy and somatosensory evoked potentials for the detection of cerebral ischemia during carotid endarterectomy. Stroke. 1998;29(10):2032–7.
68. De Letter JAM, Sie HT, Thomas BMJH, Moll FL, Algra A, Eikelboom BC, et al. Near-infrared reflected spectroscopy and electroencephalography during carotid endarterectomy—in search of a new shunt criterion. Neurol Res. 1998;20(Suppl 1):S23–7.
69. Mille T, Tachimiri ME, Klersy C, Ticozzelli G, Bellinzona G, Blangetti I, et al. Near infrared spectroscopy monitoring during carotid endarterectomy: which threshold value is critical? Eur J Vasc Endovasc Surg. 2004;27(6):646–50.
70. Schwartz ML, Panetta TF, Kaplan BJ, Legatt AD, Suggs WD, Wengerter KR, et al. Somatosensory evoked potential monitoring during carotid surgery. Vascular. 1996;4(1):77–80.
71. Kearse LA, Brown EN, Mcpeck K. Somatosensory evoked potentials sensitivity relative to electroencephalography for cerebral ischemia during carotid endarterectomy. Stroke. 1992;23(4):498–505.
72. Sbarigia E, Schioppa A, Misuraca M, Panico MA, Battocchio C, Maraglino C, et al. Somatosensory evoked potentials versus locoregional anaesthesia in the monitoring of cerebral function during carotid artery surgery: preliminary results of a prospective study. Eur J Vasc Endovasc Surg. 2001;21(5):413–6.
73. Nwachuku EL, Balzer JR, Yabes JG, Habeych ME, Crammond DJ, Thirumala PD. Diagnostic value of somatosensory evoked potential changes during carotid endarterectomy: a systematic review and meta-analysis. JAMA Neurol. 2015;72(1):73–80.
74. Endo S, Kuwayama N, Hirashima Y, Akai T, Nishijima M, Takaku A. Results of urgent thrombolysis in patients with major stroke and atherothrombotic occlusion of the cervical internal carotid artery. AJNR Am J Neuroradiol. 1998;19(6):1169–75.

Arterial Thromboembolic Complications 6

Ramyar Gilani

Scope

Despite recent advances in perioperative care, pharmacology, and technology, acute thromboembolic (TE) complications remain a challenging constellation of clinical entities that have potential for serious negative consequences for patients [1, 2]. The common final pathways for acute TE complication are the resulting downstream hypoperfusion and tissue hypoxemia. Progression leads to the cellular inability to regulate the environment and buildup of toxic radicals. Severe hypoperfusion and hypoxemia can lead to such changes within minutes to hours of insult. Continued hypoxemia ultimately leads to cellular death. Cell death manifests itself locally as tissue necrosis with release of anaerobic metabolism by-products and intracellular toxins into the systemic circulation. It is these manifestations that provide signs, symptoms, laboratory derangements, and imaging findings that allow detection and may guide management. Also, cellular perfusion must be restored to halt the process. However, there is a point at which tissue viability and sometimes even patient viability can no longer be fully restored and only a salvage operation is feasible. Patients who require salvage procedures have high mortality rates regardless of pathophysiology and treatment strategy.

TE foci can occur at any point within the vascular system and consequently affect to varying degrees the highly variable distal bed depending on location and size. The two major causative mechanisms are arterial embolism and in situ arterial thrombosis. Although the final common pathway is similar, it is important to understand the nuances that exist between the two. Cardiac emboli secondary to atrial fibrillation, ventricular dysfunction, or valvular disease account for up to 90% of embolic cases [3, 4]. However, other significant sources of emboli should be considered such as more proximal atherosclerotic plaque and/or arterial aneurysm. A

R. Gilani (✉)
Michael E. DeBakey Department of Surgery, Baylor College of Medicine, Houston, TX, USA
e-mail: rgilani@bcm.edu

R. Gilani, J. L. Mills Sr. (eds.), *Vascular Complications of Surgery and Intervention*, https://doi.org/10.1007/978-3-030-86713-3_6

history of prior embolization is common. Regardless of source, the embolus will migrate via arterial flow to a point at which the vessel lumen becomes too small for further migration, where it then lodges and causes vessel occlusion and blood stasis.

In contrast, thrombosis is initially an in situ process, commonly secondary to worsening native atherosclerotic burden or previous instrumentation/intervention, or the development of a systemic low-flow state. These insidious de novo lesions lead to significant stenosis or occlusion over a longer period of time or more acutely with instrumentation, and their significance can be heightened in times such as critical illness where overall flow is reduced. However, a critical lesion will result in similar stasis and thrombus formation as with embolic etiology. This time course allows for the recruitment of collaterals to provide some degree of distal perfusion in the setting of thrombosis and therefore a more gradual onset of symptoms as well as lesser degree of ischemia distally. However, severe ischemia may result if thrombosis continues to a point at which collaterals are also involved or if pre-existing collaterals were not well developed.

The ultimate impact of acute TE complications lies in the associated limb loss and mortality rates. Although some instances, albeit few, of witnessed thromboemboli can be observed or at the most require anticoagulation, the more severe end of the spectrum requires prompt detection and expeditious therapeutic intervention to avoid limb loss and/or death. Advanced mesenteric ischemia (Fig. 6.1) requiring

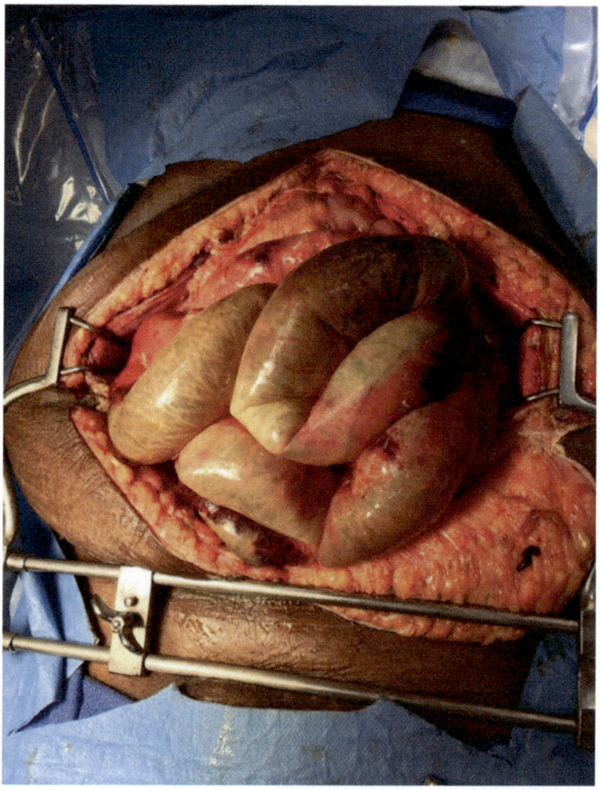

Fig. 6.1 Diffuse irreversible ischemic bowel necrosis

bowel resection is associated with a 15-fold increase in mortality, and overall mortality for mesenteric ischemia requiring surgical intervention exceeds 50% [4, 5]. Similarly documented rates of limb loss and mortality for acute limb ischemia are in the order of 20% and 25%, respectively [6]. These figures quite possibly may be higher if only evaluating already compromised patients in an intensive care setting afflicted with these complications.

Regions

As previously mentioned, TE complications may present in any distribution within the vascular tree; however, our focus for the purpose of this chapter will be limited to those instances affecting the extremities or abdominal viscera. Regardless of location, although the ultimate pathophysiology is similar, the road traveled can be quite different based on location.

Arteries within the extremities often occur as pairs separated into arteries of conduction such as the superficial femoral artery and parallel arteries of conduction such as the deep femoral artery. In certain locations, for example, the popliteal artery, flow is nearly completely dependent upon a single artery. As a result various degrees of severity can be expected based on the location of the thromboembolus.

As a general rule, the upper extremity is more resistant to severe ischemia compared to the lower extremity [2]. This is felt to be due to a more robust collateral circulation, particularly around the joints, as well as decreased perfusion distances. Nonetheless, the upper extremity can certainly be afflicted by TE complications. Upper extremity emboli classically occur in three distinct locations: distal axillary artery, distal brachial artery at the bifurcation, and distal radial and ulnar arteries at the level of the wrist. The source is most commonly cardiac [3, 4] in origin whether associated with a cardiac chamber (atrial fibrillation) or valve abnormality (endocarditis). However, primary thrombi of proximal vessels due to infection, malignancy, aneurysm, or idiopathic causes are also well-known culprits (Fig. 6.2). Therefore, when evaluating for etiology, the entire arterial tree from location of embolism retrograde to the heart must be interrogated.

Conversely, acute thrombotic events in the upper extremity are most commonly due to instrumentation (tourniquet) with background peripheral vascular disease (vascular access) in the setting of systemic illness (thrombosed arterial line). This is a consequence of the upper extremity being a major location for achieving vascular access (Fig. 6.3) and placement of monitoring devices, and as a result many iatrogenic thrombotic events occur here. Therefore, it is imperative to place the upper extremity under surveillance with some frequency monitoring for potential TE complications.

In similar fashion, the lower extremity is vulnerable to TE complications with perhaps less protection from severe ischemia. Embolism to the lower extremity (Fig. 6.4) typically occurs at the aortic bifurcation (saddle embolus with bilateral iliac artery involvement), distal common iliac artery, common femoral artery bifurcation, and popliteal artery or its trifurcation. Sources of emboli are similar to those of the upper extremity with the addition of pathology that may occur anywhere

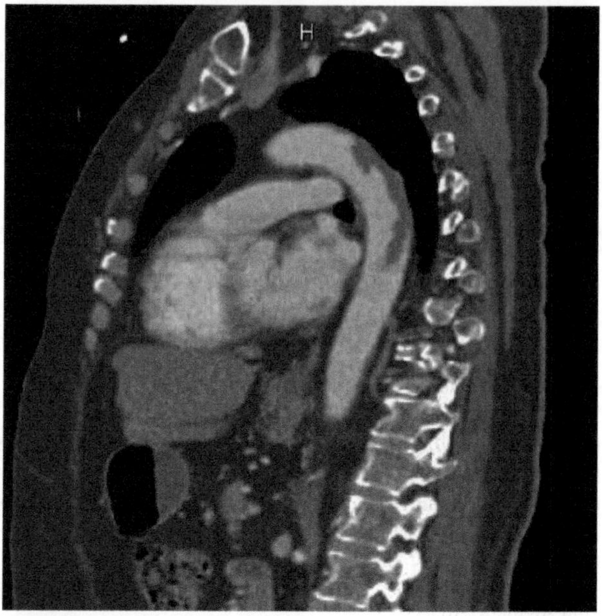

Fig. 6.2 CTA demonstrating pedunculated proximal aortic thrombus

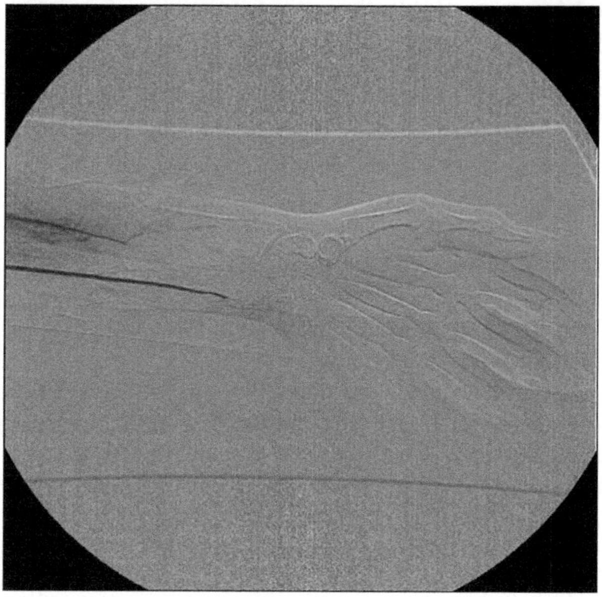

Fig. 6.3 Acute arterial thrombosis of the upper extremity secondary to arterial access

along the entire length of the aorta. In suspected cases of lower extremity TE, the arterial tree from the embolism location retrograde to the heart must be evaluated.

Unlike the upper extremity, pre-existing peripheral artery disease is more common in the lower extremity, and acute thrombosis of de novo lesions exacerbated by low-flow state or vasopressor use should be suspected in such conditions. Although

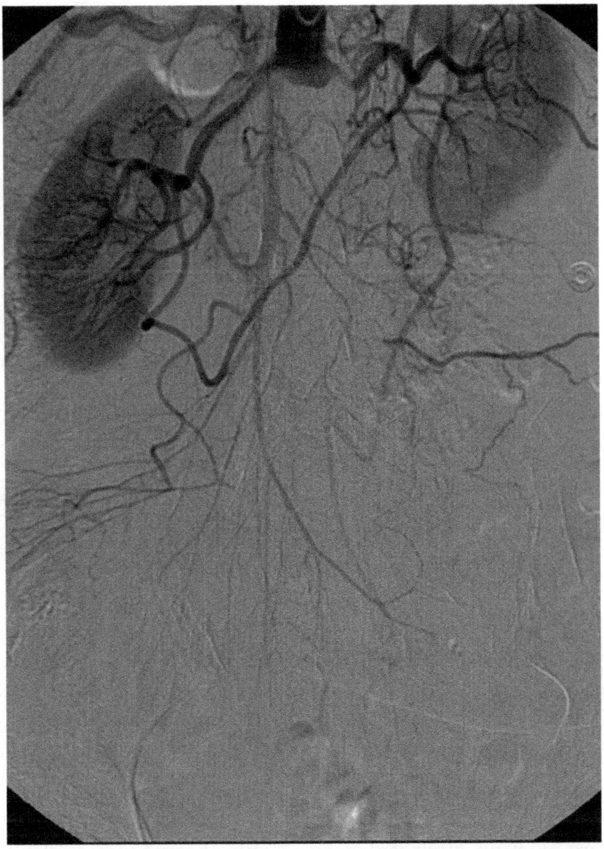

Fig. 6.4 Angiogram for acute aortic occlusion via brachial access

vascular access for patient monitoring is less common, lower extremity arterial access is often used for invasive diagnostics or interventions with significant device diameters that are associated with acute limb ischemia. Much like the upper extremities, the lower extremities are readily accessible and must undergo routine surveillance to assess for possible ischemic compromise due to TE complication.

The major etiologies of TE complication occurring in the mesentery are mesenteric arterial embolism and mesenteric arterial thrombosis in a ratio of 1.4:1 [5]. Embolism to the mesenteric arteries, which may partially or completely occlude the arterial lumen, is most frequently due to dislodged thrombus from the left atrium, left ventricle, cardiac valves, or proximal aorta. Systemic embolization occurs in 22–50% of cases of infected endocarditis, with embolization to the viscera second only to cerebral embolism [3, 7]. A history of prior embolization is common. Emboli tend to lodge at points of normal anatomical narrowing such as an arterial branch point. The large diameter and downward takeoff angle of the superior mesenteric artery (SMA) make it anatomically most susceptible to embolism. The embolus usually lodges 3–10 cm distal to the origin of the SMA (Fig. 6.5), in a tapered segment distal to the takeoff of the middle colic artery and sparing the first few jejunal

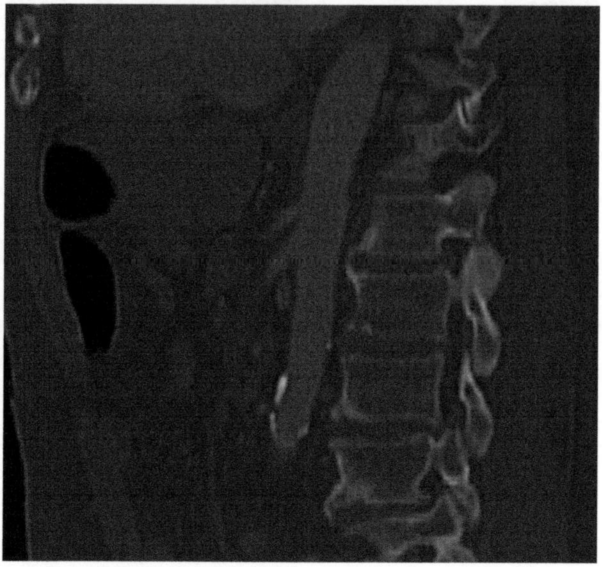

Fig. 6.5 CTA showing embolism to the SMA

branches, but approximately 15% of emboli lodge at the origin of the SMA. Because the onset is sudden without any prior obstruction, collateralization is poor and ischemia often profound although the first few centimeters of jejunum are usually preserved. Jejunal sparing suggests an embolic etiology rather than thrombotic occlusion of the SMA related to atherosclerotic disease as the underlying cause of acute mesenteric ischemia.

Arterial thrombosis occurs at areas of severe narrowing most typically due to pre-existing atherosclerosis. Acute thrombosis of the mesenteric circulation often occurs as a superimposed phenomenon in patients with a history of chronic mesenteric ischemia from progressive stenosis due to atherosclerotic aortic plaque that involves the takeoff of the celiac axis and SMA, also referred to as acute-on-chronic ischemia. Therefore, thrombosis of the SMA or celiac axis usually occurs at the origin of the vessel (Fig. 6.6), and involvement of at least two major mesenteric arteries is generally needed for the patient to have significant symptoms because of the development of the collateral circulation over time. Mesenteric arterial thrombosis can also occur in the setting of vascular injury related to abdominal trauma, infection, or mesenteric dissection. Thrombosis of a previous mesenteric revascularization can also occur, and such history should heighten concern if one suspected mesenteric ischemia.

Presentations

When discussing presentation of TE events in the abdomen and extremity, it is important to consider several fundamental similarities and differences. Since the final common pathway is similar, findings typically associated with ischemia such

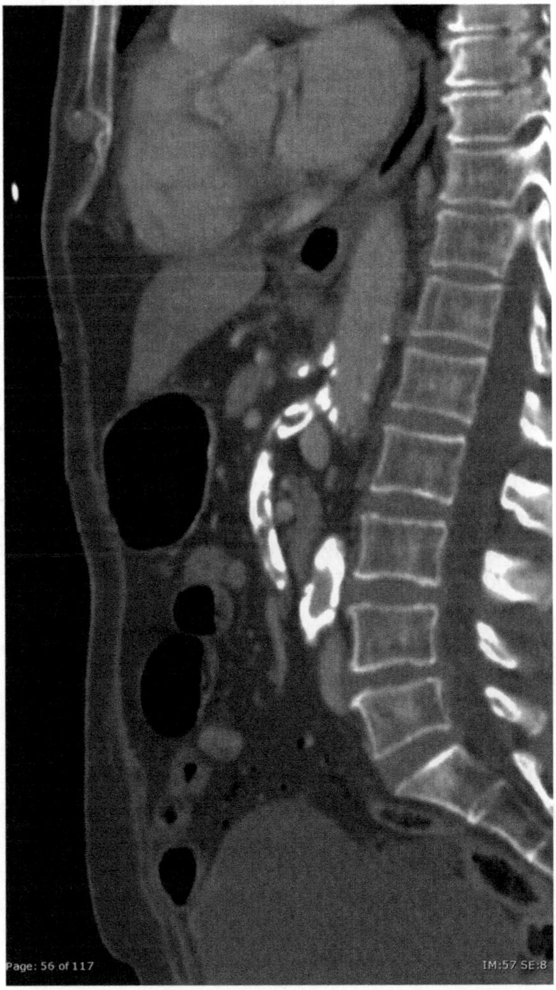

Fig. 6.6 CTA showing acute on chronic occlusion of SMA

as pain, acidosis, and systemic illness may occur in both regions. However, two important differences should be recognized that dictate somewhat different pathways to detection. First, the extremities are readily visualized, and vascular status is relatively straightforward to assess whereas the viscera are located within a so-called black box, and aside from patient complaint and tenderness, much more that is significant can't be ascertained through clinical assessment. Second, the contents most vulnerable to TE ischemia of the extremity are skin, muscle, and nerve tissue which produces a constellation of clinical findings readily detectable by the astute clinician. On the contrary, the visceral organs and their wide range of metabolic functions provide very little in terms of clinical findings, and suggestion of ongoing ischemia is much more reliant upon laboratory evaluation and imaging modalities.

Classically, determination of acute limb ischemia (ALI) is investigated through the application of the "5 Ps": pulselessness, pain, pallor, paresthesia, and paralysis occurring in that order [8]. A sixth "P" poikilothermia is sometimes added and is an ominous sign. Attention should be focused on the onset, location, and severity of pain, prior history of claudication or interventions, risk factors for atherosclerosis, and any history suggesting embolic phenomenon.

It should be reiterated that embolic events produce severe symptoms rather suddenly whereas thrombotic pathology may be more gradual in onset and progression. History of claudication and/or intervention, particularly in the setting of atherosclerotic risk factors, suggests thrombosis.

Physical examination should obviously include a complete pulse exam as well as attention to cardiac rhythm and the possible presence of aneurysmal disease (aortic, femoral, and popliteal). The presence of normal pulses, an aneurysm, and cardiac arrhythmia are suggestive of embolic disease. The level at which a pulse or Doppler signal is no longer appreciated aids in determining the location of pathology. Provocative maneuvers such as elevation and lowering of the limb can serve to intensify and alleviate findings respectfully in some patients with ALI.

Determining the degree of ischemia is clinically useful as a guide for timing of appropriate intervention. The Rutherford classification (Table 6.1) serves as a reference for categorizing degrees of severity in ALI [8]. This grading scale is intended to be applied at the bedside through physical examination and use of a handheld Doppler.

The signs and symptoms of visceral TE ischemia are more subtle and less specific; early detection often includes laboratory studies and imaging studies. Regardless, any patient with acute-onset abdominal pain, minimal findings on abdominal examination (classically described as pain out of proportion to the exam), and metabolic acidosis should be regarded as having intestinal ischemia until proven otherwise. Risk factors for arterial embolism or for atherosclerosis may be present. Symptoms of chronic mesenteric ischemia such as pain with meals and weight loss may be noted on the history. Plain films and cross-sectional abdominal imaging do not exclude mesenteric ischemia but may identify complications related to

Table 6.1 Clinical categories of acute limb ischemia

		Findings		Doppler signals	
Category	Description/prognosis	Sensory loss	Muscle weakness	Arterial	Venous
I. Viable	Not immediately threatened	None	None	Audible	Audible
II. Threatened					
(a) Marginally	Salvageable if promptly treated	Minimal (toes) or none	None	Inaudible	Audible
(b) Immediately	Salvageable with immediate revascularization	More than toes, associated with rest pain	Mild, moderate	Inaudible	Audible
III. Irreversible	Major tissue loss or permanent nerve damage inevitables	Profound, anesthetic	Profound, paralysis (rigor)	Inaudible	Audible

mesenteric ischemia (bowel wall thickening, pneumatosis, portal air, free air) and may indicate the need for immediate abdominal exploration while also helping to exclude other obvious causes of abdominal pain (e.g., volvulus, small bowel obstruction) [9–11].

The typical clinical triad of acute embolic occlusion in an older adult patient with atrial fibrillation (or other known embolic) and severe abdominal pain out of proportion to the physical examination is present in one-third to one-half of patients. Bowel emptying, nausea, and vomiting are also common, but bloody bowel movements are less frequent, unless advanced ischemia is present. The patient may be subtherapeutic on previously prescribed antithrombotic therapy, or the therapy may even have been recently discontinued. A prior embolic event is present in approximately one-third of patients. It is particularly important in these patients to perform a complete vascular examination including the carotid, upper extremity, and lower extremity pulses for evidence of reduced perfusion related to synchronous embolism. Over 20% of acute mesenteric emboli are multiple [12].

For patients with a history of infective endocarditis, most emboli (cerebral most common, followed by visceral, then lower extremity) occur within the first 2–4 weeks of antimicrobial therapy and may be more common in patients with mitral valve involvement, larger vegetation size (the largest are associated with streptococcus), staphylococcus independent of vegetation size, and increasing vegetation size while on treatment [3, 7].

The typical patient with acute mesenteric arterial thrombotic occlusion is one with established atherosclerotic risk factors and possibly known peripheral artery disease who may or may not have an established diagnosis of chronic mesenteric ischemia based upon symptoms of chronic postprandial abdominal pain, food aversion, and weight loss. However, in contrast to the classic description, one study noted that patients may not be cachectic, possibly due to earlier diagnosis or a relatively high proportion of patients who were overweight before the onset of symptoms. However, obtaining an antecedent history of chronic mesenteric ischemic symptoms may help differentiate thrombotic versus embolic occlusion and may potentially influence the choice of initial treatment [13].

Routine laboratory evaluation for abdominal pathology is performed, including complete blood count, arterial blood gas, and lactate. Classically, patients have leukocytosis, acidosis, and elevated lactate; however, these all occur in a minority of patients, and may reflect late findings associated with bowel infarction. Normal laboratory findings do not exclude the diagnosis of acute mesenteric arterial occlusion.

Imaging

Once a diagnosis of ALI has been formulated, further characterization of arterial anatomy is best obtained by diagnostic imaging. The dominant imaging modalities utilized in this assessment are computed tomographic angiography (CTA) and traditional contrast angiography, with a somewhat limited role for duplex ultrasound.

CTA is becoming the preferred initial imaging exam for ALI due to several attributes. Due to systemic delivery of contrast, CTA effectively delineates arterial anatomy simultaneously. This is useful for identifying the extent of thrombosis as well as proximal and distal vessel targets for intervention. Sluggish flow, particularly within the tibial and distal vessels, can limit the delivery of contrast and therefore reduce the amount of information provided by the exam. Additional information readily available via CTA includes vessel calcification, vessel diameter, collateralization, and presence of previous stents or bypass grafts. CTA is however a static study providing very little information about flow dynamics. It also requires radiation and potentially nephrotoxic contrast.

Contrast angiography is considered by many the gold-standard imaging modality for ALI. Angiography has the indisputable advantage of being both diagnostic and potentially therapeutic. It also provides information regarding flow characteristics. It however only provides information available through opacification of the vessel lumen and therefore does not provide extraluminal assessment. Collateral pathways can be quite variable in ALI, and the ability to opacify vessels distal to the affected region requires catheter selection of the appropriate supplying collateral pathway as well as adequate timing to allow for contrast to be delivered. Although conventional angiography also uses potentially nephrotoxic contrast, the required volume administered is often less than CTA. Additional risks are associated with arterial cannulation and intraluminal manipulation but are relatively minimal.

Duplex ultrasound (US), although not as frequently used for ALI, can expeditiously provide valuable information, especially if readily performed by the vascular consultant. In cases of strongly suspected arterial embolism, the location of embolus can be quickly confirmed via US. Visualizing the pulsatility within the limb arteries is a useful tool, and identifying a visible change within pulsation can be a tip-off of a significant embolism. Often, the actual embolic material may not be seen via ultrasound, but changes in pulsatility and color flow can be reliable surrogate markers. Also, potential access points for arterial cannulation can be quickly assessed for feasibility. Lastly, availability of venous conduit for arterial reconstruction can be ascertained.

As with all forms of mesenteric ischemia, the diagnosis of acute mesenteric arterial occlusion depends upon a high level of clinical suspicion, particularly in patients with known risk factors for peripheral embolization (e.g., atrial fibrillation, recent myocardial infarction, valvular disease) or a history of peripheral artery disease with or without a history of chronic abdominal pain. Rapid diagnosis is essential to prevent the catastrophic events associated with intestinal infarction [14].

A definitive diagnosis of mesenteric arterial occlusion relies upon demonstrating the occlusion within the mesenteric arteries on imaging studies. High-resolution CTA is highly diagnostic for acute mesenteric ischemia. In addition, based upon the appearance of vessels in the abdomen, it is often possible to differentiate between embolic and thrombotic etiologies. Further information for operative planning, such as distal arterial reconstitution and choice of inflow vessel for surgical bypass, can also be obtained. In the setting of equivocal CTA findings, catheter-based angiography may be needed. The contrast requirement for abdominal CTA may be

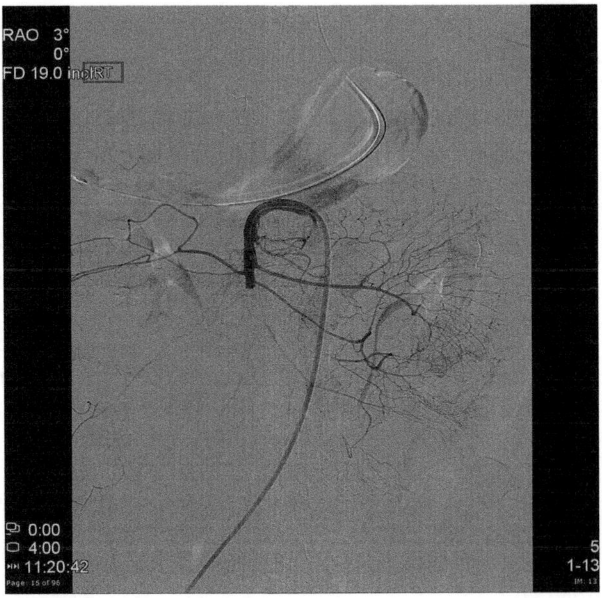

Fig. 6.7 Selective angiogram of the SMA consistent with embolism

prohibitive in some patients. Catheter-based angiography can be performed relatively safely with much lower contrast volume than CTA and is a good alternative in patients with renal compromise (Fig. 6.7). For patients who present with advanced ischemia (bowel perforation and peritonitis) and hemodynamic instability, a diagnosis will necessarily be made in the operating room.

Embolic occlusion often appears as an oval-shaped thrombus (Fig. 6.5) surrounded by contrast in a noncalcified arterial segment located in the middle and distal portion of the proximal superior mesenteric artery (SMA). In contrast, thrombotic occlusion (Fig. 6.6) usually appears as thrombus superimposed on a heavily calcified occlusive lesion at the ostium of the SMA. In addition to determining the type of mesenteric arterial occlusion (i.e., embolism or thrombus), CTA identifies the collateral circulation and potential sources of inflow and avoidable sites with extensive atherosclerotic lesions in cases that might require revascularization.

Treatment

Clinical evaluation and vascular imaging determine whether the patient is a candidate for vascular intervention and whether the occlusion is embolic or thrombotic which has a bearing on the type of intervention offered. The goal of vascular intervention is to restore blood flow as rapidly as possible. The specific treatment chosen depends upon the clinical status of the patient and the etiology and location of the occlusion. Optimal treatment may include open, endovascular, or a combined or hybrid approach. The ability to offer an endovascular approach depends upon local resources and the availability of vascular specialists. A hybrid interventional suite/

operating room may be the ideal setting to manage acute mesenteric arterial occlusion, but these are generally available only at large vascular centers.

Once a diagnosis of thromboembolism has been established, further management should be expeditious. Treatment strategies can be divided into two arms: anticoagulation and revascularization. Early anticoagulation via systemic heparinization is the initial management step in cases of TE as long as no contraindication to anticoagulation exists. Systemic anticoagulation serves several purposes. Most importantly, it reduces the risk of further clot propagation, especially in small distal run-off vessels where flow can be become quite static. In the case of embolism, anticoagulation reduces the risk of recurrent embolism. Lastly, through anti-inflammatory and microcirculation properties, heparin may improve symptoms and even restore some degree of perfusion, allowing more time for further evaluation.

In the lower extremity typically, Rutherford Class I ischemia management with anticoagulation alone is appropriate allowing time for more thorough evaluation. On the other hand, for Class IIA and IIB ischemia, anticoagulation alone is not sufficient, and prompt revascularization is warranted to prevent further ischemic damage. Class III ischemia implies irreversible damage requiring some level of amputation; however, treatment may be incorporated to lower the level of amputation [8].

Similarly, for the patient with mesenteric ischemia, those patients (e.g., acute-on-chronic occlusion) who are hemodynamically stable and do not have clinical signs of advanced bowel ischemia can be observed while on heparin anticoagulation, if there is evidence of good collateral blood flow on vascular imaging studies. Antiplatelet therapy may be justified in this setting if the risk of progressive ischemia appears to be greater than the risk of bleeding [15]. The patient should have serial clinical assessments (laboratory, physical examination) with a low threshold to repeat abdominal imaging studies or, if abdominal symptoms progress, proceed with surgical or endovascular intervention.

Patients who are good-risk surgical candidates with indications for immediate laparotomy such as peritonitis or radiologic features of advanced bowel ischemia (free air, extensive pneumatosis) should be taken directly to the operating room for exploration. Resection of the bowel should ideally be delayed until after mesenteric arterial revascularization can be performed to salvage as much bowel as possible (Fig. 6.8). The traditional treatment for mesenteric embolism is open surgical embolectomy (Fig. 6.9), which, in addition to expeditiously clearing the thrombus, allows direct assessment of bowel viability. Open surgical treatment of mesenteric artery thrombosis is treated principally with mesenteric bypass. Thrombectomy alone is unlikely to offer a durable solution due to the presence of pre-existing thrombogenic atherosclerotic plaques. Intraoperative retrograde superior mesenteric artery angioplasty and stenting is another hybrid option, particularly in the presence of gross contamination where bypass is more problematic. Patients who are hemodynamically stable and who do not have clinical or radiologic signs of advanced intestinal ischemia may be candidates for a primary endovascular approach (Fig. 6.10).

A palliative approach may be the best option for poor-risk surgical candidates with extensive transmural infarction (e.g., small bowel up to the mid-transverse

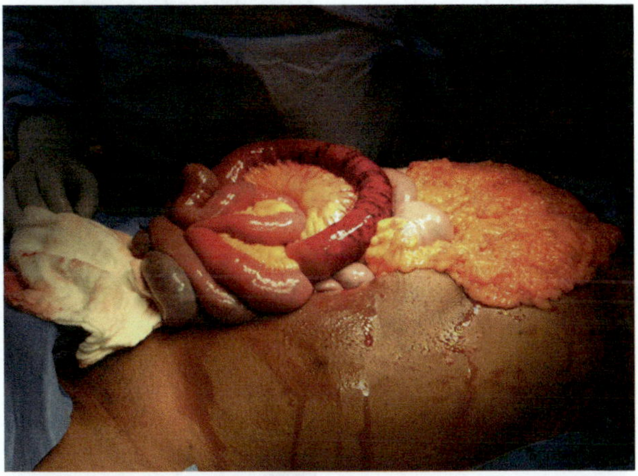

Fig. 6.8 Focal segment bowel necrosis after revascularization

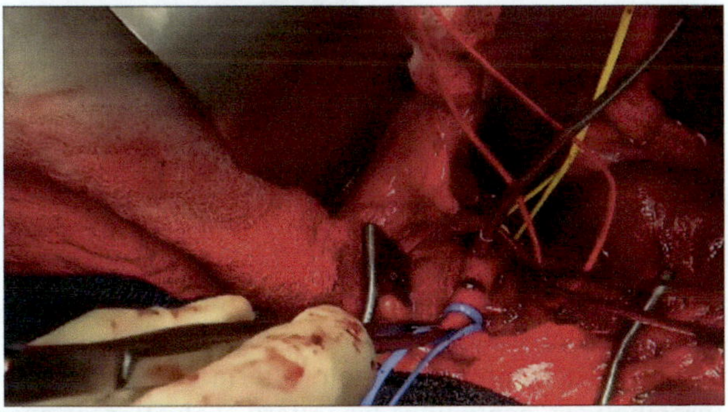

Fig. 6.9 Transverse arteriotomy for SMA embolectomy

colon). Extensive bowel resection would be inappropriate for these patients and may also be inappropriate for a subset of patients who might otherwise be expected to tolerate the procedure but for whom lifelong parenteral nutrition would be unacceptable.

Surveillance

Patients with TE complications are often very ill post-intervention, requiring intensive care management and support. The typical patient often has some degree of comorbidity and therefore is already at increased risk for complications. Close observation in a monitored clinical setting with attention to detail and appropriate treatment selection are the best methods for mitigation of complications in the perioperative setting.

Endovascular and open vascular procedures always carry a certain level of risk for standard procedural complications such bleeding, hematoma, infection, poor wound healing, etc. However, severe bleeding complications (10%) of a different variety are a potential complication with exposure to thrombolytic agents,

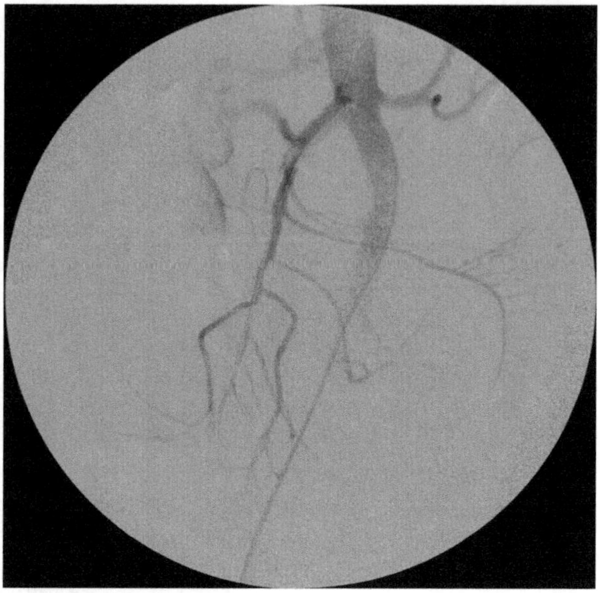

Fig. 6.10 Endovascular therapy for thrombotic mesenteric ischemia

particularly noncompressible hemorrhage. Bleeding into the central nervous system (CNS), gastrointestinal (GI) tract, eye, or body cavity can have serious consequences, with CNS bleeds (1–2%) being the most devastating [16–18]. Careful questioning concerning any recent surgery (especially within the CNS), recent stroke, recent trauma, history of bleeding, malignancy, and any other condition which might complicate systemic fibrinolysis should be elucidated. During ongoing thrombolysis, continuous laboratory evaluation of coagulation including PT, PTT, INR, fibrinogen, and CBC should be performed. Evidence of systemic fibrinolysis or bleeding should prompt cessation of thrombolytic therapy. Also close monitoring of arterial blood pressure and aggressive treatment of hypertension are good practices.

Given the degree of comorbidity in these patients, it is not surprising that cardiopulmonary complications such as myocardial infarction, congestive heart failure exacerbation, and pulmonary failure remain a real threat to desirable outcomes. What is less intuitive is the effect of revascularization on the cardiopulmonary system. After revascularization, the accumulated toxins and metabolites within the previously ischemic tissue bed become systemic with potential deleterious effects such as cardiac arrhythmias, shock, and full-blown SIRS (systemic inflammatory response syndrome). Treatment is purely supportive; however, anticipation of these outcomes can initiate preparedness and early therapy.

Limb loss is a real possibility for patients with ALI, even in the setting of a successful technical outcome. Furthermore, delayed treatment may ultimately keep a limb viable but dysfunctional secondary to nerve and/or muscle injury. Revascularized limbs are at risk for developing severe edema and secondary compartment syndrome. Limbs noted to have increasing pressures clinically and/or via compartment pressures (>30 mmHg) should undergo immediate fasciotomy. Significant degrees of muscle necrosis can lead to myoglobinemia with negative consequences on renal function. Although significant permanent renal dysfunction can usually be avoided with appropriate supportive care, severe continuous myoglobinemia can precipitate permanent renal dysfunction forcing the decision of life over limb.

Following revascularization, the viscera should be carefully assessed for areas of irreversible ischemic injury, which may require resection. Restoration of bowel continuity can be performed during the index surgery for well-demarcated, clearly viable bowel segments. If bowel viability is in question or the patient is hemodynamically unstable, a damage control approach can be undertaken by resecting the nonviable segments and stapling the small bowel closed, awaiting a second-look procedure to restore bowel continuity. The abdominal wall is left open when repeat laparotomy is planned, which is particularly likely if there has been a significant interval of ischemia that leads to bowel edema with reperfusion. If closure is elected (e.g., no necrotic bowel, minimal ischemic time), abdominal compartment pressures should be monitored. A second-look laparotomy is needed for most patients after mesenteric revascularization for acute mesenteric arterial occlusion to reevaluate the bowel 24–48 h after the initial operation. At the time of definitive abdominal closure, intravenous injection of fluorescein dye with inspection of the intestine illuminated via a Wood's lamp can assist in determining remaining bowel viability.

Summary

- Patients are at risk for TE complications during the course of their care, particularly those with underlying cardiovascular disease, abnormal coagulation, and undergoing instrumentation.
- Providers must maintain constant vigilant surveillance to detect these complications occurring in the extremity and viscera. Suspicion of an acute TE complication should lead to a prompt but orderly evaluation.
- Treatment of TE complications must be prompt to reduce significant morbidity and mortality. Treatment consists of observation, anticoagulation, endovascular therapy, and open revascularization.
- Even after treatment, patients can experience significant deleterious sequelae, and persistent observation and supportive care is required.

References

1. Blaisdell FW, Steele M, Allen RE. Management of acute lower extremity arterial ischemia due to embolism and thrombosis. Surgery. 1978;84(6):822–34.
2. Jivegård L, Holm J, Scherstén T. Acute limb ischemia due to arterial embolism or thrombosis: influence of limb ischemia versus pre-existing cardiac disease on postoperative mortality rate. J Cardiovasc Surg. 1988;29(1):32–6.

3. Baddour LM, Wilson WR, Bayer AS, et al. Infective endocarditis: diagnosis, antimicrobial therapy, and management of complications: a statement for healthcare professionals from the Committee on Rheumatic Fever, Endocarditis, and Kawasaki Disease, Council on Cardiovascular Disease in the Young, and the Councils on Clinical Cardiology, Stroke, and Cardiovascular Surgery and Anesthesia, American Heart Association: endorsed by the Infectious Diseases Society of America. Circulation. 2005;111:e394.
4. Gupta PK, Natarajan B, Gupta H, et al. Morbidity and mortality after bowel resection for acute mesenteric ischemia. Surgery. 2011;150:779.
5. Acosta S, Ogren M, Sternby NH, et al. Clinical implications for the management of acute thromboembolic occlusion of the superior mesenteric artery: autopsy findings in 213 patients. Ann Surg. 2005;241:516.
6. Kashyap VS, Gilani R, Bena JF, et al. Endovascular therapy for acute limb ischemia. J Vasc Surg. 2011;53(2):340–6.
7. Baddour LM, Wilson WR, Bayer AS, et al. Infective endocarditis in adults: diagnosis, antimicrobial therapy, and management of complications: a scientific statement for healthcare professionals from the American Heart Association. Circulation. 2015;132:1435.
8. Rutherford RB, Baker JD, Ernst C, Johnston KW, Porter JM, Ahn S, Jones DN. Recommended standards for reports dealing with lower extremity ischemia: revised version. J Vasc Surg. 1997;26(3):517–38.
9. Cappell MS. Intestinal (mesenteric) vasculopathy. I Acute superior mesenteric arteriopathy and venopathy. Gastroenterol Clin North Am. 1998;27:783.
10. McKinsey JF, Gewertz BL. Acute mesenteric ischemia. Surg Clin North Am. 1997;77:307.
11. Boley SJ, Brandt LJ, Sammartano RJ. History of mesenteric ischemia. The evolution of a diagnosis and management. Surg Clin North Am. 1997;77:275.
12. Yamada T, Yoshii T, Yoshimura H, et al. Upper limb amputation due to a brachial arterial embolism associated with a superior mesenteric arterial embolism: a case report. BMC Res Notes. 2012;5:372.
13. Björnsson S, Resch T, Acosta S. Symptomatic mesenteric atherosclerotic disease-lessons learned from the diagnostic workup. J Gastrointest Surg. 2013;17:973.
14. Kougias P, Lau D, El Sayed HF, et al. Determinants of mortality and treatment outcome following surgical interventions for acute mesenteric ischemia. J Vasc Surg. 2007;46:467.
15. Alhan E, Usta A, Çekiç A, et al. A study on 107 patients with acute mesenteric ischemia over 30 years. Int J Surg. 2012;10:510.
16. Ouriel K, Shortell CK, DeWeese JA, Green RM, Francis CW, Azodo MV, Gutierrez OH, Manzione JV, Cox C, Marder VJ. A comparison of thrombolytic therapy with operative revascularization in the initial treatment of acute peripheral arterial ischemia. J Vasc Surg. 1994;19(6):1021–30.
17. Results of a prospective randomized trial evaluating surgery versus thrombolysis for ischemia of the lower extremity. The STILE trial. Ann Surg. 1994;220(3):251–66; discussion 266–8.
18. Ouriel K, Veith FJ, Sasahara AA. A comparison of recombinant urokinase with vascular surgery as initial treatment for acute arterial occlusion of the legs. Thrombolysis or Peripheral Arterial Surgery (TOPAS) Investigators. N Engl J Med. 1998;338(16):1105–11.

Vascular Injuries in Children

7

Bindi Naik-Mathuria and Sara C. Fallon

Introduction

Vascular injuries are rare in children, occurring in approximately 1% of all pediatric trauma patients and representing about 1% of all vascular trauma [1]. Data regarding vascular injuries in pediatric patients are limited to database studies, single-center reviews and case reports, and reports of war-time experience. Management guidelines specific to pediatric patients are lacking; therefore, adult guidelines are often followed, although key differences exist between adult and pediatric vascular injuries. Vascular injuries can present in a variety of ways, from obvious bleeding due to a transection to occult intimal flaps, dissections, thrombosis, pseudoaneurysms, or fistulas. Traditionally, pediatric surgeons almost always managed pediatric vascular injuries; however, with the advent of endovascular techniques in adult vascular trauma, vascular surgeons and vascular interventionalists are called upon more frequently to manage pediatric injuries, even at freestanding children's hospitals [2]. As a result, pediatric surgical training lacks vascular cases, and pediatric vascular injuries are not a focus of training during vascular surgery fellowship, leaving a practice gap and an opportunity to progress and enhance the field of pediatric vascular trauma.

Differences in Adult and Pediatric Trauma

The injury patterns in children are fundamentally different than those seen in adult trauma. The elastic recoil of the child's body compared to adults, combined with a reduced overall rate of penetrating trauma, predisposes children to a lower rate of large vessel injury. In a National Trauma Data Bank (NTDB) study spanning the

B. Naik-Mathuria (✉) · S. C. Fallon
Pediatric Surgery, Texas Children's Hospital/Baylor College of Medicine, Houston, TX, USA
e-mail: bjnaikma@texaschildrens.org; scfallon@texaschildrens.org

R. Gilani, J. L. Mills Sr. (eds.), *Vascular Complications of Surgery and Intervention*, https://doi.org/10.1007/978-3-030-86713-3_7

years 2002–2006, compared to adults, children had lower rates of chest and abdominal penetrating injury and higher rates of blunt and penetrating upper extremity injury [1] (Fig. 7.1). Outcomes were also different, with adults having higher mortality (23% vs. 13%, $p = 0.01$), suffering from higher amputation rates after upper extremity trauma (2.5% vs. 0.7%, $p = 0.03$), and requiring fasciotomy more often (31% vs. 20%) [1]. Children were found to have shorter hospital and ICU lengths of stay than adults [1]. Mortality outcomes for children remained improved after adjustment for confounding factors, including injury severity score (ISS), Glasgow coma score (GCS), and hemodynamic parameters, likely reflecting the general better health of the pediatric compared to the adult trauma patient [1].

Children have smaller vessels, which are more prone to vasospasm, reported in up to 26% of extremity injuries in one series [3]. Vasospasm may improve with time and/or anticoagulation, which can alter the management strategy. They are also more prone to having asymptomatic vascular injuries than adults [4]. Smaller vessel diameter may increase the technical difficulty, especially for vascular surgeons who lack experience with pediatric vascular repairs. Endovascular therapy can also have its challenges, as arterial access can be difficult and could lead to thrombosis, and there is a lack of commercially available endovascular stents for smaller-sized patients.

Epidemiology

A recent study of the NTDB of 3408 pediatric trauma patients with vascular injury from 2002 to 2012 reported that patients were most commonly male (74%), were Caucasian (53%), and had a mean age of 10.5 ± 4.5 years [5]. National database studies report that children more frequently sustain vascular injuries secondary to blunt (60%) compared to penetrating (40%) mechanisms [1, 5]. However, multiple single-center level I trauma center series have reported a higher incidence of penetrating vascular injuries compared to blunt [3, 4, 6]. This may be due to regional referral patterns, as pediatric patients with penetrating vascular injuries are generally more likely to be transferred to level I pediatric trauma centers.

The most commonly reported mechanisms of injury in national database studies are motor vehicle collisions (MVC), firearm injuries, stab wounds, and falls [1, 5]. In the most recent NTDB study, mortality was reported as 7.9%, with no difference between blunt and penetrating injuries [5]. On multiple variable regression, patient-specific factors including, age, gender, and race were not associated with mortality, although a higher ISS, GCS <9, and a systolic blood pressure <9 were independently associated with an increased mortality risk [5]. The highest incidence of mortality was for those children injured via firearms (36%) [5].

The most common site of vessel injury for penetrating injuries in children is the upper extremity (43%), followed by the abdomen (23%), the lower extremity (26%), and then thoracic and neck injuries (15%). Blunt injury follows a similar pattern [1]. The incidence of thoracic aortic injuries increases with age, reaching as high as 15% in the teenage years [1].

Operative rates for vascular trauma in children are variable, ranging from 25% to 75%. In the 2002–2012 NTDB study, 42% underwent open repair, while 3% had

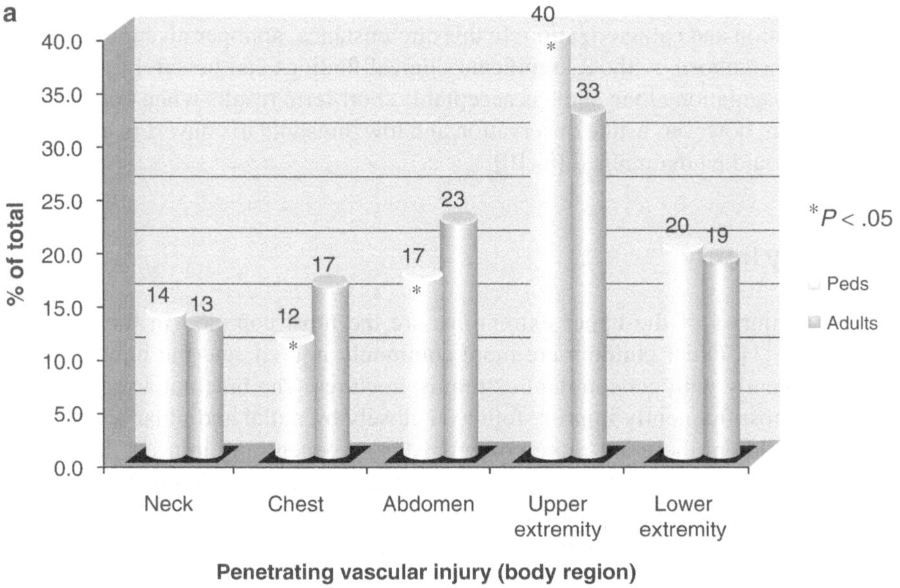

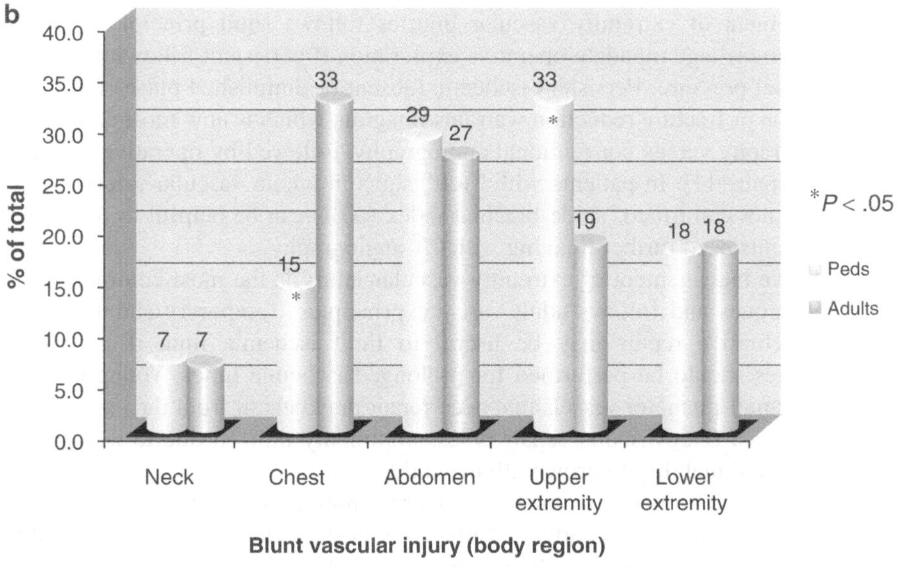

Fig. 7.1 (**a**) Distribution of vascular injuries according to body region for pediatric and adult patients with penetrating injuries. (**b**) Distribution of vascular injuries according to body region for pediatric and adult patients with blunt injuries. (From Ref. [1])

endovascular repair [5]. The use of endovascular therapy has increased in pediatric patients since 2007. Another review of the NTDB including 2007–2014 reported increase in this technique from 7% to 12% [7].

Additionally, vessel thrombosis secondary to iatrogenic trauma is a unique circumstance of injury in a child. Although infrequent, this complication can lead to limb loss and lifelong manifestations. Most commonly the occurrence is due to vessel cannulation and catheterization. In this circumstance, nonoperative management of vessel thrombosis without significant clinical findings can be safely performed with anticoagulation alone and has acceptable short-term results when compared to intervention; however, astute observation and low threshold to convert to alternative strategy should be maintained [8–10].

Extremity Injury

Vascular injuries of the upper extremities are the most common in the pediatric population [1]. Older children are more commonly injured, and the injuries occur most frequently with concomitant extremity fractures. The brachial artery appears to be the most frequently injured, followed closely by radial and ulnar arteries [3]. In older children, these are more commonly from penetrating injuries than blunt, which account for the majority of other vascular injuries in children. Mechanisms such as landing on broken glass are more common than stab wounds or gunshot wounds. Younger children more commonly have blunt upper extremity injury associated with supracondylar fractures of the humerus (elbow), often the result of falls [3].

Management of extremity vascular injuries follows adult principles. "Hard" signs of hemorrhage mandate operative exploration if persistent following manual or tourniquet pressure. Persistent ischemia (absent or diminished pulse) following resuscitation or fracture reduction warrants imaging, which is now most commonly CT angiography versus conventional angiography, followed by operative or endovascular repair [11]. In patients with "soft" signs in whom vascular injury is suspected but not confirmed, ankle-brachial index (ABI) can be helpful to determine which patients need further imaging with CT angiography.

Operative management of extremity vascular injury is the most common using open techniques and follows adult vascular principles. Temporary shunting with delayed definitive repair may be useful to limit ischemia time if necessary. Fasciotomies should be performed for prolonged ischemia times. Young patients with very small-diameter vessels that need repair may benefit from the expertise of microsurgeons. Endovascular repair is less commonly utilized due to device size availability and inability to grow with the child.

Supracondylar humeral fractures, which are common in children, can be associated with persistent brachial artery compromise postreduction which is referred to as the "pink, pulseless hand." Although this is a "hard" sign, controversy exists as to whether such cases mandate operative exploration, as many have vasospasm which improves with observation alone. Imaging generally does not help, as flow is not visible within a small vessel with severe vasospasm. In one series of 12 cases that had operative exploration, 8 had focal brachial artery thrombosis, and 4 brachial arteries were entrapped with the median nerve, with band lysis restoring flow [12]. Long-term patency has been shown to be excellent [13]. A systematic review of the literature reported that 70% of pink, pulseless hands had documented brachial artery injury rather than vasospasm. The same study reported survey results of pediatric orthopedic surgeons, who believed that only 17% of these cases would actually have brachial artery injury [13]. This study indicates that the prevalent current dogma of observation of these injuries should be questioned and operative exploration or short-term follow-up imaging should be recommended as it is low risk, is high-reward, and may avoid long-term complications such as Volkmann's contracture and limb-length deformity [13].

Carotid Injury

Penetrating carotid injury is managed according to the same principles as for adults; blunt cerebrovascular injury (BCVI) in children is more controversial, and guidelines for screening and management are still in development. These injuries are rare, occurring in less than 1% of patients. Currently, there are no clearly delineated risk factors for injury. The screening tool is a computerized tomography scan, which is generally avoided as much as possible in children; however, patients may be asymptomatic at presentation, and missed injuries can result in devastating neurologic sequelae. Furthermore, the use of standard criteria for screening has been found to decrease both the time to diagnosis and additional neurologic insult, advocating for the development of evidence-based practice [14]. In a recent KIDS database study, the incidence of BCVI was 0.2% with a male predominance (69%) and a mean age of 15 years [14]. The carotid artery was the most frequently injured vessel (59%), followed by multiple vessel injury (15%), and the vertebral artery (13%). [14] An additional KIDS study found that the incidence had doubled from 2000 (0.24%) to 2012 (0.49%), although this may be related to a detection bias from increased awareness and use of screening protocols [15].

Screening guidelines remain controversial, although recent efforts have begun to clarify this topic for children. Some data have suggested that screening criteria used for adults have a poor correlation with injury patterns that are higher risk for children, identifying <50% of children with injuries [16]. The original Eastern Association of Trauma (EAST) guideline in 2010 recommended that pediatric trauma patients should be screened using adult criteria [17]. The Denver criteria for screening included hard signs of vascular injury such as arterial hemorrhage from the neck or oropharynx, enlarging cervical hematoma, cervical bruits in age >50, focal neurologic deficits, and strokes or neurologic deficits that are not explained by the initial imaging. Increased risk criteria in asymptomatic patients included a low GCS score, C1–C3 fracture, cervical fracture with subluxation, LeFort II or III fractures, and diffuse axonal injury [18]. These criteria were then expanded in 2012 to include mandibular fractures, complex skull fractures, associated thoracic injuries, and extensive scalp degloving after a 20% false-negative rate was reported [18, 19]. A follow-up report found that the expanded criteria resulted in an increase in detection of injuries from 2.3% to 2.9% [20]. The Memphis criteria additionally added the findings of Horner's syndrome and a petrous bone fracture to the list of high risk factors, as well as soft tissue injury of the neck [21]. When the expanded Denver and the Memphis criteria were applied to pediatric patients at a single institution, it was reported that this would have resulted in an 11.9% (332 patients) rate of CT scanning with only one injury detected (0.3%) [22]. The study applied similar logic to pediatric patients in the NTDB, finding that almost 80,000 patients would have been screened for injury using the Denver and Memphis criteria, with a negative CTA in 97% [22]. A recent study examining the association of the seat belt sign to a subsequent carotid artery injury found that of 13,000 patients, only 0.5% had a carotid artery injury, and as a result this is not currently used as a high-risk criterion in children [23]. Due to concerns over the lack of generalizability of these criteria to the pediatric patient, the Utah and McGovern scores were developed. The Utah score gives points for a low GCS (1), a focal neurologic deficit (2), carotid canal fracture (2), petrous temporal bone fracture (3), or cerebral infarct on CT scan (3); those with a score > or equal to 3 should receive an angiography [24]. The McGovern score adds mechanism of injury (2) to the same scoring criteria, including high-speed MVC as a risk factor. The McGovern score was found to incorrectly classify only 19% of children as low risk, whereas the Denver, Memphis, EAST, and Utah scores had incorrect assignations in 28–48% of patients [25]. Based on recent pediatric data from the NTDB, screening is recommended in patients with skull base fractures, cervical spine fractures with and without cord injury, jugular vein injury, and cranial nerve injury [22]. Despite many proposed screening algorithms with variations in the content, there is no national consensus on the optimal protocol that limits CT use while reducing missed injuries. This topic will benefit from dedicated prospective multiple institutional study that focuses specifically on the pediatric patient, and would aim to clarify which injuries place children at a higher risk for injury. With regard to the screening modality for injury, CTA is the preferred method; however, this may overestimate injury, and cerebral angiography remains the gold standard for final diagnosis [22, 26].

Treatment recommendations are still based on adult data, and are guided by the grade of injury as listed in the Denver Grading Scale [27]. In children, no prospective study exists to validate whether these treatment recommendations result in improved clinical outcomes. Generally, patients with a grade IV injury (occlusion) are not treated, and initial therapy usually consists of a continuous heparin infusion with a goal aPTT 1.5–2.0 times the normal range. There are no specific recommendations for the duration of therapy or follow-up imaging after therapy.

A recent study from Nashville found that the majority of children had grade 1 (58%) and grade 2 (23%) injuries and that the two most common treatment modalities were no treatment (38%) and antiplatelet therapy (33%) [28]. There were no identified complications from medical management. Those with a GCS <8 and a higher-grade injury were found to have worsening injury with time, and were also found to have an increased mortality [28]. The overall mortality rate was 12%; all patients who died had a low GCS at presentation and a concomitant intracranial injury. Of those discharged, 67% underwent follow-up imaging with either a CTA, MRA, or angiography, and the majority were found to have improvement (52%), compared with no change (26%) or injury progression (19%) [28]. Due to the heterogeneity of the patient population and treatment allocations, no superior therapy is able to be recommended, although the authors comment that there were no apparent direct complications from anticoagulation. They do recommend repeat imaging at 3 months after the injury when cessation of anticoagulation would be planned [28]. Similarly, in a recent KIDS inpatient database study, mortality was 10%, and younger patients <11 years were found to have a higher stroke rate (29%) compared to older children (15%) [29]. Some data have suggested that there may be differential outcomes based on the age of the child, although this question warrants more dedicated study.

In summary, the management of blunt cerebrovascular injury in children largely borrows from adult data, although multiple studies have demonstrated the fundamental inadequacy of this approach. The development of a screening tool that has a low false-negative rate (to avoid a devastating missed injury) and a reasonable true-negative rate (to avoid unnecessary radiation) will require dedicated prospective, multicenter efforts. Commentary on the efficacy of management protocols is difficult at this time due to limited pediatric data, although at this time the risks of anticoagulation seem to be minimal. Follow-up imaging and duration of therapy have similarly not been standardized or based on any high-quality data. Given the low incidence of these types of injuries, coordinated efforts among pediatric trauma centers will be necessary to accomplish these goals.

Aortic Injury

Although aortic injury is rare in children, it does occur and is associated with high mortality [30]. A review of the KIDS inpatient database (1991–2009) reported 468 cases; the most common cause was motor vehicle crash, and overall survival was 65%. Shock at presentation and need for exploratory laparotomy were associated with the highest mortality [30]. Survival increased over the study period [30]. The diagnosis of aortic injury in children who survive to the hospital can be difficult as findings can be subtle. Approximately half of pediatric patients with blunt truncal injury demonstrate no external signs of chest trauma; therefore, a high index of suspicion is necessary when evaluating children with high-impact thoracic trauma [31]. Chest radiograph with an indistinct aortic knob or periaortic hematoma causing a widened mediastinum should prompt chest CT with angiography, which has essentially replaced conventional angiography for diagnosis of aortic injury [31]. Presence of a scapular fracture has been shown to be associated with thoracic aortic injury [32]. Abdominal aortic injury can occur in conjunction with the "seat belt syndrome," which also includes abdominal organ injury and lumbar (Chance) fracture [33].

The majority of aortic injuries require repair, although there have been reports of nonoperative management of stable injuries, which is supported by recent data from adult patients that recommends nonoperative management for low-grade injuries [33, 34]. The risk of free rupture is highest in the first few hours after injury, and strict blood pressure control (anti-impulse therapy) is important; however, this is complicated in children with concomitant traumatic brain injury that requires

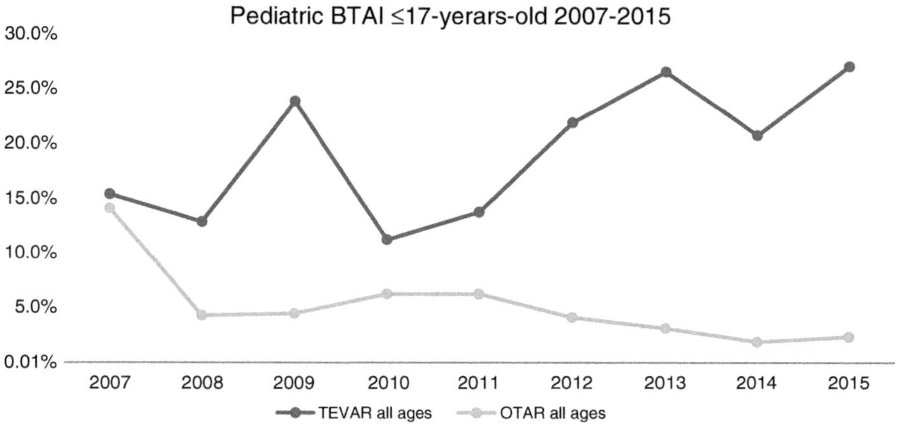

Fig. 7.2 Blunt thoracic aortic injury for patients ≤17 years from 2007 to 2015. (From Ref. [36])

adequate blood pressure to optimize cerebral perfusion pressure. Aortic repair can be delayed as long as impulse control is possible, and more pressing life-threatening injuries need to be addressed via craniotomy or laparotomy. Traditional open operative repair includes primary repair, patch repair, or an interposition graft. Autologous grafts are not large enough in young children, and prosthetic grafts have a higher thrombosis rate and don't grow with the child, leading to potential stricture. Other feared complications include paraplegia and renal failure. Intraoperative ultrasound may be useful to determine the exact extent of the injury and not sacrifice any normal aorta [35]. Thoracic endovascular aortic repair (TEVAR) has gained popularity in the past two decades. A review of the NTDB between 2007 and 15 reported that the rate of TEVAR use nearly doubled over this time period in pediatric patients [36] (Fig. 7.2). Considerations specific to pediatric patients, however, are that pediatric-sized thoracic grafts are not readily available, and nonideal sizes can lead to complications such as obstruction of important aortic branches and stent migration when non-thoracic stents are used [37]. Utilizing expandable stents helps with growth adjustments, although stent-related complications remain high despite improvements. If an adequate thoracic stent is not available, then balloon-expandable covered stents used by pediatric cardiologists to treat coarctation of the aorta may be considered and have been used successfully [38].

Anticoagulation

Anticoagulation management following vascular injury remains varied without high-quality evidence or national recommendations to guide therapy. Shahi et al. recently reported their anticoagulation practices in 99 pediatric vascular injury patients with 80% sustaining arterial injuries [39]. The majority of patients were managed in the inpatient setting with a heparin drip, and depending on the location of the injury were most commonly discharged on either aspirin or enoxaparin, although there was heterogeneity through the study including the recommended duration of anticoagulation [39]. The complication rate in this study was 17% and included vascular thrombosis and arterial stenosis, emphasizing the need for identifying optimal treatment guidelines to mitigate these sequelae [39]. This strategy appears to be more acceptable should thrombosis follow an occurrence of iatrogenic injury most likely being catheterization. In this setting, intravenous anticoagulation has been shown to have favorable clinical outcomes to intervention with correlating radiographic improvement or even resolution of thrombus. However, an approach with anticoagulation alone should be coupled with continuous clinical monitoring and interval radiographic assessment to ensure appropriate response [8–10].

Outcomes

Acute, short-term outcomes of pediatric vascular injury are similar to those in adults, including pseudoaneurysm, hemorrhage, or arteriovenous fistula of untreated injuries and thrombosis and stricture of treated injuries. Long-term follow-up of pediatric vascular injuries is rarely reported. A single-center series of 176 patients reported follow-up in 65. Two patients who also had fractures developed growth plate arrest, manifesting as a varus deformity and limb-length discrepancy [6]. One patient with vertebral artery dissection suffered a stroke, one with carotid artery injury developed aphasia with dysarthria, and one died. There were no recorded readmissions for patients with extremity vascular injuries [6]. Limb-length deformity is a feared complication in children because inadequate limb revascularization may not be able to support future limb growth despite collateral development; however, these are rarely reported. This may be due to inadequate routine surveillance in children with vascular injury. This problem is most commonly reported after femoral artery injury/occlusion, which can be reversed with revascularization prior to closure of the metaphyseal plates [40]. Prospective studies are required to understand the true incidence of limb-length discrepancy following extremity vascular injury in children and the optimal timing of revascularization.

Another delayed complication is Volkmann's ischemic contracture, which results from ischemia secondary to arm fractures (most commonly supracondylar humerus fractures) that causes compartment syndrome with subsequent muscle necrosis and severe scarring, leading to "claw hand." This is an extremely rare complication, reported in <1% of cases, only described in case reports, and with modern techniques of supracondylar humerus fracture management, should be largely preventable [41]. Prospective follow-up studies would also be helpful to understand the true incidence of this particular complication.

Conclusion

Pediatric vascular trauma is rare; however, special considerations exist such as propensity for vasospasm and vessel size, and management and follow-up may differ from that of adult patients. Endovascular options are gaining popularity and usage, although pediatric-sized device availability is still not prevalent. Anticoagulation alone may be a suitable strategy in circumstance of thrombosis secondary to iatrogenic trauma. Collaboration among pediatric trauma surgeons and vascular surgeons is of utmost importance to optimize care and ensure vascular surveillance. Prospective studies are necessary to understand outcomes.

References

1. Barmparas G, Inaba K, Talving P, David JS, Lam L, Plurad D, et al. Pediatric vs adult vascular trauma: a National Trauma Databank review. J Pediatr Surg. 2010;45(7):1404–12.
2. Gurien LA, Maxson RT, Dassinger MS, et al. Pediatric vascular injuries: are we preparing trainees appropriately to meet our needs? Am J Surg. 2017;214(2):336–40.
3. Shah SR, Wearden PD, Gaines BA. Pediatric peripheral vascular injuries: a review of our experience. J Surg Res. 2009;153(1):162–6.
4. Corneille MG, Gallup TM, Villa C, et al. Pediatric vascular injuries: acute management and early outcomes. J Trauma. 2011;70(4):823–8.
5. Eslami MH, Saadeddin ZM, Rybin DV, et al. Trends and outcomes of pediatric vascular injuries in the United States: an analysis of the National Trauma Data Bank. Ann Vasc Surg. 2019;56:52–61.
6. Klinkner DB, Arca MJ, Lewis BD, et al. Pediatric vascular injuries: patterns of injury, morbidity and mortality. J Pediatr Surg. 2007;42(1):178–82.
7. Branco BC, Naik-Mathuria B, Montero-Baker M, et al. Increasing use of endovascular therapy in pediatric arterial trauma. J Vasc Surg. 2017;66(4):1175–83.e1.
8. Kayssi A, Shaikh F, Roche-Nagle G, Brandao LR, Williams SA, Rubin BB. Management of acute limb ischemia in the pediatric population. J Vasc Surg. 2014;60(1):106–10.
9. Ramirez JL, Kuhrau CR, Wu B, Zarkowsky DS, Conte MS, Oskowitz AZ, Nijagal A, Vartanian SM. Natural history of acute pediatric iliofemoral artery thrombosis treated with anticoagulation. J Vasc Surg. 2020;72(6):2027–34.
10. Jaffray J, Goldenberg N. Current approaches in the treatment of catheter-related deep venous thrombosis in children. Expert Rev Hematol. 2020;13(6):607–17.
11. Conrad MF, Patton JH Jr, Parikshak M, Kralovich KA. Evaluation of vascular injury in penetrating extremity trauma: angiographers stay home. Am Surg. 2002;68(3):269–74.
12. Brahmamdam P, Plummer M, Modrall JG, et al. Hand ischemia associated with elbow trauma in children. J Vasc Surg. 2011;54(3):773–8.
13. White L, Mehlman CT, Crawford AH. Perfused, pulseless, and puzzling: a systematic review of vascular injuries in pediatric supracondylar humerus fractures and results of a POSNA questionnaire. J Pediatr Orthop. 2010;30(4):328–35.
14. Marenco CW, Do WS, Lammers DT, Morte KR, Eckert MJ, Eckert CM, et al. Big problems in little patients: Nationwide blunt cerebrovascular injury outcomes in the pediatric population. J Trauma Acute Care Surg. 2019;87(5):1088–95.
15. Harris DA, Sorte DE, Lam SK, Carlson AP. Blunt cerebrovascular injury in pediatric trauma: a national database study. J Neurosurg Pediatr. 2019;24:1–10.
16. Jones TS, Burlew CC, Kornblith LZ, Biffl WL, Partrick DA, Johnson JL, et al. Blunt cerebrovascular injuries in the child. Am J Surg. 2012;204(1):7–10.
17. Bromberg WJ, Collier BC, Diebel LN, Dwyer KM, Holevar MR, Jacobs DG, et al. Blunt cerebrovascular injury practice management guidelines: the Eastern Association for the Surgery of Trauma. J Trauma. 2010;68(2):471–7.
18. Burlew CC, Biffl WL, Moore EE. Blunt cerebrovascular injuries in children: broadened screening guidelines are warranted. J Trauma Acute Care Surg. 2012;72(4):1120–1.
19. Burlew CC, Biffl WL, Moore EE, Barnett CC, Johnson JL, Bensard DD. Blunt cerebrovascular injuries: redefining screening criteria in the era of noninvasive diagnosis. J Trauma Acute Care Surg. 2012;72(2):330–5; discussion 6-7, quiz 539.

20. Geddes AE, Burlew CC, Wagenaar AE, Biffl WL, Johnson JL, Pieracci FM, et al. Expanded screening criteria for blunt cerebrovascular injury: a bigger impact than anticipated. Am J Surg. 2016;212(6):1167–74.
21. Miller PR, Fabian TC, Croce MA, Cagiannos C, Williams JS, Vang M, et al. Prospective screening for blunt cerebrovascular injuries: analysis of diagnostic modalities and outcomes. Ann Surg. 2002;236(3):386–93; discussion 93-5.
22. Mallicote MU, Isani MA, Golden J, Ford HR, Upperman JS, Gayer CP. Screening for blunt cerebrovascular injuries in pediatric trauma patients. J Pediatr Surg. 2019;54(9):1861–5.
23. Ugalde IT, Claiborne MK, Cardenas-Turanzas M, Shah MN, Langabeer JR 2nd, Patel R. Risk factors in pediatric blunt cervical vascular injury and significance of seatbelt sign. West J Emerg Med. 2018;19(6):961–9.
24. Ravindra VM, Bollo RJ, Sivakumar W, Akbari H, Naftel RP, Limbrick DD Jr, et al. Predicting blunt cerebrovascular injury in pediatric trauma: validation of the "Utah Score". J Neurotrauma. 2017;34(2):391–9.
25. Herbert JP, Venkataraman SS, Turkmani AH, Zhu L, Kerr ML, Patel RP, et al. Pediatric blunt cerebrovascular injury: the McGovern screening score. J Neurosurg Pediatr. 2018;21(6):639–49.
26. Grandhi R, Weiner GM, Agarwal N, Panczykowski DM, Ares WJ, Rodriguez JS, et al. Limitations of multidetector computed tomography angiography for the diagnosis of blunt cerebrovascular injury. J Neurosurg. 2018;128(6):1642–7.
27. Biffl WL, Moore EE, Offner PJ, Brega KE, Franciose RJ, Burch JM. Blunt carotid arterial injuries: implications of a new grading scale. J Trauma. 1999;47(5):845–53.
28. Dewan MC, Ravindra VM, Gannon S, Prather CT, Yang GL, Jordan LC, et al. Treatment practices and outcomes after blunt cerebrovascular injury in children. Neurosurgery. 2016;79(6):872–8.
29. Marenco CW, Do WS, Lammers DT, et al. Big problems in little patients: nationwide blunt cerebrovascular injury outcomes in the pediatric population. J Trauma Acute Care Surg. 2019;87(5):1088–95.
30. Tashiro J, Hannay WM, Naves C, et al. Mechanism and mortality of pediatric aortic injuries. J Surg Res. 2015;198(2):456–61.
31. Pabon-Ramos WM, Williams DM, Strouse PJ. Radiologic evaluation of blunt thoracic aortic injury in pediatric patients. AJR Am J Roentgenol. 2010;194(5):1197–203.
32. Abd El-Shafy I, Rosen LM, Prince JM, Letton RW, Rosen NG. Blunt traumatic scapular fractures are associated with great vessel injuries in children. J Trauma Acute Care Surg. 2018;85(5):932–5.
33. Parrish DW, Barnhorst A, Trebska-McGowan K, et al. Nonoperative management of pediatric aortic injury with seat belt syndrome. Ann Vasc Surg. 2015;29(6):1316.e1–6. https://doi.org/10.1016/j.avsg.2015.02.019. Epub 2015 May 28. Review
34. Starnes BW, Lundgren RS, Gunn M, et al. A new classification scheme for treating blunt aortic injury. J Vasc Surg. 2012;55(1):47–54.
35. Bairdain S, Modi BP, Kim HB, et al. Pediatric blunt abdominal aortic injury and the use of intraoperative aortic ultrasound for surgical decision making. J Pediatr Surg. 2013;48(7):1584–7.
36. Hasjim BJ, Grigorian A, Barrios C Jr, et al. National trends of thoracic endovascular aortic repair versus open thoracic aortic repair in pediatric blunt thoracic aortic injury. Ann Vasc Surg. 2019;59:150–7.
37. Diez AA, Monteiro EM, Hoyos YG, et al. Management and evolution of a wallstent migration in a pediatric blunt traumatic abdominal aortic injury. Ann Vasc Surg. 2018;47:281.e15–9.
38. Goldstein BH, Hirsch R, Zussman ME, et al. Percutaneous balloon-expandable covered stent implantation for treatment of traumatic aortic injury in children and adolescents. Am J Cardiol. 2012;110(10):1541–5.
39. Shahi N, Phillips R, Meier M, et al. Anti-coagulation management in pediatric traumatic vascular injuries. J Pediatr Surg. 2020;55(2):324–30.
40. Rubinstein RA Jr, et al. Limb growth after late bypass graft for occlusion of the femoral artery. A case report. J Bone Joint Surg Am. 1990;72(6):935–7.
41. Copley LA, Dormans JP, Davidson RS. Vascular injuries and their sequelae in pediatric supracondylar humerus fractures: toward a goal of prevention. J Pediatr Orthop. 1996;16(1):99–103.

Part III

Operation and Intervention

Principles of Vascular Access and Complications

8

Amir Pezeshkmehr

Introduction

Vascular access has undergone a slow but gradual evolution, with nearly a five-century span from the historic documentation of the first attempted intravenous (IV) therapy in 1492 [2] to the introduction of the first polyurethane plastic catheter for IV infusion in 1945 [1]. However, in the past 75 years, there has been an exponential growth and innovation in vascular access and techniques. The most pivotal achievement in vascular access was the introduction of the Seldinger technique in 1952. As originally described by Dr. Sven Ivar Seldinger, a Swedish radiologist, the technique involves using a hollow needle and guidewire to establish and secure the vascular access, followed by catheter placement over the wire (Fig. 8.1). Nowadays there are a myriad of vascular access devices intended for a variety of purposes, which are available in different sizes, lengths, and hub numbers. The goal of this chapter is to provide a concise review of the principles of vascular access and the potential complications.

General Principles

The landmark technique [10], commonly used by intensivists and surgeons for vascular access, is gradually being replaced by image guidance, especially with the widespread adoption of ultrasound. Anatomic variations and the presence of vessel thrombus or occlusion (Fig. 8.2) can create unforeseen challenges for the landmark technique. On the contrary ultrasound is a great tool, enabling visualization of the anatomic structures and evaluation of the target vessel for patency and thrombosis

A. Pezeshkmehr (✉)
Division of Interventional Radiology, Department of Radiology, Texas Children's Hospital/Baylor College of Medicine, Houston, TX, USA
e-mail: ahpezesh@texaschildrens.org

R. Gilani, J. L. Mills Sr. (eds.), *Vascular Complications of Surgery and Intervention*, https://doi.org/10.1007/978-3-030-86713-3_8

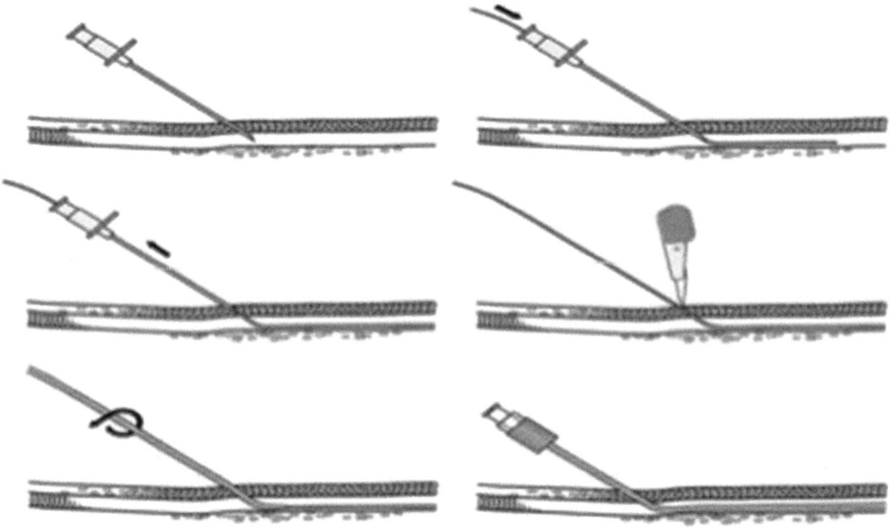

Fig. 8.1 Seldinger technique: Needle placement followed by wire and eventually catheter placement

Fig. 8.2 Internal jugular vein containing thrombus

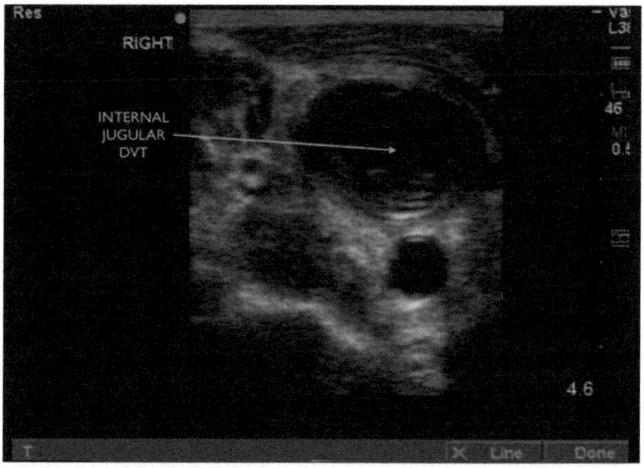

[4]. One caveat about ultrasound is that it is an operator-dependent modality. However, the required skill set could be easily achieved with time. In addition to ultrasound, fluoroscopy is usually needed for proper positioning of some central lines with longer catheters. The combination of image guidance with the Seldinger technique has significantly improved the technical success, safety, and quality of the procedure and decreased potential complications [2, 5].

Supporting the argument for image guidance are numerous studies showing that US reduces complications, improves cannulation rates, and decreases time for cannulation. In 2006, a prospective study by Karakitsos prospectively compared internal jugular vein (IJV) catheterization with real-time US versus using landmark techniques [16]. Significant differences (*P* < 0.001) were found between the two groups in regard to overall success rate (100% vs. 94%), inadvertent arterial puncture (1% vs. 10.6%), hematoma formation (0.4% vs. 8.4%), pneumothorax (0% vs. 2.4%), and hemothorax (0% vs. 1.7%), all favoring US-guided access. Furthermore, 7.6% of patients were noted to have ipsilateral thrombus, and the contralateral IJV was accessed. Also, 25 patients that had unsuccessful attempts using landmark techniques were successfully accessed with US. Reasons for failure were presence of thrombus in 20 patients and aberrant anatomy in 5 patients. Further supporting the use of US is a meta-analysis published in 2003 consisting of 18 randomized control trials [17]. Once again, the use of US demonstrated significantly improved success, reduced complications, and decreased procedural times.

Access procedures in pediatric patients, especially premature infants, can be a humbling endeavor largely due to small vessel size and variant anatomy. A study by Verghese evaluated use of US for IJV cannulation in infants [18]. US significantly improved procedural success (100% vs. 77%) and decreased arterial punctures (0% vs. 25%). US was also shown to improve overall procedural times. These findings have been reproduced in similar patients by numerous other investigators [19, 20].

Certain vascular access procedures, such peripheral intravenous (PIV) access, do not amend well to landmark techniques but rather are performed via palpation and visualization. The utility of US for insertion of PIV access has been documented. A study by Gregg in 2010 evaluated PIV insertion with US in patients that were otherwise unable to have PIV access placed by standard means [21]. They reported a 99% overall success rate of which 71% were placed on the first attempt. As a result of the 147 PIVs placed, 40 central venous catheters (CVCs) and 34 were avoided, a much-welcomed indirect benefit.

Much like venous access, arterial access can also pose significant obstacles to performing a successful procedure without complication such as hemorrhage, thrombosis, dissection, and nerve injury. The secondary effects of arterial access complications can result in significant morbidity and mortality by way of amputation, stroke, need for open surgery, and death [22]. The use of US for arterial access has been validated through prospective randomized trials demonstrating improved success rates, decreased complications, and shorter procedural times [23, 24]. Also compelling is data published within a pediatric population. Once again US use correlates significantly with increased success (100% vs. 80%), decreased number of attempts (1.3 vs. 2.3), and shorter procedural times (*P* < 0.05) [25].

As one can see, there is much data supporting use of US for vascular access within the literature as prefaced above. Furthermore, an apparent observation is that the potential for benefit with US-guided vascular access increases with incremental increase in difficulty. However, the possibilities for US use remain more expansive than that which has been touched on by the literature. A sampling of challenges to access would include obesity, hypovolemia, coagulopathy, need for anticoagulation, and previous access procedures, all of which are routinely encountered by acute care surgeons. US-guided vascular access is not a requirement for success; however, the facile physician must be readily prepared to implement its use reliably when traditional access methods appear to be insufficient.

Based on the Centers for Disease Control and Prevention (CDC) guidelines, maximum sterile barrier precautions should be used for vascular access. Exceptions to this rule are peripheral intravenous (IV) lines. The procedure should preferably be performed in a sterile environment such as the interventional radiology suite or the operating room. Other less favored alternatives include the patient room or a designated space with minimal human traffic [8]. The insertion site is usually prepped with a 2% chlorhexidine solution, or Betadine in case of chlorhexidine allergy, and draped with sterile towel and covers. The operator should be wearing a cap, mask, gown, and sterile gloves during the procedure. A sterile ultrasound probe cover should be used for all lines requiring maximum sterility. The sterile field should not be compromised until the procedure has been completed and an appropriate sterile dressing has been applied. The skin entry site is usually covered by a protective antimicrobial disk such as Biopatch, which contains chlorhexidine gluconate (CHG). These catheters are usually secured in place with stitches or a securing device such as StatLock and covered with a clear tape (Figs. 8.3 and 8.4).

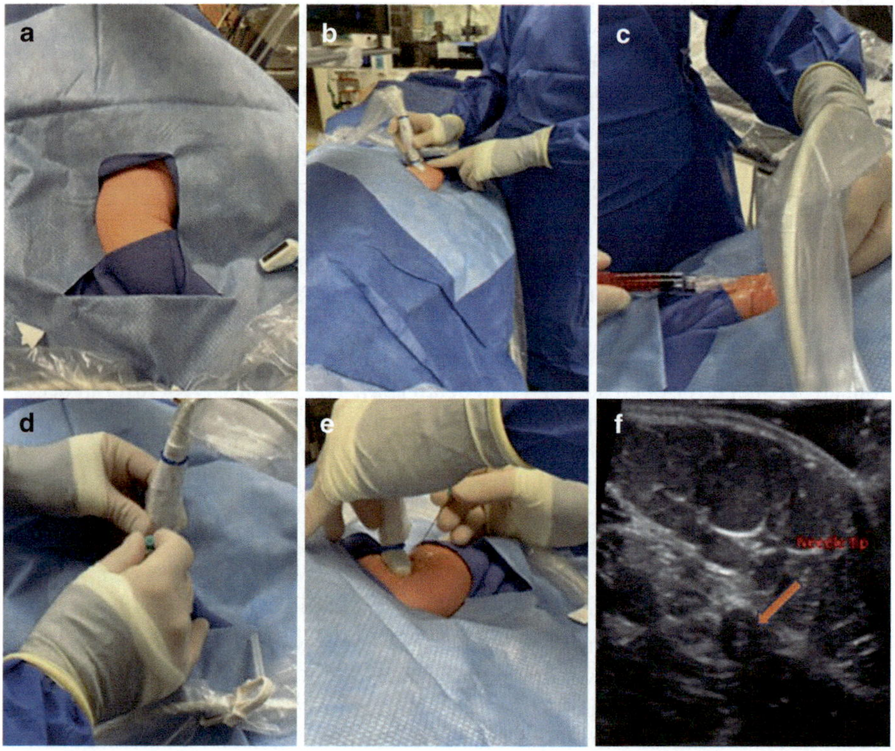

Fig. 8.3 Steps of an image guided vascular access using an aseptic Seldinger technique (part 1). (**a**) Prepped and draped sterile field (**b**) Evaluation of the target vein and choosing entry site with ultrasound (**c**) Administration of local anesthesia (**d**) Venous access (Long-axis technique) (**e**) Venous access (Short-axis technique) (**f**) US image demonstrating the needle tip in the target vein

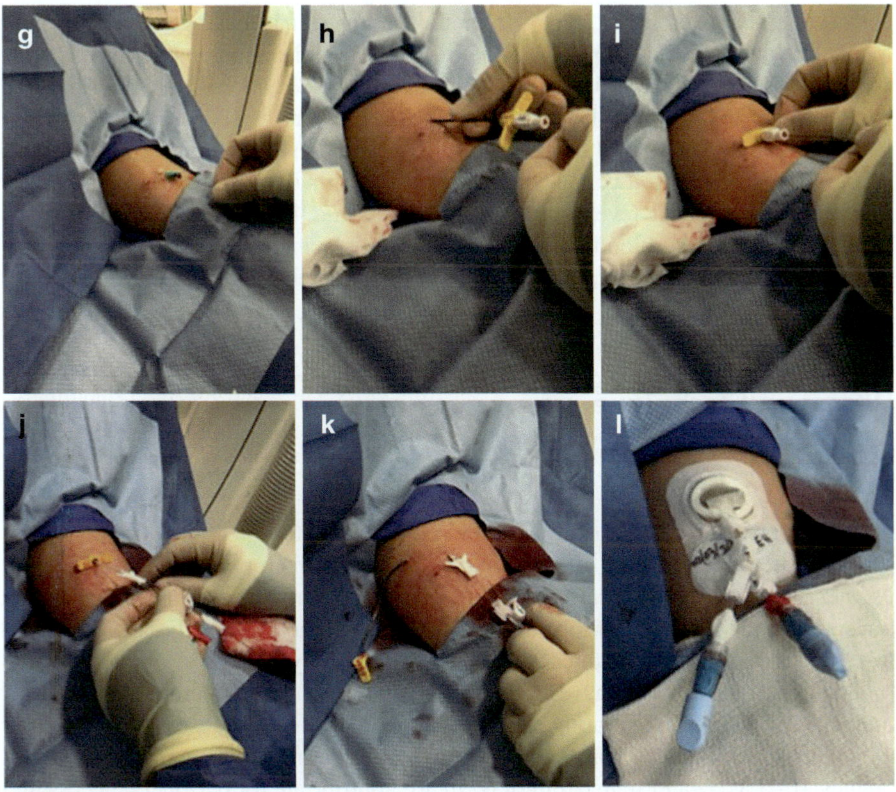

Fig. 8.4 Steps of an image guided vascular access using an aseptic (Seldinger) technique (part 2). (**g**) Insertion of wire through hollow needle (**h**) Needle exchange with eel away dilator (**i**) Final position of peel away prior to dilator removal (**j**) Catheter insertion (**k**) Removal of eel away (**l**) Completion of procedure and application of sterile dressing

Routine antibiotic therapy is usually not recommended for arterial lines and non-tunneled temporary central venous lines. Use of antibiotics for tunneled-cuffed central lines and ports has been a controversial subject. Regardless of the recent data demonstrating no significant benefit in antibiotic therapy, many physicians continue to use periprocedural antibiotics for skin flora coverage for these lines [6].

Baseline preprocedural laboratory tests such as CBC, PT/INR, and PTT are usually obtained to rule out coagulopathy. Historically the acceptable laboratory values of platelet count >50,000 and INR <1.5 were used for central line placement. Markedly abnormal values are usually corrected with platelet or fresh frozen plasma (FFP). However, newer guidelines by the Society of Interventional Radiology classify the arterial and all central venous lines in the low bleeding risk category, for which a platelet count >20,000 and an INR <2 are considered as acceptable levels. Based on the same guidelines, screening laboratory tests are not routinely recommended, and withholding of anticoagulation medication is not warranted for arterial or venous lines, with the exception of patients on warfarin, who should have a corrected INR of less than 3 [14]. It should be noted that these guidelines are not meant to supersede the judgment of the treating physician, and deviations based on specific patient needs and risk assessments should be considered on a case-by-case basis in order to minimize the risk of significant bleeding.

Special emphasis should be made to rule out the presence of blood-borne bacteria before placing central venous lines, especially ports or tunneled lines. Therefore, in patients with recent fever or suspected bacteremia, having documentation of at least 48 h of negative blood cultures prior to line placement is necessary to reduce the risk of bacterial colonization of the line. Patients with urgent need for a central line are exempt of this rule.

Ultrasound Technique

Equipment

Advances in technology have made US nearly ubiquitous within hospitals today. Furthermore, machines are often mobile or portable which makes US available for use nearly anywhere vascular access procedures are performed. Linear-array transducers, so-called because of the parallel alignment of the contained crystals, in contrast to curved-array transducers are most commonly used for vascular access procedures. Each transducer, regardless of crystal orientation, operates within a frequency range. It is the operating frequency that determines the resolution and depth of penetration which are inversely related. Linear-array transducers with a frequency 10–5 MHz and scan depth of 6 cm are appropriate for peripheral access and IJV cannulation. Curved-array transducers (5–2 MHz and scan depth of 30 cm) may be more appropriate for femoral access in obese patients; however, resolution is diminished. The ideal probe utilized achieves the required depth of penetration at the highest possible frequency, thereby providing the best resolution.

Scanning

Vascular ultrasonographic evaluation utilizes three separate imaging modalities while scanning in order to perform a complete exam. These are 2D grayscale B-mode imaging, color-flow imaging, and pulsed-Doppler spectral waveform analysis. Regardless of exam performed, adequate skin-transducer interface is required while performing surface US. This is facilitated with the use of ultrasound gel applied on the skin as well as within a probe cover during sterile procedures. Sufficient pressure is applied to the transducer to maintain proper interface while not excessive to compress venous or arterial structures.

Examination begins with 2D grayscale imaging which is also used while performing access procedures. The monitor should be readily visible throughout the exam and procedure. Appropriate depth of penetration is selected to visualize structures of interest while maximizing resolution, and minor adjustments are made to far and near gain knobs to optimize image quality. Grayscale imaging allows the operator to visualize access site anatomy, visualize the lumen and wall of the access vessel (looking for thrombus or calcification), evaluate for compressibility of veins (the presence of echolucent thrombus may render the vein noncompressible), and assess for arterial pulsation (non-pulsatility may indicate more proximal obstruction). After grayscale, color flow is selected within the region of interest. The presence of flow helps to ensure patency of the lumen. Flow may be sluggish, and distal compression and Valsalva can be used to modulate venous flow. The exam is completed with Doppler waveform analysis. An area of sampling is selected within the vessel of interest and pulsed analysis is initiated. Veins should display phasic flow and arteries pulsatile phasic flow. Lack of phasic flow may indicate more central obstruction. Using this information, the access site can be confirmed as appropriate, or if unsatisfactory another site can be selected for evaluation.

Access Technique

Access Site Selection

After assessing a patient for vascular access, a point of access must be selected. Generally, PIV sites are evaluated from distal to proximal. Common central venous access sites are IJV, common femoral vein (CFV), subclavian vein, and basilic vein for peripherally inserted central catheter (PICC) line. Arterial access points are selected where manual pressure can be adequately applied over bony landmarks to ensure hemostasis during decannulation such brachial artery, radial artery, and common femoral artery. The access site is then evaluated via US (see scanning) prior to initiating the access procedure to confirm adequacy of the access site.

Preparation

The patient is positioned for comfort and adequate exposure of the access site must be ensured. Venous dilation can be enhanced through by positioning into a gravity-dependent position or through the use of a proximal tourniquet for PIV placement. The access site is then prepped and draped using sterile technique. The ultrasound monitor is placed in direct view of the operator. The probe is placed into a sterile glove or sterile probe cover containing ultrasound gel. Sterile gel is necessary on the field to ensure proper skin-transducer interface.

Cannulation

Prior to cannulation the access vessel is visualized along the transverse axis (Fig. 8.5). During transverse reference, visualized vessels will appear round. Furthermore, veins can be identified as being compressible and arteries as pulsatile. Center the vessel in the field of view, and identify a point on the skin overlying the vessel by gently probing with a 21-ga needle supplied in a micropuncture set (21-ga needle, 0.018″ wire, 4-Fr sheath) attached to a syringe. A micropuncture set is used

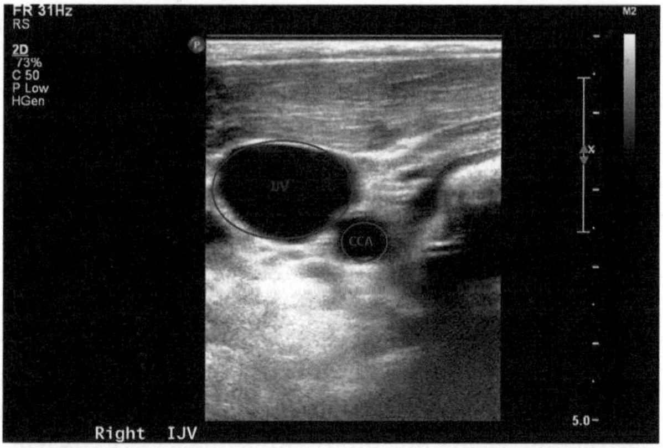

Fig. 8.5 Tranverse axis visualization of neck anatomy

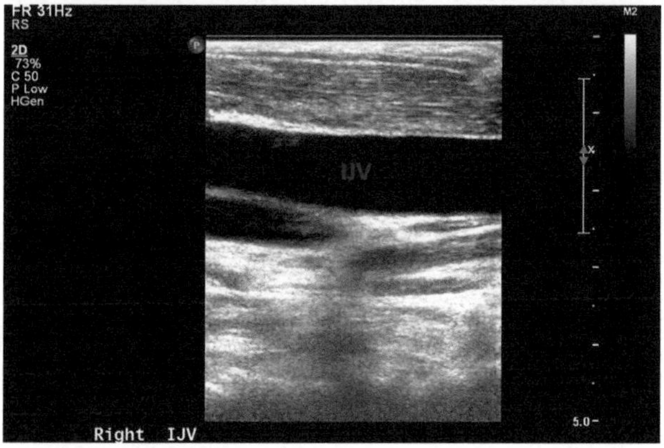

Fig. 8.6 Long axis visualization of internal jugular vein.

during difficult access to mitigate complications from inadvertent or unsuccessful cannulation. While maintaining the position of the needle, turn the probe 90° into the long axis. The vessel should now appear rectangular along the length of the screen (Fig. 8.6). Long reference visualization allows for more precise assessment of penetration depth with the tip of the needle helping to avoid accidental back wall penetration. Slowly advance the needle to identify the tip. Once the tip is located, gently advance the needle until the vessel is cannulated under direct vision, visualizing the tip at all times (Fig. 8.7). A 0.018″ guidewire is threaded through the needle and should pass without difficulty. Failure to easily pass the wire indicates a potential problem such extravascular position, central obstruction, or placement within a dissection plane. The probe is returned to the transverse axis and guidewire placement within the lumen is confirmed. The wire will appear as an echogenic dot within the lumen. The needle is exchanged for a 4-Fr sheath that will allow passage of 0.035″ and 0.038″ guidewires that are supplied in most vascular access kits. The guidewire and inner cannula are removed, and blood return through the sheath is assessed whether as being venous or arterial. If satisfactory, the procedure is then completed in standard fashion using over-the-wire technique.

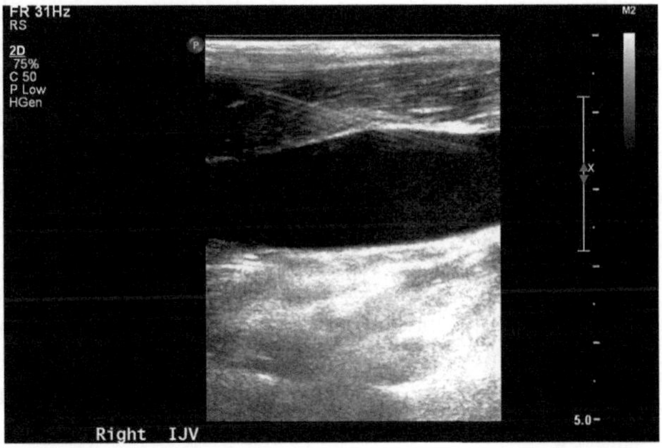

Fig. 8.7 Needle cannulation of internal jugular vein in long axis

Summary

1. Perform ultrasonographic evaluation of access site.
↓
2. Position and prep.
↓
3. Identify overlying skin position in transverse axis.
↓
4. Cannulate vessel in long axis under direct vision.
↓
5. Confirm position of the wire in transverse axis.
↓
6. Place a 4-Fr sheath and assess blood return.
↓
7. Place standard wire and complete procedure.

Vascular Access Types

Arterial Access

Arterial access is essential for monitoring of critically ill patients and is commonly performed in intensive care and operative room settings. It is also obtained for diagnostic angiography and interventional procedures. Arterial line placement is one of the most commonly performed procedures with major complication rates of less than 1% [15]. There are some technical challenges as it requires knowledge of the anatomy and certain skill sets.

Multiple upper and lower extremity arteries could be used for this purpose, but radial and femoral arteries are the most commonly used access sites for both patient monitoring and also diagnostic and interventional purposes, with comparable complication rates [15]. Historically the common femoral artery has been the main access site for diagnostic and interventional radiology procedures; however, the radial access is gaining momentum in most adults and older pediatric patients. Brachial artery access has a limited role for the non-interventionalist due to high complication rates and should be avoided by in large. As an alternative for the difficult patient, axillary artery cannulation for hemodynamic monitoring is quite safe, however should be limited to smaller-diameter catheters due to challenges with hemostasis after decannulation. The procedure is done with or without image guidance, using either a catheter-over-needle or catheter over-the-wire technique. Sedation is not required for peripheral access; however, some level of sedation may be needed for central arterial access.

Most common indications include continuous arterial pressure monitoring, arteriovenous hemoperfusion or dialysis, access for cardiac catheterization and interventional procedures, manual or automated exchange transfusions, plasmapheresis, and extracorporeal membrane oxygenation.

Absolute and relative contraindications are absent pulse; full-thickness burn; peripheral or distal arterial vascular insufficiency; peripheral arterial diseases, such as medium to small vessel arteritis; anticoagulation or coagulopathy; anatomical variants in which there may be a lack of collateral circulation such as absence of the ulnar artery; and infection at the catheter insertion site.

Serious complications are rare and include bleeding, hematoma, arterial dissection, pseudoaneurysm, thrombosis, distal ischemia, arteriovenous (AV) fistula, compartment syndrome, and infection.

Pseudoaneurysms with a narrow neck are initially addressed with manual compression or ultrasound-guided thrombin injection if compression fails. Large necked pseudoaneurysms, AV fistulas, and vessel dissection require surgical or endovascular intervention. Thrombosis and distal emboli are usually managed with either systemic anticoagulation or catheter-directed thrombolysis.

There has been a small decline in the number of arterial lines, due to the potential complications and most importantly the development of new, less invasive tools and techniques that enable more accurate hemodynamic monitoring without the need for catheter placement.

Venous Access

Venous access is the most commonly performed procedure in a hospital or ambulatory setting. These catheters and lines are intended for therapeutic or diagnostic purposes. There are several types of vascular access devices (VAD) in the market, which could be used for either peripheral or central intravenous access. Device selection requires meticulous clinical workup. Multiple factors including patient's clinical condition, type, and duration of treatment and even caregiver or patient's intellectual status and family dynamics should be taken into consideration for better device selection.

The peripheral access mainly consisted of conventional peripheral intravenous (PIV) lines and midlines. Peripherally inserted central catheters, also known as PICC lines, tunneled and non-tunneled central lines, and Port-a-Catheters are the different types of central venous lines (Fig. 8.8).

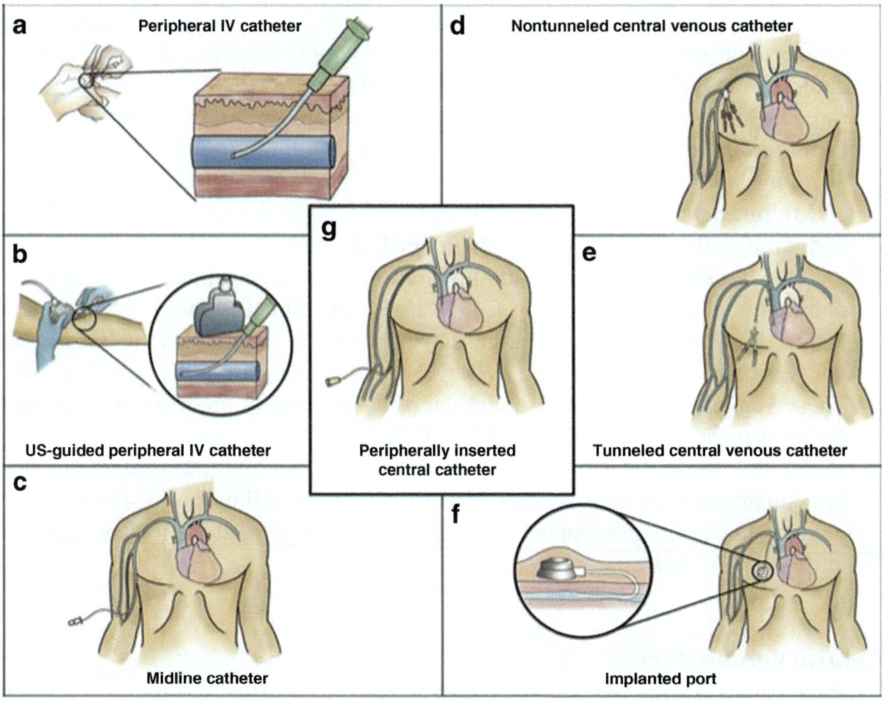

Fig. 8.8 Different types of venous access. (The Michigan Appropriateness Guide for Intravenous Catheters). (**a**) Peripheral IV catheter (**b**) US guided IV cathteter placement (**c**) Midline catheter (**d**) Nontunneled central venous catheter (**e**) Tunneled central venous catheter (**f**) Implanted Por-A-cath

Peripheral Venous Access

1. *Peripheral IV Lines*

   The conventional peripheral intravenous (PIV) catheter is by far the most commonly performed vascular access with more than 230 million IV lines placed annually in the United States, and more than one billion worldwide [12]. PIV placement is usually performed using the palpation and visualization technique, with ultrasound guidance usually reserved for patients with difficult IV access [13]. They are usually placed using an over-the-needle catheter technique and are available in ported and non-ported versions. Needle sizes range from 14 to 24 gauge and catheter lengths range from 25 to 44 mm.

   Indications include frequent lab draws, short-term IV therapies such as IV hydration, antibiotics, peripheral parenteral nutrition (PPN), and administration of IV contrast for diagnostic MRI and CT studies. There are no absolute contraindications, and the relative contraindications include infection, phlebitis, venous thrombosis, infiltration, burn injuries, and vesicant and irritant medications.

   Known complications include catheter dislodgment and soft tissue infiltration, swelling, phlebitis, inadvertent arterial puncture and injury, and infection. Despite new evidence arguing against routine peripheral IV-line replacements, current CDC guidelines continue to recommend close catheter monitoring and replacement every 72–96 h [7]. The local complications usually resolve with catheter removal, limb elevation, and application of a warm or cold compress. In rare cases a compartment syndrome may develop from a large volume or vesicant fluid infiltration, which is usually managed with fasciotomy.

2. *Midlines*

   Midlines are an alternative for peripherally inserted central catheter (PICC) and are usually suitable of patients in need of a peripheral IV access for more than 5 days and less than a month in duration. They are available as a single- or double-lumen catheter, ranging from 3 to 5 French in size and 3 to 8 inches in length. Since the tip is not central, they are suitable only for IV hydration and non-vesicant medications with PH levels of 5–9 and osmolarity less than 500. These venous catheters are usually placed at the level of antecubital fossa, and the tip is positioned proximal to the axillary line [7]. Midlines have been associated with lower phlebitis rates than peripheral IV lines and lower infection rates in comparison with central lines. However, usage is falling out of favor due to increased complications such as venous thrombosis [3] and the increased popularity of PICC lines.

Central Venous Access

By definition a central venous access is placement of a catheter within a vein that does not have valves, and ideally from the upper extremity, its tip is positioned in the inferior third of the superior vena cava, the right atrium, or the inferior vena cava. Over five million central venous catheters are placed every year in the United States alone, accounting for 15 million central venous catheter days [5]. These lines are usually indicated for patients in need of a secure and large-bore central access in an emergent or acute care setting. Administration of vesicant and irritant solutions such as chemotherapy agents, total parenteral nutrition, trauma or intraoperative resuscitation, hemodialysis, and also extracorporeal membrane oxygenation (ECMO) access are common indications for central venous lines. They are usually placed percutaneously either directly into a large vein, such as internal jugular, subclavian, or femoral veins, or via a smaller peripheral vein, most commonly the basilic, brachial, or cephalic veins with the catheter tip terminating in a central location. Other methods of central access, such as intrahepatic or translumbar, are usually reserved for patients with no other available veins. There are a variety of central vascular access devices (CVAD) available in the market, with catheter materials predominantly consisting of polyurethane or silicone. These catheters are available in different diameters and lengths and may contain multiple lumens to allow simultaneous infusions through a single catheter. As mentioned previously, device selection requires meticulous clinical evaluation, with catheter selection dependent on multiple factors, including therapy requirements, acuity of the patient's condition, and psychosocial conditions.

Implementation of a strict aseptic technique is mandatory to minimize catheter-related infections, with extra caution toward long-term devices such as ports and cuffed-tunneled central lines.

Central lines are usually placed under image guidance, with a technical success rate of nearly 100%. A heparin lock is placed immediately after placement to prevent catheter thrombosis.

Depending on the patient's age, clinical condition and type, and location of central line, various levels of sedation may be necessary to ensure technical success and improve patient comfort.

At minimum, a local anesthetic such as plain or buffered 1% lidocaine should be used to minimize pain during and immediately after the procedure.

Complications result in increased mortality and morbidity and subsequently an increased financial burden on healthcare system. Therefore, it is very crucial to recognize and manage these complications as soon as possible [5]. Complications are generally divided into immediate, early, and delayed subtypes, with minimal overlapping features.

Immediate complications, which usually happen during catheter placement, include procedural failure, pneumothorax and hemothorax for internal jugular and subclavian vein lines, retroperitoneal hematoma for femoral lines, arterial puncture, guidewire-induced arrythmia, and air embolism. There is a direct correlation between number of attempts and immediate complications [5]. Expeditious recognition of immediate complications is crucial for preventing worsening of the situation and can often be remedied with simple maneuvers. For example, when attempting to cannulate during central line placement, inadvertent arterial puncture via brisk return of bright red blood with a needle is recognized. The needle can be removed and pressure applied for hemostasis. Pressure control of inadvertent arterial puncture and even dilation up to 7 Fr can be controlled with pressure if the location can undergo effective application of pressure. Larger devices regardless of location will require more advanced technique for removal and often require additional consultation. At times, confirmation of arterial placement can be more insidious as in a hypotensive or hypoxic patient. Under the circumstances, if there is any uncertainty, a segment of arterial line tubing can be connected to an 18-gauge catheter and a pressure transduced. Alternatively, an arterial blood gas sample can be analyzed to make the determination. Finally, verification of line position upon completion is readily achieved via plain X-ray of the site and serves as documentation into the medical record. Careful review of line placement X-ray must be methodical to ensure accurate interpretation as inadvertent line placement findings can be rather subtle.

Early complications which may happen immediately after catheter placement include catheter malposition and malfunction, thrombosis, and arrythmia.

Late complications are venous and catheter thrombosis, venous stenosis, and infection.

Catheter-related infections are one of the most dreaded complications with the most significant impact on the healthcare system. The central line-associated bloodstream infection (CLABSI) is defined as a laboratory-confirmed bloodstream infection not related to an infection at another site, which develops within 48 h of a central line placement. An estimated 250,000 bloodstream infections occur annually, which are mostly related to the presence of intravascular devices. The common pathogens are gram-positive organisms such as coagulase-negative Staphylococci, Enterococci, and *Staphylococcus aureus*, followed by gram-negative organisms, and candida species. Patients' underlying illnesses and especially chronic conditions, such as hemodialysis, malignancy, gastrointestinal tract disorders, pulmonary hypertension, and immune-compromised states such as bone marrow transplant, end-stage renal disease, diabetes mellitus, malnutrition, total parenteral nutrition (TPN), extremes of age, loss of skin integrity (burns), and prolonged hospitalization before line insertion, have a major role in increased CLABSI numbers. Other important factors include catheter type and location (femoral line has the highest, followed by internal jugular, then subclavian), conditions of insertion (emergent versus elective and use of full versus limited barrier precautions), catheter site care, and skill of the line operator.

Most cases are preventable with proper aseptic techniques, surveillance, and management strategies [9].

Management of catheter-related complications can be as simple as applying pressure to cease bleeding, but at times other advanced interventions such as chest tube placement, angiogram, endovascular repair, and open surgical procedure may be warranted (Fig. 8.9). Catheter or intravascular thrombosis is usually managed with anticoagulation and catheter removal. Based on a recent meta-analysis, the use of anticoagulant prophylaxis for prevention of catheter-related thrombosis is not recommended [11].

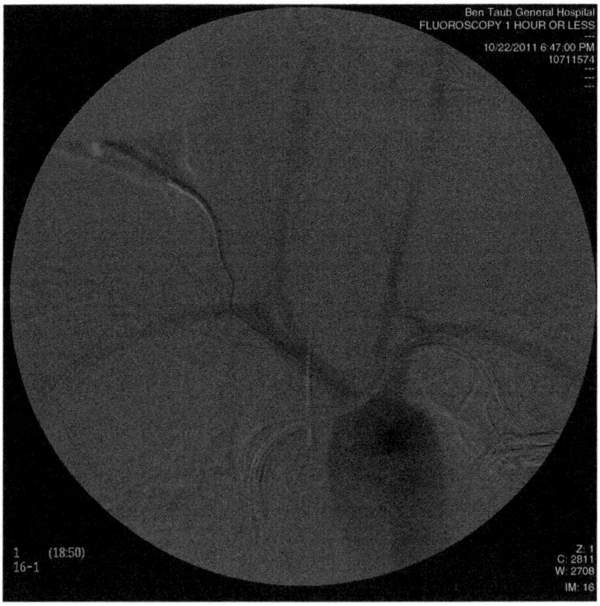

Fig. 8.9 Inadvertent catheter placement into subclavian artery during attempted cannulation of internal jugular vein. Puncture site was closed via deployment of an endovascular closure device

Catheter-related infections are usually managed with antibiotics and in most cases with catheter removal. Patients will require a line holiday and clearance of bacteremia, before a new catheter could be placed.

Attempts should be made to use the smallest catheter size possible and to limit catheter dwelling time also known as catheter-day time to reduce catheter-related complications such as thrombosis, vessel stenosis, and most importantly CLABSI cases.

As mentioned earlier, the use of periprocedural antibiotics is controversial; despite the new conflicting data, most physicians prefer to continue using antibiotics for tunneled-cuffed central lines and chest ports. The other debated subject is the use of antibiotic- or chlorhexidine-impregnated catheters. These catheters are expensive and are prone to antimicrobial resistance; therefore, their use should be limited to a specific subset of patients with compromised immunity and recurrent infections and also centers with higher catheter-related infection rates. Ethanol locks have been shown to be effective in reducing catheter-related infections and should be only used with compatible catheters [6]. Other important measures that will help reduce bloodstream infections include utilization of closed infusion systems, cleansing of the port site with 2% chlorhexidine instead of alcohol, appropriate site selection, nursing education on proper catheter management, and most importantly early catheter removal [6].

The catheter care and management instructions should be provided to patients or caregivers before they are discharged home.

The common types of central access include PICC lines, tunneled or non-tunneled central lines, and chest ports. Vascular sheaths are non-tunneled temporary central lines and are generally used for diagnostic or interventional purposes and will be discussed briefly later in this chapter (Table 8.1).

Peripherally Inserted Central Catheter (PICC)

PICC lines are the second most commonly placed venous lines following PIVs. This catheter is usually recommended for patients requiring IV therapy for up to 6 months. The arm veins including basilic, brachial, and cephalic are the common access sites in adults and older pediatric patients. The tip of the arm PICC line is usually positioned at the SVC and right atrial junction. The femoral vein is the access of choice in smaller children, and the catheter tip is positioned at IVC and right atrial junction. PICC placement usually requires no sedation in adult and older pediatric patients; however, sedation is usually needed in younger patients. These catheters come in different diameters ranging from 1.9 to 7 French and may have one to three ports.

Placement of leg PICC lines in younger patients can be performed at the bedside with ultrasound guidance. However, upper extremity or femoral access for larger pediatric patients will require fluoroscopy for proper catheter tip positioning. The complications are similar to other central lines.

Table 8.1 Common types of central venous access. CVC: central venous lines

Catheter type	Entry site	Duration of use	Advantages	Disadvantages	Comments
Non-tunneled CVCs	Percutaneously inserted into central line	Short-term	Percutaneous insertion relatively safe and inexpensive	Require local anesthesia May be inserted in the operating room or interventional radiology suite dressing required over site. Risk of infection	Account for the majority of CLABSIs. More commonly used than long-term CVCs
Tunneled CVCs	Implanted into the internal jugular, subclavian, or femoral vein	Long-term	Dressing not needed after healed	Require surgical or interventional insertion and removal May require general anesthesia Increased cost	Lower rate of infection than non-tunneled CVCs Cuff is a stabilizing component and also inhibits migration of organisms into catheter tract
Implantable ports	Inserted in the internal jugular or subclavian vein. Tunneled beneath the skin; subcutaneous port accessed with a non-coring needle	Long-term	Improved body image (low visibility of port). Patient comfort. Local catheter site care and dressing not needed when not in use	Require surgical or interventional insertion and removal May require general anesthesia increased cost	Lowest risk of CLABSI
Peripherally inserted central catheter	Inserted percutaneously into the basilic, brachial, or cephalic vein and enters the superior vena cava, or the saphenous, popliteal, or femoral vein and enters the inferior vena cava	Usually short-term to intermediate	Ease of insertion Could be performed at the bedside relatively inexpensive and safe	Can be difficult to position in central vein potential for occlusion	Lower rate of infection than non-tunneled CVCs

Central Venous Catheters

(a) *Non-tunneled Central Lines*

These temporary lines are used in patients in need for a central access up to 3 weeks. These catheters may have up to five ports and are usually placed in the internal jugular or femoral veins for emergent or nonemergent large volume IV therapy and resuscitation, central venous pressure monitoring, hemodialysis, ECMO, and stem cell retrieval. They usually have the highest.

CLABSI rates among other central lines. Vascular sheaths are a different type of temporary non-tunneled catheters and are mainly used for diagnostic imaging studies and interventional procedures. These catheters are available in different lengths and diameters ranging from 3 to 24 French. The side port of the sheath enables blood draw, administration of IV fluids, and also contrast injection for diagnostic studies. The sheaths are usually removed after completion of the imaging study or procedure. These temporary lines should always be placed using an aseptic technique either with or without image guidance. The complications are similar to other arterial or venous central lines (Fig. 8.10).

(b) *Tunneled Catheters*

Tunneled lines are indicated for patients who require frequent long-term IV access. These catheters can be either uncuffed or cuffed. The Dacron cuff is mainly intended to stabilize the catheter but also helps to prevent spread of infection and bleeding along the tract. The initial venous access is similar to other central lines, but the catheter is tunneled from a skin insertion site (usually 5–7 cm away from the venous access site) to the venotomy site, and the tip is positioned in the right atrium. At the end the venotomy site is closed, and the catheter is secured to the skin. The interal jugular and subclavian veins are the most common access sites. The catheter is placed in the tunnel, which is created in the upper chest from the skin insertion site to the venotomy site. These lines are usually available in single or double lumens with similar indications of use as the non-tunneled catheters.

(c) *Ports*

Ports, also known as Port-a-Cath or Infuse-a-Port, are indicated for long-term intermittent IV access. They consist of two parts: a reservoir and a catheter which attaches to the reservoir hub. The reservoir is implanted within a subcutaneous pocket. It can be single or double chambered and is usually made of a titanium or plastic base with a silicone dome. The dome is accessed percutaneously for intermittent IV infusion. The catheter is connected to the reservoir hub and tunneled under the skin from the subcutaneous pocket to the venotomy site, and the tip is positioned in the right atrium. Upon completion of the procedure, there are no exposed components. The port is accessed percutaneously after identification of the silicone dome by palpation. A non-coring needle, such as a Huber needle, is passed percutaneously through the dome and into the reservoir. The most common venous access site for ports is the internal jugular vein, with placement of the subcutaneous pocket in the upper chest (or upper abdomen in some pediatric cases). Arm ports have fallen out of favor due to complications such as catheter

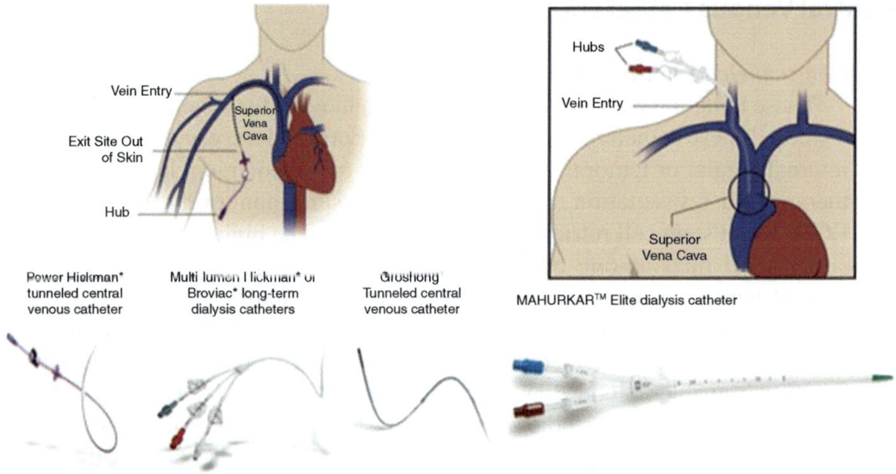

Fig. 8.10 Tunneled and non-tunneled central lines

fracture and adhesions at the port pocket. The primary advantages of ports, compared to other central lines, include lower infection rates and allowance of the patient to bathe or swim after the skin incision has healed. Aside from the aforementioned complications of all central lines, the ports are also prone to pocket infection, wound dehiscence, reservoir extrusion, and port malfunction. Port pocket infections are usually managed with oral or IV antibiotics first but may eventually necessitate removal if antibiotic therapy fails. The most common culprits for port malfunction are thrombosis and formation of fibrin sheath around the catheter tip. Other possibilities include catheter fracture, detachment of the catheter from the reservoir hub, catheter migration, and at times the catheter tip position abutting the vessel wall or a heart valve. An image-guided port check with contrast injection of the port under fluoroscopy can be performed to diagnose the issue. Reservoir or catheter thrombosis and fibrin sheaths can be alleviated with alteplase. Fibrin sheath stripping can also be performed by an interventional radiologist. Other issues may require port replacement (Fig. 8.11).

Decannulation

Success with decannulation begins with proper cannulation. For venous access the margin for error is quite large for decannulation. Assuring that the access has been placed in the desired compressible location and assuming normal coagulation, venous access can be aborted with relatively little consequence. However, when holding pressure, the amount of pressure applied is significantly less when compared to arterial decannulation to avoid venous thrombosis. Sufficient pressure is such that no external hemorrhage occurs. Time of compression can be

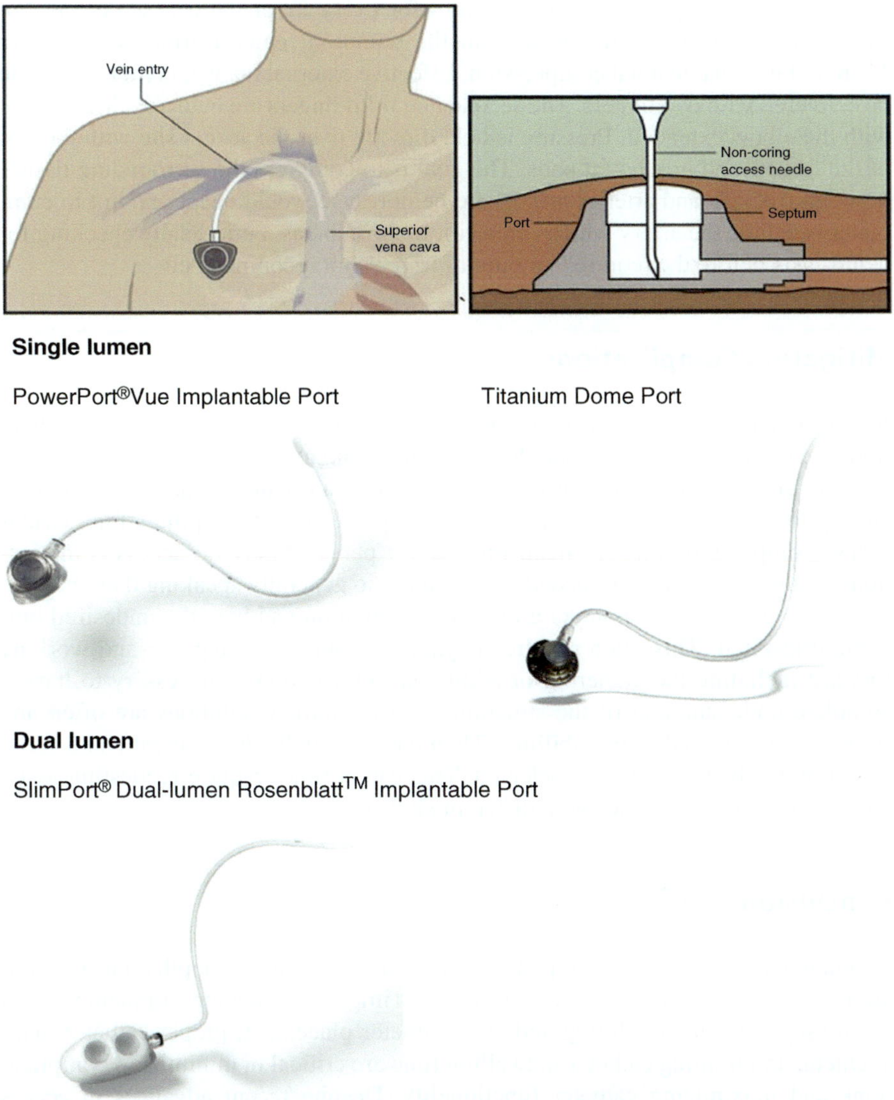

Fig. 8.11 Single- and dual-lumen Port-A-Caths

determined by evidence of thrombus formation in the blood that has escaped externally during decannulation.

In terms of arterial decannulation, the margin for error is significantly lessened, and adherence to proper technique is mandatory. External manual pressure can be successful for decannulation in properly selected sites and normal coagulation for up to 9-Fr devices. Larger devices, noncompressible locations, and coagulopathy should prompt to consider operative decannulation and repair. As a general rule, direct manual compression is held 3 min for every Fr of the access device. For example, a 5-Fr sheath removed from the common femoral artery will require 15 min of external manual compression. Effective external manual compression can be delivered with two fingers. The second and third fingers are held together straight with the elbow extended. Pressure is held directly over the access site with the tips of the fingers and not the fat pads. The goal is to compress the surrounding tissues between the skin and arteriotomy where hemorrhage would occur and not to completely occlude the artery which can result in thrombosis. Periodically checking for hemostasis before the required amount of time is not recommended.

Mitigating Complications

It is to remember that like with any invasive procedure, vascular access complications are going to occur. One should always maintain a vigilant posture before, during, and after the procedure for assessing and mitigating unintended circumstance. During this surveillance, there are three concepts to be used as pillars for vascular access complication management. First, don't panic. Rarely do access complications require rescue within seconds or minutes, so generally speaking there is time. Next, it is important to conduct a thorough evaluation and how the undesired outcome transpired. This often requires beginning again from step one and working forward including the gathering of additional information as necessary to have a complete understanding of the situation. Lastly, multiple solutions are often and should be considered as possibilities. Then based on individual patient characteristics, a more "better" option is selected. This can at times require requesting assistance from other specialties with different skill sets.

Conclusion

Vascular access is the vital component of modern medicine. In-depth clinical evaluation is essential for proper device selection and improved outcomes. Implementation of an aseptic technique during and after catheter placement, proper catheter management, and limiting catheter indwelling time are critical in minimizing complications and maximizing catheter functionality. Despite recent advances in access technique, development of newer medical devices, and utilization of image guidance, major complications such as infection and thrombosis still do occur. Perhaps the best way to ensure clinical success when obtaining vascular access is to observe the following mantra, "Right patient, right line, and right time."

References

1. Dudrick SJ. History of vascular access. J Parenter Enteral Nutr. 2006;30(1, Suppl):S47–56.

2. Rivera AM, Strauss KW, van Zundert A, Mortier E. The history of peripheral intravenous catheters: how little plastic tubes revolutionized medicine. Acta Anaesthesiol Belg. 2005;56:271–82.
3. Bahl A, Karabon P, Chu D. Comparison of venous thrombosis complications in midlines versus peripherally inserted central catheters: are midlines the safer option? Clin Appl Thromb Hemost. 2019;25:1076029619839150. https://doi.org/10.1177/1076029619839150.
4. Seto AH, Abu-Fadel MS, Sparling JM, et al. Real-time ultrasound guidance facilitates femoral arterial access and reduces vascular complications: FAUST (Femoral Arterial Access With Ultrasound Trial). JACC Cardiovasc Interv. 2010;3:751–8. https://doi.org/10.1016/j.jcin.2010.04.015.
5. Kornbau C, Lee KC, Hughes GD, Firstenberg MS. Central line complications. Int J Crit Illn Inj Sci. 2015;5(3):170–8. https://doi.org/10.4103/2229-5151.164940.
6. Chehab MA, et al. Adult and pediatric antibiotic prophylaxis during vascular and IR procedures: a Society of Interventional Radiology Practice Parameter Update Endorsed by the Cardiovascular and Interventional Radiological Society of Europe and the Canadian Association for Interventional Radiology. J Vasc Interv Radiol. 2018;29(11):1483–1501.e2.
7. Adams DZ, et al. The midline catheter: a clinical review. J Emerg Med. 2016;51(3):252–8.
8. Practice guidelines for central venous access 2020: an updated report by the American Society of Anesthesiologists Task Force on Central Venous Access. Anesthesiology. 2020;132(1):8–43. https://doi.org/10.1097/ALN.0000000000002864.
9. Haddadin Y, Regunath H. Central line associated blood stream infections (CLABSI) [Updated 2019 Dec 22]. In: StatPearls [Internet]. Treasure Island: StatPearls Publishing; 2020. Available from: https://www.ncbi.nlm.nih.gov/books/NBK430891/.
10. Brass P, Hellmich M, Kolodziej L, Schick G, Smith AF. Ultrasound guidance versus anatomical landmarks for subclavian or femoral vein catheterization. Cochrane Database Syst Rev. 2015;1(1):CD011447. https://doi.org/10.1002/14651858.CD011447.
11. Smith RN, Nolan JP. Central venous catheters. BMJ. 2013;347:f6570. https://doi.org/10.1136/bmj.f6570.
12. Alexandrou E, et al. International prevalence of the use of peripheral intravenous catheters. J Hosp Med. 2015;10(8):530–3.
13. Franco-Sadud R, Schnobrich D, Mathews BK, Candotti C, Abdel-Ghani S, Perez MG, Rodgers SC, Mader MJ, Haro EK, Dancel R, Cho J, Grikis L, Lucas BP, SHM POCUS Task Force, Soni NJ. Recommendations on the use of ultrasound guidance for central and peripheral vascular access in adults: a position statement of the Society of Hospital Medicine. Published Online Only September 6, 2019. https://doi.org/10.12788/jhm.3287.
14. Patel IJ, et al. Society of Interventional Radiology consensus guidelines for the periprocedural management of thrombotic and bleeding risk in patients undergoing percutaneous image-guided interventions—part II: recommendations. J Vasc Interv Radiol. 2019;30(8):1168–1184.e1.
15. Scheer B, Perel A, Pfeiffer UJ. Clinical review: complications and risk factors of peripheral arterial catheters used for haemodynamic monitoring in anaesthesia and intensive care medicine. Crit Care. 2002;6(3):199–204.
16. Karakitsos D, Labropoulos N, De Groot E, Patrianakos AP, Kouraklis G, Poularas J, Samonis G, Tsoutsos DA, Konstadoulakis MM, Karabinis A. Real-time ultrasound-guided catheterisation of the internal jugular vein: a prospective comparison with the landmark technique in critical care patients. Crit Care. 2006;10(6):R162.
17. Hind D, Calvert N, McWilliams R, Davidson A, Paisley S, Beverley C, Thomas S. Ultrasonic locating devices for central venous cannulation: meta-analysis. BMJ. 2003;327(7411):361.
18. Verghese ST, McGill WA, Patel RI, Sell JE, Midgley FM, Ruttimann UE. Ultrasound-guided internal jugular venous cannulation in infants: a prospective comparison with the traditional palpation method. Anesthesiology. 1999;91(1):71–7.
19. Leyvi G, Taylor DG, Reith E, Wasnick JD. Utility of ultrasound-guided central venous cannulation in pediatric surgical patients: a clinical series. Paediatr Anaesth. 2005;15(11):953–8.

20. Tercan F, Oguzkurt L, Ozkan U, Eker HE. Comparison of ultrasonography-guided central venous catheterization between adult and pediatric populations. Cardiovasc Intervent Radiol. 2008;31(3):575–80. Epub 2008 Mar 11.
21. Gregg SC, Murthi SB, Sisley AC, Stein DM, Scalea TM. Ultrasound-guided peripheral intravenous access in the intensive care unit. J Crit Care. 2010;25(3):514–9. Epub 2009 Oct 15.
22. Bhananker SM, Liau DW, Kooner PK, Posner KL, Caplan RA, Domino KB. Liability related to peripheral venous and arterial catheterization: a closed claims analysis. Anesth Analg. 2009;109(1):124–9. Epub 2009 Apr 17.
23. Levin PD, Sheinin O, Gozal Y. Use of ultrasound guidance in the insertion of radial artery catheters. Crit Care Med. 2003;31(2):481–4.
24. Shiver S, Blaivas M, Lyon M. A prospective comparison of ultrasound-guided and blindly placed radial arterial catheters. Acad Emerg Med. 2006;13(12):1275–9. Epub 2006 Nov 1.
25. Schwemmer U, Arzet HA, Trautner H, Rauch S, Roewer N, Greim CA. Ultrasound-guided arterial cannulation in infants improves success rate. Eur J Anaesthesiol. 2006;23(6):476–80. Epub 2006 Mar 2.

Procedural Checklist/Situational Awareness

9

George E. Anton

Procedural Checklist/Situational Awareness

I grew up on Long Island and first flew a floatplane at age 14. Long Island has a rich aviation history: Charles Lindbergh departed on his transatlantic flight from Garden City, only10 minutes from my home. By age 19, I earned a commercial rating for land and seaplanes, but I stopped flying after my second year in medical school as I felt I could not devote the time to remain safe and current. I offer a unique perspective as I was a pilot before becoming a surgeon. I learned early on the value of planning, discipline, and critical thinking. I will explore the analogies between aviation and surgery by providing a surgeon's view from the cockpit.

I have found many similarities between piloting an aircraft and performing a surgical procedure in the operating room. I frequently tell the O.R. staff that I operate the way I used to fly. I share the "flight plan" with the surgical and anesthesia staff. There is no hierarchy, so that everyone may speak up, contribute, and maintain situational awareness. I always try to instill an atmosphere of cognitive ease, communication, and cooperation because I recognize that this will improve situational awareness.

There are two specific aviation practices that have served me well as a surgeon: (1) the value of checklists to prevent missing steps as a result of faulty memory or distraction during a complex intervention or surgical procedure and (2) the use of Crew Resource Management (CRM) a codified set of training procedures employed to improve air safety by focusing on interpersonal communication, leadership, and decision-making in the cockpit. CRM in the O.R. fosters enhanced communication and teamwork resulting in improved problem-solving and increased safety.

G. E. Anton (✉)
Department of Vascular Surgery, Cleveland Clinic, Heart, Vascular and Thoracic Institute, Mayfield Heights, OH, USA
e-mail: ANTONG@ccf.org

R. Gilani, J. L. Mills Sr. (eds.), *Vascular Complications of Surgery and Intervention*, https://doi.org/10.1007/978-3-030-86713-3_9

My First Checklist. Why I Made My Checklist and Why Every Surgeon Should Too!

I recognized early in my career that there was a way to improve ruptured abdominal aortic aneurysm (AAA) mortality figures. At that time, it became clear that the legal community was measuring time to diagnosis and time to treatment for surgical emergencies. Establishing the diagnosis of a leaking AAA can be quite challenging. I felt it would be unreasonable for an E.R. physician to absolutely clinch the diagnosis. Quite often, the E.R. physicians are busy diagnosing and treating multiple patients with complex and varied diagnoses. This task saturation can lead to delay in diagnosis and treatment. I simply wanted them to suspect the diagnosis and get the wheels in motion for surgical repair.

In 1985, I developed a ruptured aneurysm protocol for the emergency room (Fig. 9.1). This checklist was introduced to be a no-fault process thereby relieving the E.R. physician of the burden of proof. They were not reprimanded if the final diagnosis turned out to be something other than a ruptured AAA. My intention was to lower the threshold to notify a vascular surgeon and the operating room of the suspected diagnosis to better prepare all of our resources should the patient require them.

My next task was to introduce the checklist to the nursing and physician staff of all three emergency room shifts. I call this the "installation phase." The educational process included the introduction of the checklist as well as reviewing signs, symptoms, and physical findings of typical presentations as well as unusual ruptured AAA presentations. For example, a 70-year-old man presents to the E.R. complaining of unilateral testicular pain. The E.R. staff is now aware that this unusual presentation of a ruptured AAA is the result of compression of the ilioinguinal nerve or the genitofemoral nerve as it courses along the psoas muscle.

The next part of this educational process is what I call the "maintenance phase." The plan was to review our performance and outcomes at six-month intervals. I would review the clinical presentations as a form of scenario-based learning. This was particularly important to sustain a high level of interest as well as introduce the concept to newly hired staff, nurses, and physicians as there is always some element of staff turnover. This resulted in a surgical mortality rate of 25% matched against the national average mortality rate of 50% for ruptured AAAs. The improved outcome was the result of a combination of a culture shift, having a local Champion and an educational process. I also credit my incredibly talented and dedicated O.R. team and great instruments.

Successful Checklist Implementation

Peter Pronovost et al. [1] reported a dramatic and sustained reduction in catheter-related bloodstream infections while employing a checklist. In addition to the checklist, the highly motivated teams actively improved the safety culture when physicians and nurses were designated as team leaders. A strong educational

COMMUNITY HOSPITAL QUALITY MANAGEMENT SERVICES

EMERGENCY DEPARTMENT

1985 Aneurysm/ TQI Monitoring Tool

Name__________________ **#**_____________ **Admin Date**_________ **Time to OR**________

Arrival Time_________ **Time vascular surgeon notified or time diagnosis made**_________

The following are ordered or per protocol

OBTAIN BLOOD FOR:	**YES**	**NO**	**NA**
1. CBC	____	____	____
2. SMA-7, SMA-12	____	____	____
3. Amylase	____	____	____
4. PT, PTT, Platelets	____	____	____
5. Type and Cross Match for 8 units of PRBC's, 8 FFP, 20 Platelets	____	____	____
6. ABG after-ALine	____	____	____
OBTAIN:			
1. Chest X Ray	____	____	____
2. KUB	____	____	____
3. Cross Table KUB	____	____	____
4. EKG	____	____	____
5. Previous Medical Records	____	____	____
NOTIFY:			
1. Notify attending physician for referral	____	____	____
2. If no response within 5 minutes, notify Vascular surgeon on call	____	____	____
3. If High probability or if vascular instability, Notify anesthesia and operating room	____	____	____
OTHER:			
1. Insert large bore (14, 16 or 18 gauge) IV access x 2. Hang IV's with blood tubing & extension tubing.	____	____	____
2. Assess timing for central venous placement with Cordis introducer.	____	____	____
3. Monitor vital signs and cardiac status	____	____	____
4. Prepare for surgery per hospital policy			
a. Complete pre-op check list	____	____	____
b. Notify Nursing Supervisor	____	____	____
c. Notify family	____	____	____
6. Administer antibiotic per surgeon's order	____	____	____
7. Insert foley catheter	____	____	____

Signature of reviewer____ Date_________

Fig. 9.1 1985 Community Hospital AAA Checklist Protocol

process was established so that all clinicians would fully understand and appreciate the importance of sterile technique and infection control. The ultimate success was due to more than just a checklist; it required a change to organizational culture.

Haynes et al. [2] also recognized that a surgical safety checklist dramatically reduced surgical morbidity and mortality in a global population. They also reported that implementation of the checklist as well as associated culture changes were responsible for the outcome. They understood the importance of establishing high functioning teams that would introduce the checklist to the operating room staff by providing an educational process that included lectures, written materials, and direct guidance from the designated study team. In essence, this was a multifactorial process requiring a culture shift, identifying local champions/leaders, as well as offering structured educational and training opportunities.

The challenge now is how to make a checklist succeed beyond the surgical environment by improving patient safety and outcome in various hospital and outpatient settings. Haynes et al. [2], Harvard School of Public Health [3], Anthes [5], White [6], Clay-Williams and Collogan [7], and Treadwill et al. [4] report the challenges of implementing a checklist and ultimately realizing the perceived benefits of improved surgical morbidity and mortality. Concerns are many, such as creating and implementing the checklist, developing institutional/local leadership, improving surgeon and staff engagement, developing a culture shift, and providing sustained educational and training opportunities. Organizations must also recognize the toxic effect of top-down management schemes and steep hierarchical cultures within the operating room as they can disengage the staff and prevent successful completion of the surgical safety checklist.

A checklist alone will fail to produce a meaningful and sustained impact in aviation or medicine without a significant culture shift, commitment to education and training, as well as establishing hands-on local leadership. Giving a checklist to a dysfunctional team is doomed to failure.

Cultural Shift

Leadership, education, and culture are the three most important areas of direct and meaningful individual impact. You don't need to have a position of authority or a title to become a leader in any organization; the goal is to create a work environment that empowers an individual in any role to lead from the top, middle, or bottom of an organization. As a leader, one needs to read and present information to the staff. I recognized early on the importance of organizational behavior and leadership in the workplace and how it can have a direct impact on staff and patient safety. As a result, I developed a series of presentations that I give to hospital staff, physicians, and medical students because a good leader shares information and knowledge. The leader sets the tone in the operating room and inspires others to become leaders.

We know that typical operating room culture has been identified as one of the barriers to successful implementation of a surgical checklist. However, little attention has been given as to how that culture can be improved. What are the mechanisms that we can employ to break through those barriers? With that in mind, I will review some of the basic concepts with recommended references to support a culture of empathy, empowerment, engagement, and reduction of stress.

Paul Zak [10] delineates the management behaviors that foster employee engagement in *The Neuroscience of Trust.* His neuroscience research demonstrates the importance of increased levels of oxytocin, a neurochemical that increases a person's empathy and allows them to develop strong bonds of trust and friendship. It is important to point out that cortisol is a potent oxytocin inhibitor. Therefore, commitment to decreasing stress in the operating room produces cognitive ease and improves social skills and decision-making ability.

In *The Culture Code*, Daniel Coyle [8] discusses the importance creating a culture where everyone feels safe and connected allowing the staff to think and act spontaneously without intimidation or humiliation. He points out that trust within an organization is preceded by vulnerability. Basically, if a surgeon demonstrates his or her vulnerability by requesting the operating room staff to help with a complex procedure, they will respond with concern and empathy. Such an approach builds trust within the organization.

In *Leaders Eat Last*, Simon Sinek [9] emphasizes the importance of empathy in the workplace. He points out that strong leaders provide a Circle of Safety so that people feel safe, valued, and cared for. This type of protection and support from a surgeon is invaluable in the operating room. I treat my operating room and office staff as my children. I provide a Circle of Safety by committing to my operating room and office staff's education, development, and psychological safety. I encourage curiosity and critical thinking with non- judgmental open dialogue. I will not allow them to bullied or marginalized. I offer protection from above as an A-10 Warthog providing close air support to troops on the ground.

Turn the Ship Around by Capt. L. David Marquet [11] is the consummate book on leadership with the goal of achieving excellence within the organization and not just simply perform tasks such as checking the boxes in a checklist to avoid errors. He describes the virtues of transitioning from Top-Down/Leader-Follower management scheme to Bottom-Up/Leader-Leader model. Under his command, every member of the crew became a teacher and a leader with shared goals and increased responsibility for their actions. For example, seasoned O.R. staff will teach and develop new staff to assume greater responsibilities such as performing checklist with confidence.

Gallup [12] State of the Global Workplace report provides a wealth of information regarding employee development and engagement. Engaged workers were found to have a higher degree of situational awareness contributing to greater safety. As a result, highly engaged business models realized 70% fewer safety incidents and 58% fewer patient safety incidents. These findings underscore the significance of improving employee engagement as it has a direct impact on safety in the workplace.

Planning, Staffing, and Checklist

Empowered employees provide the best cultural environment for a checklist to succeed, but a checklist alone cannot substitute for appropriate planning and communication on behalf of the surgeon. The surgical checklist should not become the victim of poor planning and communication by the surgeon. No surgeon should arrive at the "Time Out Step" to discover that a member of the surgical team is not familiar with the procedure or that you don't have the appropriate device. Appropriate planning includes assigning surgical staff to the room the day before the procedure. This allows everyone advanced opportunity to review the inventory as well as possible contingency plans. For example, the surgical team can prepare to convert from an endovascular procedure to an open surgical procedure. Strong planning allows the staff to approach the day with a high level of confidence and cognitive ease, resulting in elevated feelings of competence and genuine engagement in the operating room. In a properly planned environment, the checklist will not become a distraction, thereby greatly minimizing any frustration or disruption during the three-phase checklist process.

Most hospitals employ a version of the World Health Organization, *WHO Surgical Safety Checklist* [13]. The three phases of the WHO surgical checklist are as follows: Sign In (before induction of anesthesia), Time Out (before skin incision), and Sign Out (before patient leaves the operating room). The checklist may be modified to accommodate local needs of a particular specialty; however, eliminating steps is strongly discouraged. Additional checklists, either verbal or written, can be added at important junctures during a complex procedure. The additional checklist can be introduced with a formal Time Out. This additional pause will allow everyone to recalibrate and remain focused on the overall plan.

The checklist is used to prevent errors of omission and reduce adverse events by compensating for potential limits of human memory and attention. In addition, every checklist should be complemented with safe practice habits. I will next take you into the operating room and review important concepts such as communication, redundancy, closed loop communication, and situational awareness.

Entering the Operating Room

Upon entering the operating room, as a former pilot, I perform a visual "preflight" walk around inspection as you would for an aircraft. In aviation, a preflight assessment of the aircraft is performed to mitigate potential flight hazards and this assessment of the operating room mitigates surgical hazards. I assess ambient room temperature and make adjustments accordingly. I check that the circulating nurse has written the first names and functions of the all O.R. staff on the whiteboard. I inspect the overhead surgical lights to ensure that they are functioning and that they do not have dust bunnies as big as house cats. The trash bin and the laundry bin are displaced far from the table of open instruments so as not to contaminate them. I review the surgical instruments, suture material, and potential devices to be employed during the case with the scrub nurse/tech. I then round everybody up, and sometimes this can be like herding cats, but it is an opportunity to introduce each other and share the "flight plan." In my "flight plan," I review pertinent preoperative imaging, state my intentions, and discuss possible contingency plans. It is important that this is an open discussion with inquiries, not a set of directives in order to promote professional discipline but without harmful hierarchy. My goal is always to teach people how to think about what to think.

Ultimately, this systematic review enables everyone to know what I am thinking, what are my intentions and expected outcome. This creates redundancy in the operating room that allows staff to become my backup systems should I forget a step in this complex process. In engineering, redundancy is the duplication of critical components or functions of the system with the intention of increasing reliability; redundancy is an essential component of creating a highly reliable organizational culture in the operating room.

Redundancy provides backup or failsafe opportunities to improve actual system performance to enhance safety and flying. For example, most commercial aircraft have up to three redundant hydraulic systems that allow critical components such as control surfaces and landing gear to function. Should one hydraulic system fail, a second or third one will take over. In the same manner, each member of an informed surgical *team* increases reliability.

At this point, I feel comfortable and confident to perform the Sign In phase of the checklist. As a surgeon and leader, I set the tone. My presence in the operating room sends a message to the staff that this patient is important to me. I lead the Sign In with the circulating nurse at my side as she/he will be involved in the Time Out and Sign Out portions of the checklist. This practice habit demonstrates my interest and support in their development and serves to build their confidence. It is no different than attending your child's sporting event or music recital. You can just feel the oxytocin levels rise.

After the induction phase of anesthesia, I review the positioning and surgical prep of the patient. I make a point of reviewing sterile technique and the surgical service assistants enjoy being a part of it and take pride in teaching their cohorts. In a Leader-Leader management model, everyone teaches and learns from each other (Marquet 2012).

The Time Out phase is now performed with everybody's undivided attention. At this point, I extend the Time Out to review what I call "table manners." I remind everyone that in more than four decades in the operating room, I have not seen a surgical case worth getting stabbed for. I review how to pass instruments without harm, economy of motion as well as designated safe and danger zones. Some people prefer to pass scalpels on a designated sterile tray. Whatever people's preferences are, it is important to establish the ground rules so as to prevent injury.

Recall that additional timeouts and additional checklists can be employed during any complex procedure. For example, during the course of a carotid endarterectomy, I routinely employ a timeout and verbal checklist prior to clamping and performing the arteriotomy for shunt placement. This ensures that all the appropriate instruments and the shunt are readily available.

Closed loop communication is essential to my leadership in the operating room. Blood pressure is controlled and heparin will be requested in the form of a closed loop communication. For example, I state "please give 7500 units of heparin and let me know when it has been in for three minutes.". The anesthesia personnel will definitively agree to give the heparin and reaffirm the action in 3 minutes time. This completes the Sender–Receiver–Sender communication loop. There is no ambiguity and the request was verbalized in a manner that allows everyone to be aware of the proposed course of action.

Finally, the Sign Out phase can be initiated before the surgeon leaves the operating room. Importantly, the transfer "handoff" of the patient with pertinent clinical information will be directly communicated to the next hospital team accepting the patient transfer. At this point, the designated checklist leader will complete the documentation process with complete confidence.

Several years ago, I entered a procedure room performing my customary "pre-flight" walk around inspection at which point the nurse exclaimed "Oh, situational awareness." I spun around quickly and joyfully inquired how she became familiar with that phrase. She told me that she was a flight nurse on a helicopter and that they were taught to look out the windows of the helicopter to report other aircraft traffic or obstacles that may become a threat to their flight path. For her, it was a matter of self-preservation. However, she fully understood the implications as it relates to an operating room environment.

Situational awareness is fully and comprehensively understanding one's surroundings, environment, and situation by observation and remaining vigilant to any changes. Ultimately, extracting and processing information permits a surgical team to anticipate future trends or events, potentially interrupting a trend or cascade of events that could result in patient harm. Some people have a natural gift for situational awareness, but it can be learned and developed.

Loss of situational awareness may occur during periods of high workload, multitasking, distractions, periods of stress, and interactions with computers/checklists (Fig. 9.2).

NO LONGER THINKING AHEAD OF THE AIRPLANE

"The wise airman uses his superior judgment in order to avoid situations that would require the use of his superior skills"
(Frank Borman, January 8 2008)

Case Scenarios

Did you Give the Heparin?

During the course of a lower extremity angiogram/angioplasty contralateral common femoral access with placement of a sheath is often employed. The sheath surface is thrombogenic and partially occludes some of the native vessels. Therefore, heparin is infused to prevent thromboembolic complications during the course of the procedure. See the following diagram.

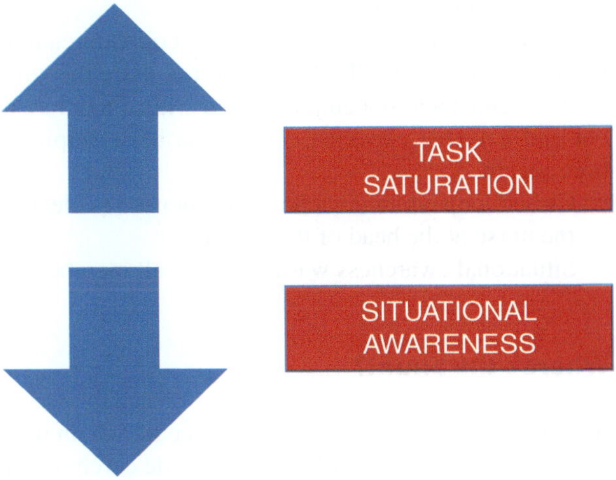

Fig. 9.2 Situational awareness compromised

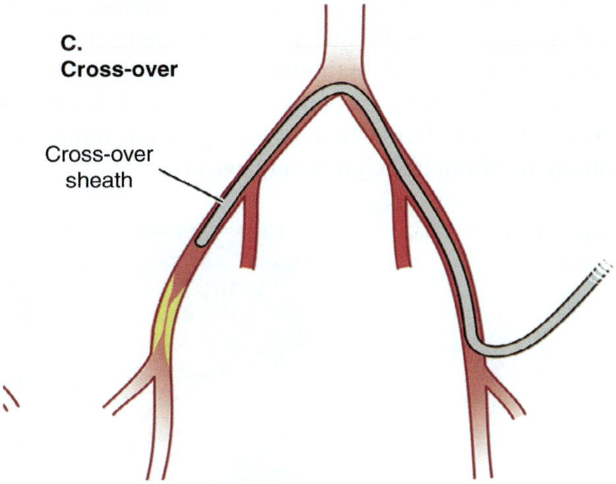

Fig. 9.3 Crossover aortogram

An elderly diabetic male presented with right lower extremity limb-threatening ischemia with angiographic evidence of right superficial femoral artery stenosis and single vessel runoff. The plan was to perform right superficial femoral artery angioplasty. Access was performed via the contralateral common femoral artery. A crossover sheath was placed, and a technically straightforward angioplasty was performed (Fig. 9.3).

Completion angiography revealed thrombus in the runoff vessel. The accomplished vascular surgeon immediately asked the nurse providing conscious monitored sedation if she had given the heparin. She replied that she did not hear the request. They were separated by a barrier drape. At that point, he had asked the other staff participating in the procedure if they had heard his request. They had heard him but the nurse above the barrier drape did not. The result was a time-consuming, complex, and costly additional limb salvage procedure.

Contributing Factors

There was a deficiency in planning and communication between the surgeon and the nurse providing the sedation. He did not share the "flight plan."

A checklist was not employed at a critical juncture during the procedure. A time-out and a verbal checklist could have been employed prior to placing the large bore sheath.

Closed loop communication was not used to clearly request the heparin be given by the nurse at the head of the O.R. table.

Situational awareness was absent for all members of the surgical team.

Where's the Shunt?

It is common practice that during the course of an open carotid endarterectomy, an intraluminal shunt is employed to provide cerebral perfusion. The following intraoperative photographs outline a typical surgical sequence (Figs. 9.4, 9.5, and 9.6).

An elderly woman was scheduled to undergo an elective carotid endarterectomy. The patient was heparinized. The common, internal and external carotid arteries were clamped and a longitudinal arteriotomy was made. The surgeon then asked for the shunt. No shunt was on the mayo stand. Further search revealed that no shunt was to be found anywhere in the operating room. The patient suffered a massive stroke resulting in a significant lawsuit.

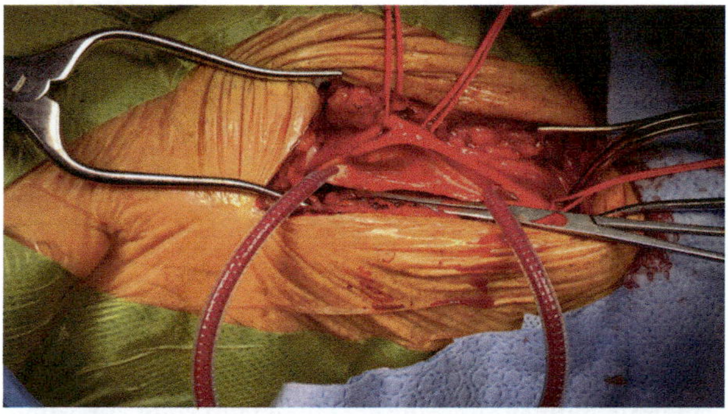

Fig. 9.4 Intraluminal shunt

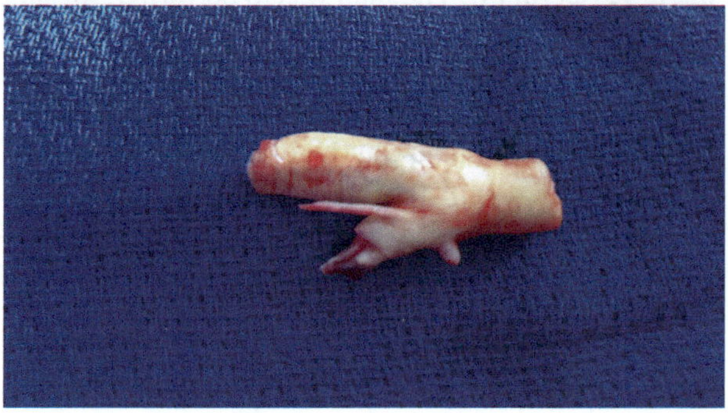

Fig. 9.5 Specimen

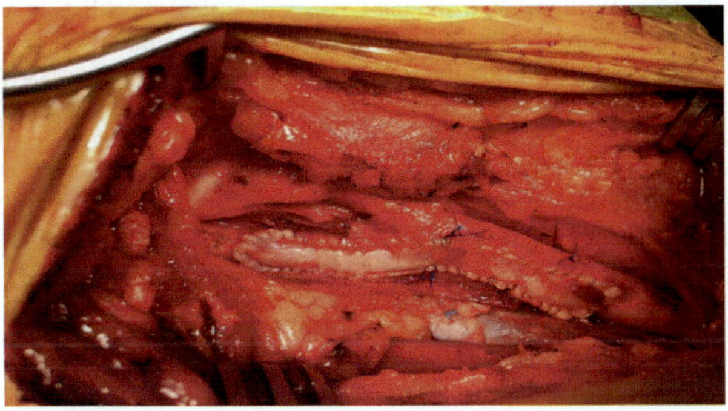

Fig. 9.6 Completion carotid endarterectomy with saphenous vein patch angioplasty

Contributing Factors

There was a deficiency in planning and communication. The surgeon did not share the "flight plan" with the surgical staff.

A timeout and checklist were not employed at a critical juncture during the procedure, both of which should have occurred prior to clamping and opening the vessel.

Situational awareness was absent among the entire operating room staff as no one anticipated the use of an intraluminal shunt.

Conclusion

Surgical safety checklists, when used correctly, have been an important tool employed to improve safety by ensuring that required actions are performed in the proper sequence and without omission. Without the appropriate institutional foundation and commitment, the checklist will simply be at the mercy of an unruly crowd. Checklists promote teamwork and communication between surgical and anesthesia staff with the additional benefit of heightened situational awareness. Successful checklist implementation can be accomplished through effective and sustained cultural improvement, dedicated leadership and education.

References

1. Pronovost P, et al. An intervention to decrease catheter-related bloodstream infections in the ICU. N Engl J Med. 2006;355:2725–32.
2. Haynes AB, et al. A surgical safety checklist to reduce morbidity and mortality in a global population. N Engl J Med. 2009;360:491–9.
3. Harvard School of Public Health. Surgical safety checklist drops deaths and complication by more than a third. Science Daily, January 15, 2009.
4. Treadwill JR, Lucas S, Tsou AY. Surgical checklists: a systematic review of impacts and implementation. The 2019 Healthcare Quality and Safety Conference, 2019.
5. Anthes E. The trouble with checklists. Nature. 2015;523(7562):561.
6. White J. Checklists improve outcomes for surgery. Healthcare Treatment & Outcomes, Feb 4, 2016.

7. Clay-Williams R, Collogan L. Back to basics: checklists in aviation and healthcare. The 2019 Healthcare Quality & Safety Conference, November 6–7, 2019.
8. Coyle D. The culture code-the secrets of highly successful groups. Bantam Books; 2018. ISBN 9780804176989.
9. Sinek S. Leaders eat last: why some teams pull together and others don't. Penguin Books; 2014.ISBN 978-1-59184-532-4.
10. Zak PJ. The neuroscience of trust. Harv Bus Rev. 2017;95(1):84–90.
11. Marquet LD. Turn the ship around!: a true story of turning followers into leaders. Penguin; 2012. ISBN 978-1-59184-640-6.
12. Gallup. State of the global workplace. Gallup Press; 2017.
13. World Alliance For Patient Safety. Implementation manual surgical safety checklist. 1st ed; 2016. p. 1–20.

Management of Iatrogenic Abdominal Vascular Injuries

10

Christopher R. Ramos and Ravi R. Rajani

Introduction

Iatrogenic intra-abdominal vascular injuries remain thankfully rare. Historically, they occurred during large, open intra-abdominal operations performed by non-vascular specialists. Laparoscopic and robotic-assisted surgeries have increased in use and are associated with intra-abdominal vascular injuries at a rate as low as 0.2–0.5/1000 cases [2]. Treatment of vascular injury following minimally invasive surgery carries special consideration, as such complications may be associated with a higher mortality rate than during open surgery. We will describe risk factors that lead to vascular injury and indicated interventions required for resuscitation and appropriate surgical management. Once an injury has occurred, prompt recognition and management remain the most important means of reducing patient morbidity and mortality.

Incidence

The global incidence of iatrogenic abdominal vascular trauma is difficult to determine. Specialty reports from gynecology, urology, orthopedics, spine, and general surgery literature [2, 11, 13, 29] suggest that the overall incidence is much less than 1 in every 1000 cases. There is no suggestion that any specific operation is associated with a significantly higher rate of injury, nor are there any data to suggest defined risk factors for iatrogenic vascular trauma. Iatrogenic abdominal vascular trauma can be divided into early and delayed presentations. Early presentation tends to be dramatic, hemorrhagic, and promptly recognized. Late presentations,

C. R. Ramos (✉) · R. R. Rajani
Division of Vascular and Endovascular Surgery, Emory University School of Medicine, Atlanta, GA, USA
e-mail: Christopher.R.Ramos@emory.edu

R. Gilani, J. L. Mills Sr. (eds.), *Vascular Complications of Surgery and Intervention*, https://doi.org/10.1007/978-3-030-86713-3_10

however, tend to be insidious in onset, can often be thrombotic, and are often not identified until later. Understandably, late presentations are rarely included in any calculation determining the total incidence of iatrogenic abdominal vascular trauma.

In the modern era, much of the available literature focuses on the risk of vascular trauma during laparoscopic surgery and how to best mitigate that risk. Vascular injury during laparoscopy leading to significant intra-abdominal hemorrhage is one of its most feared complications. The overall incidence in one large series was approximately 1 in 2500 [22] with an associated mortality as high as 23%. A review of 75 patients reported to have sustained vascular injury during initial entry revealed that 25% of the injuries involved the aorta and 21% the common iliac arteries. Vena cava injuries occurred in 11% and were associated with arterial injuries [28].

A review of 31 cases, consisting primarily of trocar injuries, demonstrated that 26/31 (83.8%) of injuries occur on the patient's right side [3]. The iliac artery was the most commonly injured vessel on the right side, and the iliac vein was the most commonly injured on the left. There were 7/31 (22.6%) fatalities, all from venous injuries involving the right or left side common/external iliac veins or hypogastric veins.

Iatrogenic vascular trauma can also occur during placement of large bore sheaths by endovascular specialists while performing endovascular aortic repair, transcatheter valve therapy, and other emerging techniques. Thankfully, through-and-through wire access is usually available, allowing for prompt treatment with endovascular techniques. The estimated incidence of such injuries is 0.5–5% [7, 12, 16, 32], and a much smaller number require open vascular repair as outlined below.

Injury Recognition

Intra-operatively identified iatrogenic vascular trauma is usually hemorrhagic as opposed to thrombotic and is often obvious. Iatrogenic vascular injuries during minimally invasive approaches require rapid recognition for immediate management as delay may lead to profound hemorrhage and death. Vascular injuries may be recognized if there is blood return into the Veress needle, fresh blood seen in the abdominal cavity at entry, blood leaking around a port site, or visualization of a rapidly expanding retroperitoneal hematoma. Sometimes the injury is not immediately seen on entry, or the gaseous pressure initially tamponades the injury. A small intraoperative injury may occur and post-operatively lead to a retroperitoneal hematoma and present later with anemia. In severe cases, retroperitoneal hematoma may lead to extensive bruising of the flank 24–48 hours later, known as Grey–Turner sign[22].

While late presentation of iatrogenic vascular trauma may be hemorrhagic (such as a ruptured pseudoaneurysm), it is more often thrombotic. Injuries during spine surgery, in particular, may not be readily identified at the index operation [11, 17]. This is due to a lack of a "bleeding space" around the damaged vessel, particularly following with posterior approaches to the spine. Such injuries may be identified incidentally years later or may cause acute hemorrhage. An unrecognized iatrogenic arteriovenous fistula represents a special case that may present in delayed fashion with signs and symptoms of high-output cardiac failure [17].

Risk Factors

No specific operation or surgical specialty is associated with an increased rate of iatrogenic vascular trauma. Distortions of normal vascular anatomy certainly place the patient at increased risk of iatrogenic injury. Large solid malignancies, bulky perivascular lymphadenopathy, and pre-operative radiation therapy can all create unique challenges during oncologic operations [25, 26]. During spine procedures, prominent scoliosis or extensive scar during redo surgery may put the patient at increased risk [5, 15, 30].

Intra-abdominal vasculature injury can also occur during dissection using powered instruments delivering thermal energy [8, 19, 27]. Understanding the specific instrument used and its limitations are essential to prevent injury. Electrosurgery during minimally invasive procedures may lead to thermal injury of vascular structures through lateral thermal spread with immediate or delayed rupture of a vessel wall. Providing enough tension on structures to elevate them off of nearby vessels is key to decrease risk of thermal spread to major vasculature.

Injury during laparoscopic surgery deserves special attention, as the literature assessing risk for vascular trauma in this setting is substantial. The use of a Veress entry seems to be associated with an increased risk of vascular trauma when compared with other options [22]. If a Veress technique is to be used, the safest point of entry seems to be at Palmer's point in the left upper quadrant. This avoids the dangers of vascular injury to the infrarenal aorta, vena cava, and iliac vessels. Once the abdomen is insufflated, a secondary port site can be placed under direct visualization. Regarding non-Veress options, optical trocar insertion appears to be associated with a lower risk of vascular injuries when compared with the open Hasson technique in a large randomized trial [31].

Body habitus may play an important role in increasing the risk of iatrogenic vascular trauma. The distance between the skin and the retroperitoneal vessels at the umbilicus is directly proportional to the body mass index (BMI) and can be as short as 2 cm in very thin patients. This can increase up to 10 times with increasing BMI. Extreme care must be used during laparoscopic entry in all patients, particularly those with low BMI. In thin patients, inserting instruments at a 45° angle aiming caudad in a flat supine position can reduce risk of injury to major vasculature. In obese patients, the length of instrument needed to achieve entry is longer, making a 90° entry a safe technique [1].

Table 10.1 summarizes vessels at risk with different operations and laparoscopic entry points.

Management

If a vascular injury is intra-operatively suspected, the primary surgeon should make an attempt to identify the bleeding vessel and control it if at all possible. In a stable patient with a minor injury, simple suture ligation may be all that is needed. In select cases, laparoscopic vascular repair may be an option.

Table 10.1 Vessels at risk with different access points and surgeries

Vessels at risk	
Associated surgery	*Injuries*
Umbilical port placement	Infrarenal aorta
	Common iliac arteries
	Inferior vena cava
	Common iliac veins
Palmer's point port placement	Celiac artery
	Left renal artery
Right upper quadrant port placement	Inferior vena cava
	Portal vein
	Celiac artery
	Hepatic artery
	Right renal artery
Pelvic surgery	Common iliac arteries/veins
	External iliac arteries/veins
	Internal iliac arteries/veins
Spine durgery	Aorta
	Inferior vena cava
	Common iliac arteries/veins
	External iliac arteries/veins
Endovascular surgery	Aorta
	Common iliac arteries
	External iliac arteries

For major injuries, pressure should be held and the surgeon should allow the anesthesia team to "catch up" while performing several adjunctive measures (Table 10.2). The nursing staff and anesthesia team should be made aware of the situation. Additional nursing and ancillary staff should be obtained to act as "runners." Adequate intravenous access is necessary in order to potentially deliver large amounts of blood products. A type and crossmatch for an appropriate amount of blood and plasma should be sent. If a massive transfusion protocol is available, it should be initiated. An arterial line should be placed to closely monitor the patient's hemodynamics. A vascular instrument set should be obtained and brought to the room. Rapid infusers should be brought into the room, and the cell saver should be obtained if possible. External warming agents should be employed and the room temperature should be increased to maintain the patient's temperature >36° C [18].

To ensure the best outcomes, one should seek help for major vascular injuries. Clear communication with the operative team regarding the plan of action and ongoing dialogue during the resuscitation is of utmost importance. The most effective maneuver for hemostasis is direct pressure at the site of injury, either digitally or with an instrument. If the injury is inaccessible or difficult to control the area can be packed or endovascular control with balloon tamponade could be obtained if endovascular skills and equipment are available [10]. Lead surgeons need to be aware of the overall situation unfolding around them, including the patient's

Table 10.2 Major vascular injury considerations

Major vascular injury considerations
Nursing
Call for vascular surgeon on call
Need for additional circulators/runners
Need for additional anesthesia assistance
Inform blood bank – Type and cross blood
Consider initiation of massive transfusion protocol
Obtain rapid transfusers
Consider calling for cell saver
Call for laparotomy tray, vascular instrument set
Obtain ICU bed for postoperative care
Anesthesia
Allow permissive hypotension
Ensure 2 large bore IVs or Cordis catheter
Frequent labs: ABG, coags, CBC, lactate, etc.
Keep patient euthermic, increase room temperature, Bair hugger
Consider arterial line, endotracheal intubation (if LMA), Foley catheter placement
Surgeon
If bleeding controlled with pressure, wait for help
If bleeding not controlled, obtain more proximal control
Consider packing, resuscitating, interval return to OR
Consider open abdomen – If massive transfusion, elevated peak airway pressures, bowel edema, extremis
Completion of index procedure if patient stable

hemodynamic status, arrival of blood products, appropriate instruments, equipment, and surgical support.

A controlled resuscitation is important. Permissive hypotension, allowing systolic blood pressure to run in the 80–90 mmHg range while maintaining a mean arterial pressure >60 mmHg, should be sufficient for end-organ perfusion and potentially decrease bleeding from arterial vascular injuries [4, 9]. As the patient starts to bleed and resuscitation is started with blood products and crystalloid, the patient will become coagulopathic. One should consider a 1:1:1 ratio of products transfused (1 unit PRBC for every 1 unit of plasma for every 1 unit of platelets) to decrease dilutional effects on clotting factors [6]. If available, rotational thomboelastometry (ROTEM) or thromboelastography (TEG) can be used to help guide resuscitation, as they are a point of care test that identify which specific factors must be transfused in order to have a normal coagulation profile within minutes [23]. These tests can also determine if there is hyperfibrinolysis which can be treated with tranexamic acid or aminocaproic acid, whereas other routine lab tests cannot readily determine if hyperfibrinolysis is occurring. During massive hemorrhage, a patient can enter a catastrophic cycle, whereby the patient becomes coagulopathic and bleeds regardless of surgical repair, leading to acidosis which causes ongoing bleeding, which makes the patient hypothermic leading to nonfunctional clotting factors, leading to worsening coagulopathy and acidosis. Maintaining a patient's PH > 7.2 and a core temperature of 36 °C will help decrease a worsening coagulopathy. Fluids and blood products should be administered through a fluid warmer when able. Additionally, calcium should be administered during the resuscitation as calcium stores become depleted due to the citrate in packed red blood cells. Chelation of calcium due to citrate leads to conformational changes of the coagulation factors V and VIII which results in loss of procoagulant activity [21].

Exploratory Laparotomy for Vascular Control and Repair

If the abdomen is not yet open, a generous midline laparotomy should be performed to immediately control the bleeding by judicious use of suction and careful placement of digital pressure if able to safely visualize the injury versus packing the area with laparotomy pads. Once temporary control has been obtained, it is then necessary to allow the anesthesia team to "catch-up," by providing adequate volume replacement through appropriate vascular access. Additionally, the measures described in the previous section should be taken to be prepared for exposure, proximal and distal control, and repair of the injury. When assessing the injury, attempts should be made to determine whether the injury site lies in the anterior abdominal wall, intra-abdominal visceral, or retroperitoneal structures. Injury to a retroperitoneal vascular structure is likely to require vascular surgery consultation.

Direct puncture of a major artery (common iliac or distal aorta) is best addressed with primary repair when possible. For more extensive injury/laceration, the artery may need to be debrided to a healthy vessel proximally and distally to allow an end to end anastomosis. Arterial injuries are readily compressible until intraoperative assistance, preferably by a vascular surgeon, can be obtained. Venous injuries can be life-threatening due to profuse bleeding from the extensive collateral blood supply. They are more difficult to manage, particularly in the pelvis. When confronted with a pelvic venous injury, the bleeding site should be carefully packed, and if this achieves control, careful consideration should be given leaving pack in place and the abdomen "open" with a temporary abdominal wall closure with negative pressure therapy [2]. Aggressive resuscitation should continue in the intensive care unit (ICU) with normalization of the patient's coagulation parameters, temperature, PH, and vital signs. The patient should return to the operating room the following day for pack removal and re-assessment. At this second procedure, a vascular surgeon should be present.

Vascular Exposures During Damage Control Laparotomies

When approaching a major vascular injury, proper exposure, focusing on safe proximal and distal control, is of utmost importance. A dedicated vascular instrument set, which includes a variety of clamps in standard configurations, is required (Table 10.3). Exposure can be achieved with any large self-retaining intra-abdominal

Table 10.3 Instruments needed for repair of major vascular injuries

Instruments needed for major vascular injury
Heparinized saline (5000 units/500 mL)
Prolene suture (5–0 C1 and 6–0 BV1 for smaller vessels, 4–0 SH and 3–0 SH for larger vessels)
Aortic clamp (potentially with soft inserts)
Angled clamps for iliac, mesenteric, renal vessels
Side-biting clamps
Allis clamps for grasping vein injuries
Sponge sticks
Self-retaining retractor
Appropriately sized tube and bifurcated prosthetic grafts

retractor. A preferred aortic clamp should be selected early in the procedure and kept readily available. Additionally, sponge sticks (large and "peanut") should be assembled and ready to use. Heparinized saline should be on the field to perform local heparinization, irrigation of open vessels, and flushing. A set of vascular sutures should be pre-loaded on needle drivers of appropriate length (longer is better when in the retroperitoneum). Double-armed 3-0 and 4-0 Prolene sutures can be used for most major intra-abdominal vascular emergencies.

Following midline laparotomy and application of direct pressure on the site of the vascular injury, one may attempt to obtain proximal and distal control above and below the injured vascular segment. If a major aortoiliac arterial injury has occurred, and control is not possible due to poor visualization, supraceliac aortic exposure may be temporarily necessary to help safely achieve proximal control. It is often helpful to have the anesthesiologist place a naso- or oro-gastric tube aid in identifying the esophagus. Concurrently, the left lobe of the liver is retracted to the right by dividing the triangular ligament. The gastrohepatic ligament is incised, taking care not to injury any major vascular structures. With the gastric tube is in place, the esophagus is retracted to the left. The fibers of the right crus are split, and a space is created using blunt dissection on each side of the aorta. This blunt dissection must be taken down to the spine to avoid inadvertent dislodgement of the vascular clamp once it has been placed. Once supraceliac control is obtained, one must monitor the time, and subsequently move the clamp to a more inferior segment, such as the infrarenal aorta as soon as it is safe, in order to allow reperfusion of the visceral segment [20].

After the abdomen is opened, the hemoperitoneum is rapidly evacuated. Exposure of the infrarenal aorta is obtained by first retracting the transverse colon cephalad. The small bowel is then retracted to the right and can be kept in a bowel bag or wrapped with laparotomy pads and retracted with a wide fence attached to the self-retaining retractor. The retroperitoneum just lateral to the duodenum above the aortic pulse is sharply dissected, caring not to injure the duodenum. The dissection can be carried out superiorly up to the left renal vein. Once again, the periaortic segment can be bluntly dissected down to the spine to place an infrarenal aortic clamp, using a long clamp. Once proximal control has been obtained, the dissection can be

Table 10.4 Intra-abdominal vessels which will tolerate ligation

Intra-abdominal vessels which tolerate ligation
Renal veins (near confluence with IVC)
Celiac artery (prior to bifurcation of splenic and common hepatic)
Internal iliac arteries (high risk of pelvic ischemia if both ligated at once)
Internal iliac veins
Splenic artery
Splenic vein

carried out distally to the aortic bifurcation and extending the retroperitoneal dissection to the iliac arteries. Care must be taken as the inferior mesenteric artery comes off in the mid infrarenal aorta to the patient's left. The retroperitoneal dissection can be extended to the patient's right common iliac artery. Care must also be taken to avoid the sympathetic nervous plexus crossing over the aortic bifurcation to the left.

If the injury is in the suprarenal visceral segment, a left medial visceral rotation (Mattox maneuver) should be performed. This will achieve exposure of the entire abdominal aorta and the origins of the visceral branches (with the exception of the right renal artery). The dissection starts very low and laterally by incising and dissecting along the avascular retroperitoneal colon attachments. This allows medial mobilization of the left colon, pancreas, spleen, and left kidney. As the left kidney is mobilized medially, care must be taken to ligate the left descending lumbar vein to prevent injury to the left renal vein.

Injuries to the infra-hepatic IVC and the right renal artery may require a right medial visceral rotation. This exposure requires retraction of the small intestine to the left, followed by incision of the peritoneal attachments lateral to the right colon to the hepatic flexure and reflecting it medially. The second and third portions of the duodenum and pancreatic head are reflected to the patient's left through a generous Kocher maneuver. The retroperitoneal exposure is then extended distally by incising the posterior parietal peritoneum parallel to the left border of the root of the mesentery. The right colon and small bowel can be eviscerated, the duodenum and pancreas retracted to the left, the liver gently retracted cephalad to expose the entire IVC and common iliac veins.

While revascularization is indicated for most intra-abdominal vessels, the patient's overall clinical status may support ligation or shunting of the injury in order to allow for subsequent definitive repair. Table 10.4 lists vessels that may be treated with ligation alone.

Special Considerations for Injuries to Specific Vessels

Aortoiliac Injuries

If there is suspicion of an aortoiliac injury during a minimally invasive approach direct pressure should be applied if able. If the patient remains hemodynamically stable, the bleeding controlled with pressure or contained in the retroperitoneum, the aforementioned measures should be taken in preparation for an exploratory laparotomy. If the patient becomes unstable and the bleeding cannot be controlled initially, an immediate exploratory laparotomy should be performed and digital pressure should be applied to the segment. It may be tempting to dissect directly into the injured segment to gain proximal and distal control, but this should only be done with the assistance of a second, capable, surgeon by dissecting well above and below the injury. Long vascular clamps should be used to clamp the aorta and common iliac vessels. If suspicion for other injuries is low, once the arterial system is clamped, one should strongly consider an intravenous heparin bolus of 50–100 units per kilogram to prevent arterial thromboembolism. Despite proximal and distal control, there may be ongoing bleeding from lumbar vessels which may be temporarily controlled using clamps. Posterior aortic wall injures may be difficult to repair from an outside in approach; therefore one must consider performing a longitudinal anterior arteriotomy and performing a posterior repair from within the artery. A transverse injury or transection can be repaired by performing an end to end anastomosis, as long as the repair is tension-free. If the vessel cannot be approximated without tension, an interposition graft will be needed. If the bowel has been opened, a prosthetic graft should be avoided due to the risk of infection. A venous autograft, such as femoral vein, would be the best solution in a controlled environment, but it requires time and tedious dissection, which may be inadvisable in patients who have had major blood loss and may be in hemorrhagic shock. In these patients, expedient repair may be necessary using a Dacron or polytetrafluoroethylene (PTFE) graft of appropriate diameter.

Aortic and common iliac artery repairs with a prosthetic should be covered with retroperitoneum or an omental flap if possible. The latter can be done by pulling the transverse colon downward and then stretching out the omentum. The splenic flexure is identified and will serve as the base of the flap. The blood supply to this flap is a branch of the left gastroepiploic artery and the left omental artery. An omental flap about 10 cm in width is created by dividing the omentum in an avascular plane in a direction perpendicular to the transverse colon. If a longer omental pedicle is needed, extra length can be obtained by extending the division plane in a transverse direction parallel to the transverse colon. The omental pedicle is allowed to fold gently over the transverse colon mesentery and is placed over the aortoiliac prosthesis. It can also be brought through the bare area of the transverse colon mesentery. The flap is secured in place to the retroperitoneum with a few interrupted sutures. An interrupted 3-0 silk suture can also be used to secure the lateral edge of the flap to the mesocolon to prevent any herniation between the omentum and the transverse colon [14].

Iliocaval Venous Injuries

The differentiation between a venous injury and arterial injury can be made readily by evaluating the quality and quantity of the extravasating blood. Dark venous blood is under lower pressure than bright red arterial blood. If an iliocaval injury occurs initial control is obtained by direct digital compression of the vena cava against the vertebral column. Similarly sponge sticks can be used to in a similar fashion to control above and below the injury following exposure. When facing uncontrolled bleeding, one should avoid blindly placing vascular clamps as this could lead to additional venous or collateral injury. Once bleeding is controlled either with pressure or after dissection with proximal and distal control, vascular clamps could be placed after dissecting the anterior inferior vena cava or common iliac segment. If the injury is in the anterior or lateral cava, a curved U-clamp can be placed to control bleeding from proximal, distal, and posterior aspects of the vein. If the posterior wall of the vena cava is also involved, an anterior venotomy can be made to expose the posterior wall and repair the vein from within. A 4-0 or 5-0 prolene suture should be used on the iliocaval segment. Injuries can be primarily repaired as long as they do not create a >50% stenosis, which would lead to a flow limiting lesion. If primary repair will cause a significant stenosis, then a patch angioplasty may be performed.

Injuries to the common iliac veins or at the caval confluence may require transverse transection of the overlying common iliac artery in order to improve exposure. Following repair of the vein, the artery can be repaired in an end to end manner. Injuries to internal iliac veins can be primarily ligated if needed as these are difficult to control and repair. Major pelvic venous bleeding may require gentle traction of the vein using Allis clamps to assist with repair. Simply picking up the transected veins with Allis clamps may be enough to stop bleeding and allow visualization, control and repair of the bleeding vein. Deep pelvic venous injuries can be life-threatening due to profuse bleeding from extensive collateral blood supply leading to difficulty in management. With a deep pelvic venous injury, the bleeding site should be carefully packed. If packing controls the bleeding, one should consider temporarily closing the abdomen, allowing resuscitation until the patient physiologically normalizes including normalization of coagulopathy, PH, and temperature. Once the patient's status improves, they may return to the OR for pack removal and re-assessment. At this second procedure, a vascular surgeon should be readily available for repair.

If the injury affects the sacral venous plexus or internal iliac veins, hemorrhage occluder pins can be directly applied to the bleeding site. These are titanium pins with 7 mm serrated screws that drill into the sacral vertebrae to compress and stop bleeding from the presacral venous plexus. These can be used when clamping, suturing, or electrocautery are not effective [2].

Mesenteric Arterial Injuries

Injury to the celiac artery at its ostium may require ligation for management, unless it can be primarily repaired either with an interposition graft, an end-to-end anastomosis, or a patch angioplasty. If the SMA is healthy and uninjured, the liver may be sufficiently perfused through collateral flow via the gastroduodenal artery and splenic artery. The proper hepatic artery can be assessed in the hepatoduodenal ligament with continuous Doppler or intraoperative ultrasound to assess if there is sufficient flow. If primary repair is not feasible due to limited exposure or destruction of the origin of the celiac artery, and there does not appear to be adequate flow, an aortoceliac or right renal-hepatic bypass can be performed. If the common hepatic artery or proper hepatic artery is injured saphenous vein interposition should be used to bypass the injury. Injuries to the superior mesenteric artery should be repaired to prevent mesenteric ischemia.

Renal Vascular Injuries

Due to some inherent redundancy, renal artery injuries can often be repaired primarily or with a primary end-to-end anastomosis. If an interposition is required, the saphenous vein is the preferred conduit. Warm ischemia time of as low as 30 minutes has been shown in the renal transplant literature to correlate with irreversible renal injury [24]. Aortorenal bypass may be necessary when the ostium of the renal artery is destroyed. If the aorta is not clampable, a hepatorenal or splenorenal bypass can be performed for the right and left renal arteries, respectively. Renal veins should be repaired when able. The left renal vein may be ligated close to inferior vena cava, as long as the gonadal, adrenal, and lumbar veins are preserved. There are few reports of ligation of the right renal vein, as this vein is shorter, and there are fewer venous collaterals for drainage of the right venous outflow if the renal vein is ligated. Remaining right renal outflow includes capsular veins which drain into the gonadal vein and inferior vena cava.

Summary

Iatrogenic abdominal injuries are associated with potentially high mortality. Direct pressure of the injury should be performed, whether this is laparoscopically or following laparotomy. Communication with OR team will allow the proper instruments and adjuncts for patient resuscitation to be available during expeditious repair of major vascular injuries. Once control is obtained, the standard vascular repair options are indicated for most intra-abdominal vessels in order to preserve organ perfusion.

References

1. Afifi Y, Raza A, Balogun M, Khan KS, Holder R. New nomogram for safe laparoscopic entry to reduce vascular injury. J Obstet Gynaecol. 2011;31:69–72.
2. Asfour V, Smythe E, Attia R. Vascular injury at laparoscopy: guide to management. J Obstet Gynaecol. 2018;38:598–606.
3. Baggish MS. Analysis of 31 cases of major-vessel injury associated with gynecologic laparoscopy operations. J Gynecol Surg. 2004;19:63–73.
4. Bickell WH, Wall MJ Jr, Pepe PE. Immediate versus delayed fluid resuscitation for hypotensive patients with penetrating torso injuries. N Engl J Med. 1994;331:1105–9.

5. Campbell RM. Spine deformities in rare congenital syndromes: clinical issues. Spine. 2009;34(17):1815–27.
6. Cannon JW, Khan MA, Raja AS, Cohen MJ, Como JJ, Cotton BA, Dubose JJ, Fox EE, Inaba K, Rodriguez CJ, Holcomb JB, Duchesne JC. Damage control resuscitation in patients with severe traumatic hemorrhage: a practice management guideline from the Eastern Association for the Surgery of Trauma. J Trauma Acute Care Surg. 2017;82(3):605–17.
7. Chan YC, Morales JP, Reidy JF, Taylor PR. Management of spontaneous and iatrogenic retroperitoneal haemorrhage: conservative management, endovascular intervention or open surgery? Int J Clin Pract. 2008;62(10):1604–13.
8. Cormier B, Nezhat F, Sternchos J, Sonoda Y, Leitao MM Jr. Electrocautery-associated vascular injury during robotic assisted surgery. Obstet Gynecol. 2012;120:491–3.
9. Dutton RP. Low-pressure resuscitation from hemorrhagic shock. Int Anesthesiol Clin. 2002;40:19–30.
10. England EC, Spear CR, Huang DD, Weinberg J, Bogert JN, Gillespie T, Mankin J. REBOA as a rescue strategy for catastrophic vascular injury during robotic surgery. J Robot Surg. 2019;14(3):473–7.
11. Erkut B, Unlü Y, Kaygın MA, Olak AC, Erdem AF. Iatrogenic vascular injury during to lumbar disc surgery. Acta Neurochir. 2007;149:511–6.
12. Farouque HM, Tremmel JA, Raissi Shabari F. Risk factors for the development of retroperitoneal hematoma after percutaneous coronary intervention in the era of glycoprotein IIb/IIIa inhibitors and vascular closure devices. J Am Coll Cardiol. 2005;45:363–8.
13. Guloglu R, Dilege S, Aksoy M, Alimoglu O, Yavuz N, Mihmanli M, Gulmen M. Major retroperitoneal vascular injuries during laparoscopic cholecystectomy and appendectomy. J Laparoendosc Adv Surg Tech A. 2004;14(2):73–6.
14. Hoballah JJ, Mohan C, Nazzal MM, Corson JD. The use of omental flaps in abdominal aortic surgery: a review and description of a simple technique. Ann Vasc Surg. 1998;12:292–5.
15. Inamasu J, G. B. Vascular injury and complication in neurosurgical spine surgery. Acta Neurochir. 2006;148(4):375–87.
16. Kent KC, Moscucci M, Mansour KA. Retroperitoneal hematoma after cardiac catheterization: prevalence, risk factors, and optimal management. J Vasc Surg. 1994;20:905–13.
17. Kim JH, Ko G-Y, Kwon TW, Nam GB, Cho YP. Endovascular treatment of an iatrogenic large vessel arteriovenous fistula presenting as high output heart failure: a case report. Vasc Endovasc Surg. 2012;46(6):495–8.
18. Lamb CM, MacGoey P, Navarro AP, Brooks AJ. Damage control surgery in the era of damage control resuscitation. Br J Anaesth. 2014;113(2):242–9.
19. Makai I. Complications of gynecologic laparoscopy. Clin Obstet Gynecol. 2009;52:401–11.
20. Mechchat A, Bagan P. Management of major vascular complications of laparoscopic surgery. J Visc Surg. 2010;147:e145–53.
21. Mikaelsson ME. The role of calcium in coagulation and anticoagulation. Hematol Immunol. 1991;26:29–37.
22. Molloy D, Kaloo P, Cooper M, Nguyen TV. Laparoscopic entry: a literature review and analysis of techniques and complications of primary port entry. Aust N Z J Obstet Gynaecol. 2002;42:246–54.
23. Moore EE, Moore H, Chapman MP, Gonzalez E, Sauaia A. Goal-directed hemostatic resuscitation for trauma induced coagulopathy: maintaining homeostasis. J Trauma Acute Care Surg. 2018;84(6):S35–40.
24. Nishikido M, Noguchi M, Koga S. Kidney transplantation from non-heart-beating donors: analysis of organ procurement and outcome. Transplant Proc. 2004;36:1888–90.
25. Oderich GS, Panneton J, Hofer J, Bower TC, Cherry KJ Jr, Sullivan T, Noel AA, Kalra M, Gloviczki P. Iatrogenic operative injuries of abdominal and pelvic veins: a potentially lethal complication. J Vasc Surg. 2004;39(5):931–6.
26. Oktar GL. Iatrogenic major venous injuries incurred during cancer surgery. Surg Today. 2007;37(5):366–9.

27. Philosophe R. Complications of laparoscopic surgery. Sexuality Reprod Menopause. 2003;1(1):30–9.
28. Pickett SD, Rodewald K, Billow MR, Giannios NM, Hurd WW. Avoiding major vessel injury during laparoscopic instrument insertion. Obstet Gynecol Clin N Am. 2010;37:387–97.
29. Sotelo R, Nunez Bragayrac L, Machuca V, Garza Cortes R, Azhar RA. Avoiding and managing vascular injury during robotic-assisted radical prostatectomy. Ther Adv Urol. 2015;7(11):41–8.
30. Stulík J, Vyskocil T, Bodlák P, Sebesta P, Kryl J, Vojácek J, Pafko P. Injury to major blood vessels in anterior thoracic and lumbar spinal surgery. Acta Chir Orthop Traumatol Cechoslov. 2006;73(2):92–8.
31. Tsin DA, Tinelli A, Malvasi A, Davila F, Jesus R, Castro-Perez R. Laparoscopy and natural orifice surgery: first entry safety surveillance step. JSLS. 2011;15:133–5.
32. Waksman R, King SI 3rd, Douglas JS. Predictors of groin complications after balloon and new-device coronary intervention. Am J Cardiol. 1995;75:886–9.

Inadvertent Ischemia Occurring with Abdominal Surgery

11

Eric Silberfein

Introduction

I am a fellowship trained surgical oncologist, but this chapter is not going to be about seeing a bunch of Kaplan–Meier survival curves, p-values, and waterfall plots. I am not going to expand on any elaborate molecular pathways of carcinogenesis, and there will be no fancy photos from the operating room on exciting new techniques in tumor extraction. Rather, this will be a chapter reflecting experiences arising from the sorrowful contemplation of errors I have both seen and committed in my own operating room as well as the operating rooms I have been called into to assist others who have unfortunately found their way into trouble secondary to vascular compromise. It is a hands-on, practical, collection of knowledge and pearls that I hope will be beneficial to all surgeons, both novice and experienced. With that, I'd like to begin with a famous quote by Douglas Adams who said, "Human beings, who are almost unique in having the ability to learn from the experience of others, are also remarkable for their apparent disinclination to do so." Let's begin…

It is Tuesday morning, early March, OR#6 and I am finishing up a cancer operation when I am paged to OR#8 where there is a laparoscopic right colectomy being performed for cecal cancer. I am greeted by the surgeon who asks me to "take a look at something." I look on the video screen and see a surgeon grasping a large vascular structure with a bowel grasper. As I look further, I see many large clips in the area and the small bowel looks dusky. Can you relate to this story? Have you been there before? Practicing where I do I cannot help but think that "Houston, we have a problem…"

E. Silberfein (✉)
Baylor College of Medicine, Houston, TX, USA

Ben Taub Hospital, Division of Surgical Oncology, Michael E. DeBakey Department of Surgery, Houston, TX, USA
e-mail: ejs@bcm.edu

R. Gilani, J. L. Mills Sr. (eds.), *Vascular Complications of Surgery and Intervention*, https://doi.org/10.1007/978-3-030-86713-3_11

Chapter Overview

- Identify three common operations performed by general surgeons which can be prone to major vascular injury.
- Illustrate common and aberrant vascular anatomy inherent to these operations.
- Review "pitfalls" that can lead to vascular injuries.
- Discuss management of vascular injuries related to these operations.

The law of the land in surgical oncology has long been attributed to Dr. Blake Cady when he stated over 20 years ago that "Biology is King; selection of cases is Queen, and the technical details of surgical procedures are princes and princesses of the realm who frequently try to overthrow the powerful forces of the King and Queen, usually to no long-term avail, although with some temporary apparent victories." [1]. I would like to take the liberty of applying and adapting this quote to what I call the law of the land when things aren't looking so good by stating, "Anatomy and technical maneuvers are King, and the Queen, Prince and Princesses can save their biology and selection for another day…." This aphorism will be illustrated by looking at three common operations performed by general surgeons which can be prone to major vascular injury.

Common Operations Prone to Vascular Injury

Case 1: The Unassuming Cholecystectomy

Cholecystectomy is one of the most common operations performed by general surgeons both in academic medical centers and in private practice. The operation has traditionally been performed open, and still can be, but the standard of care has shifted to less invasive laparoscopic and robotic approaches. Regardless of the technique, the anatomy has not changed and complications can be devastating. Knowledge of both common and aberrant vascular anatomy is the key to avoiding major morbidity and mortality.

In 1955, Nicholas Michels, M.A., D.Sc., Professor of Anatomy at Jefferson Medical College in Philadelphia, published what many consider to be the landmark text and atlas describing the blood supply and anatomy of the upper abdominal organs [2]. In his work, he defined common and aberrant anatomy of the hepatic arteries that has subsequently been named the Michels hepatic artery classification. This classification below (Table 11.1) describes ten different variations along with their frequencies [3]. Most vascular complications during cholecystectomy occur when there is an unexpected encounter with a replaced or accessory right hepatic artery. Knowledge of this vascular anatomy in the porta hepatis is key to the prevention of complication. A replaced or accessory right hepatic artery (Fig. 11.1) passes lateral to the portal vein and lies posterior and lateral to the common bile duct behind the cystic duct in the hepatoduodenal ligament [4]. Vascular injury to this area results in the most feared cycle in gallbladder surgery (Fig. 11.2). It usually

Table 11.1 Michels hepatic artery classification

Type	Frequency of occurrence (%)	Description
I	55	Right hepatic artery (RHA), middle hepatic artery (MHA), and left hepatic artery (LHA) arise from common hepatic artery
II	10	RHA, MHA, and LHA arise from common hepatic artery; replaced LHA arises from left gastric artery
III	11	RHA and MHA arise from common hepatic artery, replaced RHA arises from superior mesenteric artery
IV	1	Replaced RHA and LHA
V	8	RHA, MHA, and LHA arise from common hepatic artery; accessory LHA arises from left gastric artery
VI	7	RHA, MHA, and LHA arise from common hepatic artery; accessory RHA
VII	1	Accessory RHA and LHA
VIII	4	Replaced RHA and accessory LHA or replaced LHA and accessory RHA
IX	4.5	Entire hepatic trunk arises from superior mesenteric artery
X	0.5	Entire hepatic trunk arises from left gastric artery

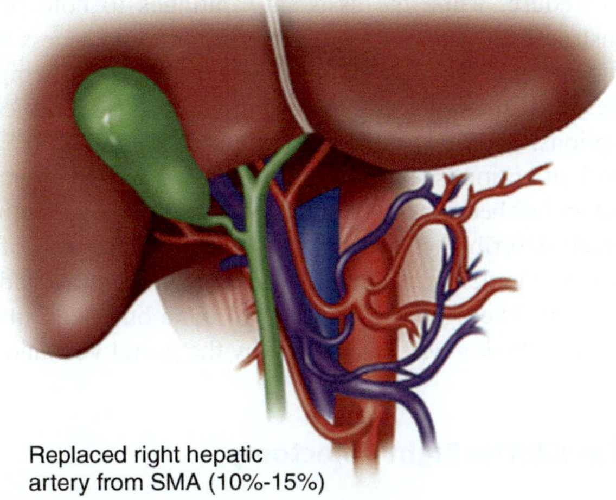

Fig. 11.1 Anatomy of a replaced right hepatic artery off the superior mesenteric artery

starts with unanticipated profuse bleeding from injury to what later will be identified as the replaced right hepatic artery. This then often leads to frantic use of the electrocautery or multiple clips being placed with less than ideal visualization of the offending vessel. Often times, these maneuvers do not completely control the bleeding so attempts at suture ligation are made which eventually control the bleeding. However, not infrequently, this cycle leads to injury to the bile ducts eventually necessitating complex biliary reconstruction.

A more controlled approach to hemorrhage in the porta hepatis would start with direct pressure to the vessel with either laparoscopic peanuts or insertion of a small sponge and pressure with a bowel grasper until calm is restored. At the same time,

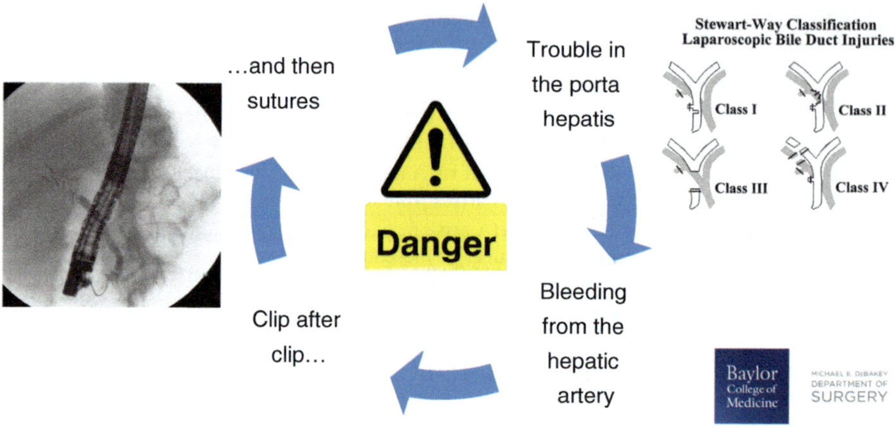

Fig. 11.2 The most feared cycle in gallbladder surgery

the surgeon should alert the anesthesiologist that there is potential for heavy blood loss and allow their team to catch up and notify the OR team that a vascular set of instruments should be obtained. A safe alternative is simply to convert to an open procedure, while the assistant continues to hold pressure with the laparoscopic instruments. The quickest and easiest way to access this area is with upper midline laparotomy. Bulldog clamps are very useful to temporarily control the identified vessel. If the replaced right hepatic artery is identified as the culprit, there are two options. The first option is to repair the vessel with 5–0 or 6–0 prolene suture. The bailout option is simply to ligate the vessel. Accidental ligation of the right hepatic artery has been described in the surgical literature dating back to 1964 when Brittain et al. described five cases of inadvertent ligation of the right hepatic artery that resulted in demarcation of the liver, transaminitis, and a low-grade hyperbilirubinemia [5]. The ligation was not fatal in an otherwise uncomplicated case as adequate liver perfusion was maintained by the portal vein and arterial collaterals.

Case 2: The Right Colectomy

Right colectomy for benign or malignant pathology is still a large part of a general surgeon's practice. Like cholecystectomy, these procedures can be performed with a minimally invasive approach, either laparoscopically or robotically or with an open approach. Vascular complications during these procedures are relatively rare but are often memorable and morbid when they do occur. An ounce of prevention in this arena is worth a pound of cure.

Let me describe a case for which I was consulted. I was called into an adjacent operating room in which a right hemicolectomy was being performed for a perforated cecal cancer. The surgeon wanted my opinion on how much small bowel should be resected. When I scrubbed in the case I saw lots of Prolene suture and metallic clips in the vicinity of the superior mesenteric vein (SMV). The small bowel was viable and a standard right colectomy was completed without events. Overnight the patient was taken back to the operating room for concern of necrotic bowel. Upon reopening the abdomen, the bowel was noted to be grossly ischemic (Fig. 11.3). The patient was immediately heparinized and a vascular surgery consult called. Thrombectomy and patch venoplasty of the SMV was performed and 3 days later when the patient went back for fascial closure the bowel was completely viable (Fig. 11.4). Upon review of the operative report, it was noted that, "While mobilizing the hepatic flexure, an injury was made in a large branch of the SMV. This was controlled and repaired with 5–0 Prolene but total EBL was about 600 mL."

Vascular pitfalls during right colectomy almost exclusively involve injury to the SMV or one of its branches. Specifically, injury most often occurs when a large collateral branch connecting the inferior pancreaticoduodenal vein with the middle colic vein/SMV is avulsed by over retracting the mobilized right colon (Fig. 11.5). The resultant bleeding is often difficult to control as the vein retracts and cannot be easily isolated. As is the case with bleeding in the porta hepatis, frantic attempts at control are often made with multiple clips and suture leading to hemostasis but unfortunately also leading to vascular injury. This injury can best be prevented by avoiding excess upward and medial traction to the right colon when mobilizing the hepatic flexure. Additionally, transillumination of the mesocolon can help to identify arcades around the SMV with early ligation to avoid the shearing force.

If injury to the SMV, or one of its major branches, does occur during colectomy, management should be stepwise and calculated. First, direct pressure should be applied until calm is restored. Again, the anesthesiology team should be alerted and vascular instruments obtained. Avoid frantically placing clips or sutures until the injury is clearly identified. The case should probably be converted to open and

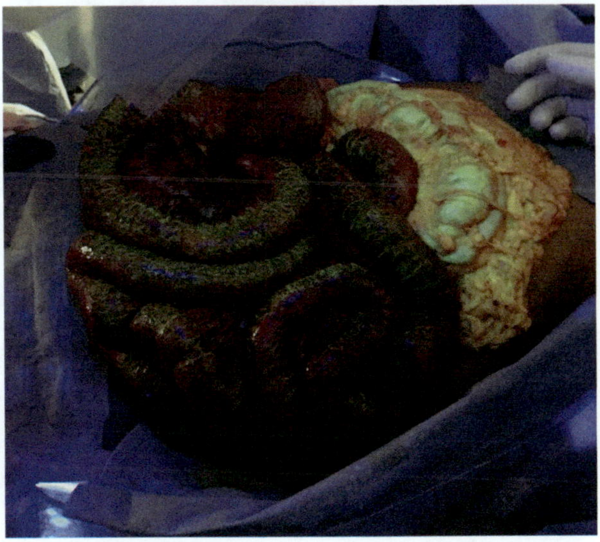

Fig. 11.3 Grossly ischemic small bowel after right colectomy

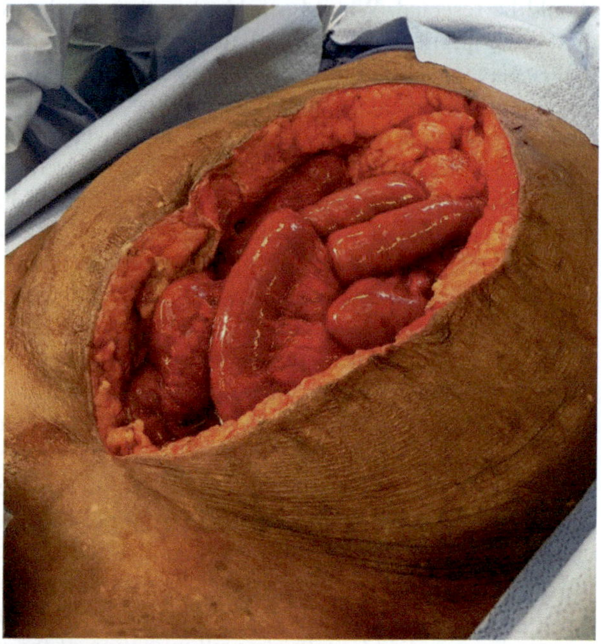

Fig. 11.4 Reperfused small bowel 3 days later after SMV thrombectomy and patch venoplasty

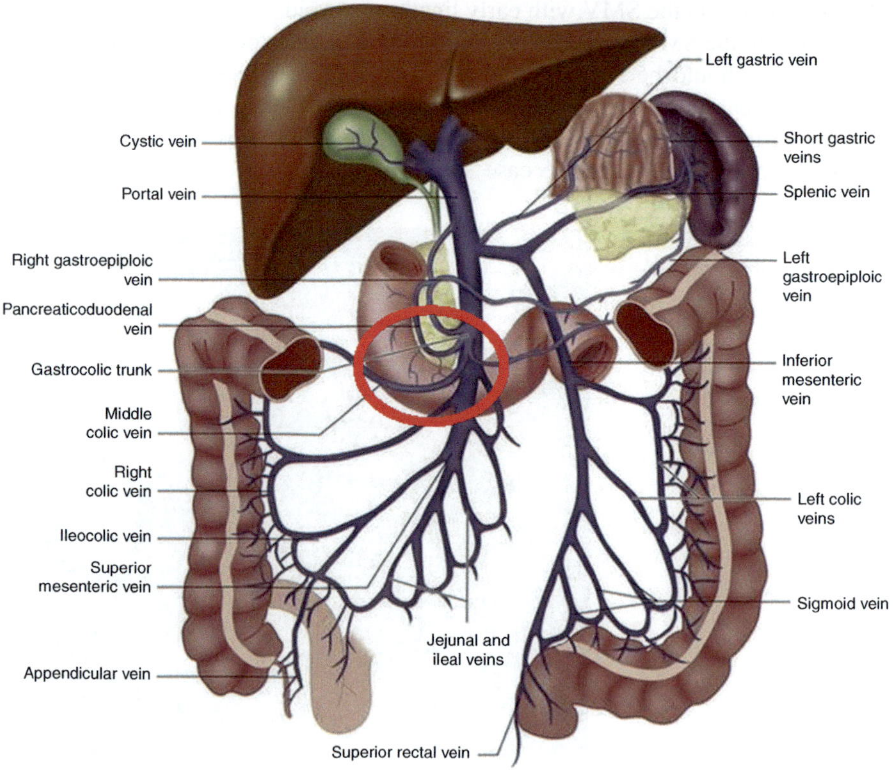

Fig. 11.5 Location of avulsed veins during excessive retraction of hepatic flexure during right colectomy

"anatomic navigation" performed to obtain proximal and distal control and the vessel repaired or patched under direct visualization. Anatomic navigation is a term that refers to navigating and dissecting outside of the disrupted anatomy and finding recognizable anatomy. In the case of SMV bleeding, this would begin with identification of the middle colic vein, the portal vein and the first jejunal branch of the SMV. Tracing the known anatomy back to the zone of damage, i.e., the so called "trail of safety," will involve moving from one key landmark to the next without getting lost or causing iatrogenic injury. This can be accomplished in the following eight steps

- Step 1 – Apply digital pressure or a sponge stick on the bleeding vessel.
- Step 2 – Perform a Kocher/Cattell–Braasch maneuver to "relax" the duodenum and the root of the mesentery.
- Step 3 – Identify the middle colic vein and gastroepiploic vein and trace them back to the gastrocolic trunk of Henle.
- Step 4 – Isolate the infrapancreatic SMV by widely incising the retroperitoneum along the length of the inferior border of the pancreas.
- Step 5 – Manually compress the root of the small bowel mesentery proximal to the injury.
- Step 6 – Trace back the proximal SMV and isolate the first jejunal branch on the right lateral SMV.
- Step 7 – Identify the injury and perform thrombectomy if needed.
- Step 8 – Heparinize if needed and repair the injury while avoiding narrowing of the vein.

Case 3: This Is Not Looking So Good…5–6 Days Later

Bowel anastomosis is inherent to general surgery practice. The principles of anastomosis are the same whether being performed with a minimally invasive technique or an open approach. A failed anastomosis almost always has a vascular component thereby making understanding of the vascular anatomy critical. Additionally, there needs to be meticulous attention to the surgical technique when performing these reconstructions. The core principle of constructing an anastomosis, whether it be blood vessels, bowel, bile duct, or skin is to bring healthy, vascularized tissue together without tension. Tension will inherently lead to ischemia and anastomotic breakdown.

There are three major watershed areas of the colon that are worth mentioning as colon resection with anastomosis is a common procedure performed by general surgeons and also inherently prone to anastomotic breakdown by the nature of the blood supply. Specifically, the areas of vascular compromise involve operations on the right colon, splenic flexure, and rectosigmoid (Fig. 11.6, [6]). There should be meticulous attention to the vascular anatomy on preoperative imaging to help plan the proper operation.

The right colon is quite vulnerable in low flow states as the marginal artery of Drummond is poorly developed in 50% of the population. This becomes particularly important if there is consideration of performing an ileocecectomy as the right colic

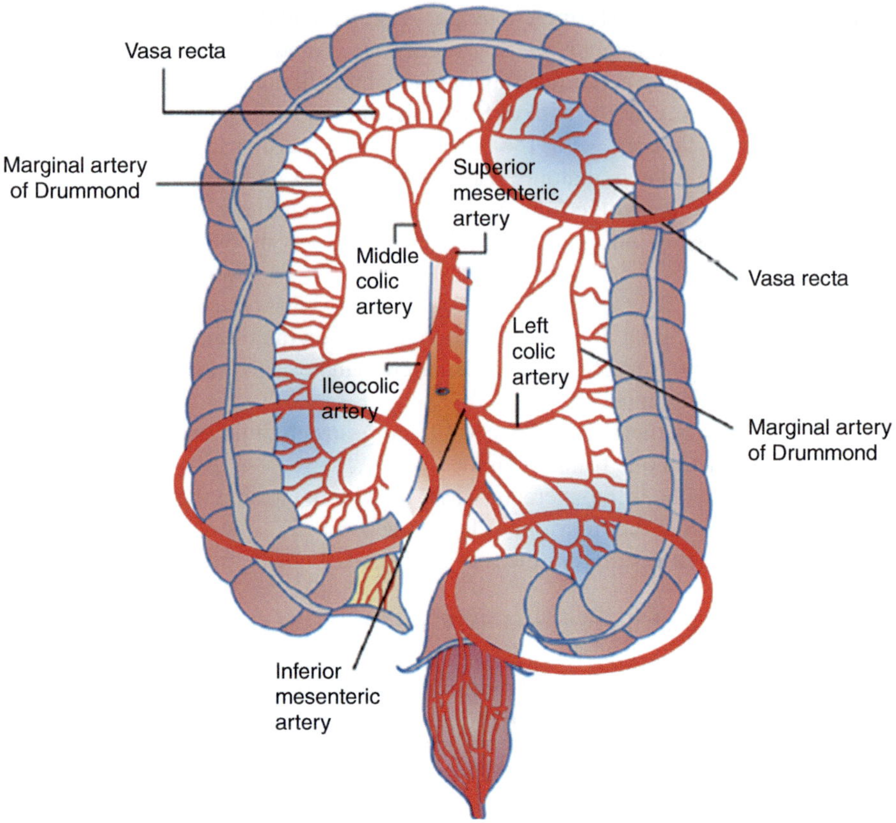

Fig. 11.6 The three watershed areas of the colon

artery branches off the ileocolic pedicle or is absent altogether. This can result in ischemia to the anastomosis and ascending colon. It is important to document that this situation is not the case prior to entertaining performing an ileocecectomy. A second consideration when operating on the right colon is circumstances where an extended right colectomy is being performed. Since the middle colic artery is ligated at its origin the anastomosis is again dependent on the marginal artery of Drummond. However, the majority of this flow will be coming from the inferior mesenteric artery (IMA), and if this artery is occluded (as is not infrequently the case in elderly patients or those with vascular disease), there may not be enough collateral flow to heal an anastomosis. There may be times, however, in which the chronicity of the occlusion of the IMA has allowed collaterals to form allowing for a healthy anastomosis.

The splenic flexure is another watershed area of the colon as there is a 3–5 cm area of the colon at this location that is devoid of the vasa recta. Furthermore, the marginal artery of Drummond is absent in up to 10% of the population. This area is also referred to as Griffith's point. This is specifically important when performing a transverse colectomy or the creation of an end colostomy. It is often necessary to extend the distal resection on a transverse colectomy until the ascending branch of the left colic artery is encountered to assure that this segment of bowel is well perfused. Performing an end colostomy at the splenic flexure with a large distance between the bowel at the abdominal wall and the vascular pedicle can be fraught with complication. Too often, I have seen end colostomies at this location become necrotic due to poor planning of bowel transection.

Finally, the rectosigmoid junction, or Sudek's point, is a watershed area as this segment of bowel is distal to the last collateral connection with proximal arteries. For this reason, the distal resection margin on a sigmoid colectomy should always be on the rectum, where the tenia coli splay out on the bowel wall, marking the anatomic end of the sigmoid colon. This assures that a portion of potentially poorly perfused sigmoid colon is not part of the anastomosis. Another consideration that merits consideration is the case when a low anterior resection is being performed and there is occlusion of the internal iliac artery which normally would supply blood to the remaining distal rectum. The anastomosis in this case would have to rely on the blood supply from the proximal bowel, specifically the marginal artery of Drummond. If this blood supply is absent or compromised, an end colostomy may be a better choice than anastomotic dehiscence and the accompanying added morbidity.

Summary

- Ischemic compromise results in significant morbidity and mortality in general surgery.
- Knowledge of common and aberrant anatomy is paramount.
  - Hepatic artery anatomy.
  - Root of the mesentery.
  - Watershed areas of the colon.
- "An ounce of prevention…."
  - Review the vascular anatomy on all preoperative studies.
- Learn from the experiences of others.

References

1. Cady B. Basic principles in surgical oncology. Arch Surg. 1997;132:338–46.
2. Michels NA. Blood supply and anatomy of the upper abdominal organs with a descriptive atlas. Philadelphia: Lippincott; 1955.
3. Michels NA. Newer anatomy of the liver and its variant blood supply and collateral circulation. Am J Surg. 1966;112(3):337–47.
4. Cheng EY, Zarrinpar A, Geller DA, Goss JA, Busuttil RW. Chapter 31: liver in Schwartz's principles of surgery, 10e, Brunicardi FC ed. New York: McGraw-Hill; 2015.
5. Brittain RS, Marchioro TL, Hermann G, Waddell WR, Starzl TE. Accidental hepatic artery ligation in humans. Am J Surg. 1964;107:822–32
6. Trotter JM, Hunt L, Peter MB. Ischaemic colitis. BMJ. 2016;355:i6600.

12 Vascular Injury During Spine Surgery

Rebecca Kelso

Anterior lumbar interbody fusion (ALIF) has been used for several decades by spine surgeons as one of several approaches to provide fusion for degenerative disc disease, scoliosis, and spondylolisthesis. It can also be an approach for infections such as discitis, osteomyelitis, and cancers of the spine. This approach is performed primary for the lumbar spine; however, similar techniques can be adopted to the thoracic spine. It is often preferred as it preserves the posterior ligaments and paravertebral muscles while providing improved visualization of the entire disc space which can improve fusion.

Approaching the anterior vertebral column of the lumbar spine can be done from either a retroperitoneal or a transabdominal approach with most favoring the retroperitoneal approach due to the natural planes in this area and avoidance of the bowel. Regardless of the surgical approach, the exposure requires knowledge of the retroperitoneal anatomy; specifically, the iliac vessels, pelvic nerves, and their common variations. The proximity to the retroperitoneal structures has led to the development of a two-team approach with an access surgeon performing the actual dissection and exposure of the anterior spine for the spine surgeons. A shrinking group of spine surgeons learn exposure as part of their training and continue to perform their own exposures in practice.

While the technical steps have similarities to other surgical procedures, spine access surgery is its own unique surgical procedure with specific nuances that a proceduralist must be aware of to perform high level safe surgery. Knowledge of the potential contraindications to anterior access and complications can help surgeons hone the specific techniques and thus prevent untoward events which can have significant consequences. It is also useful to share this knowledge with patients during preoperative risk conversations. The most common complication during anterior spine exposures is vascular injury, first reported in 1945 by Linton and White [1].

R. Kelso (✉)
Novant Health Heart and Vascular Institute, Presbyterian Hospital, Charlotte, NC, USA
e-mail: rlkelso@novanthealth.org

R. Gilani, J. L. Mills Sr. (eds.), *Vascular Complications of Surgery and Intervention*, https://doi.org/10.1007/978-3-030-86713-3_12

The incidence of vascular injury is not clear due to the wide definition used to identify injuries and ranges from 0.3% to 20% and up to 57% in redo exposures associated with hardware removal [2–6]. Management of intraoperative and postoperative complications also draws corollaries from surgery; however, the small, deep space lends to several adaptations to managing vascular complications.

Preoperative Considerations

The proverb "forewarned is forearmed" is especially apropos when considering candidacy for anterior access surgery. Knowledge of the patient's comorbidities and previous surgical history will provide important information and can be obtained during preoperative discussion. As each access surgeon gains experience, the list of contraindications for anterior exposure often shortens. Increasing experience has led to increased comfort with unique situations and awareness of pitfalls, converting some previously held absolute contraindications to relative contraindications. The main components to be considered include factors such as length of time from previous surgery, involvement of other retroperitoneal organs, associated infections, and previous surgeon experience.

It is easiest to divide comorbidities and surgical history into two categories: anterior abdominal wall vs retroperitoneum (Table 12.1). Anterior abdominal wall considerations include operations that lead to scar tissue which may obliterate the tissues planes of the rectus sheath or other factors such as an ostomy or mesh which may lead one to consider alternative incisional placement or dissection from the right vs left space. Retroperitoneal risk factors include previous surgery around the iliac vessels, sacral promontory radiation, or infections in this area. In general, retroperitoneal factors are of higher risk than anterior abdominal factors, primarily due to mobilization of the iliac vessels during the procedure.

Today's electronic medical record can both be helpful and limiting. The surgical history inputted is often overly basic and lacking in detail. It is important to tease out some of the specifics regarding an operation with specific questions to your

Table 12.1 Patient risk factors associated with increased complexity in anterior lumbar spine exposures

Anterior abdominal wall	Retroperitoneum
Laparoscopic hernias with mesh	Retroperitoneal fibrosis
Inguinal hernia repairs	Iliac lymph node dissections
Ostomy/urostomy	Iliac stents
Open prostate surgery	Open aortoiliac vascular surgery
Previous anterior spine surgery	Upper pelvic abscess (i.e., diverticular)
Abdominal wall reconstruction	Bladder sling/suspension
TRAM flap	Iliac or hypogastric aneurysms
	Pelvic radiation
	Sigmoid colon resection
	Pelvic kidney

patient. Some of these specifics include laparoscopic or open surgery and mesh or no mesh repair. One can draw inferences about the previous operation if drain or pigtail catheters were required. Many details related to a pelvic abscess, location of stents, use of mesh, or addition of a lymph node dissection to a cancer operation may have to be identified by other sources such as radiologic findings of metallic objects consistent with vascular stents, laparoscopic tacks, or a clip pattern. If the specifics of an operation truly matter, there is no better source than the operative report. This is especially useful in patient with previous anterior spine surgery to determine the laterality of retroperitoneal approach for L5/S1 or other anatomic findings during more proximal approaches.

Current discussions of *absolute* contraindications among access surgeons continue to include untreated common iliac and/or hypogastric aneurysms, known retroperitoneal fibrosis, transplanted kidneys, and bilateral transverse rectus abdominis myocutaneous (TRAM) flap reconstructions. Some surgeons have discussed performing open surgery to repair the iliac aneurysm at the time of the spine repair. It is important to be willing to recognize scar tissue during the dissection and be prepared to perform more advanced maneuvers, use radiologic guidance to minimize extent of dissection, or even abortion of access.

Potential Complications

The most dreaded anterior spine access injuries are vascular ones, as they can become quickly significant, directly affect patient hemodynamics and be difficult to repair given the small space used to provide exposure. In general, due to the differences in the wall composition between arteries and veins and the pelvic anatomy, all vessels have been shown to be susceptible [2]. In series of 269 cases with a vascular injury occurring in 37 cases, venous injuries were more common than arterial (70% vs 12.5%), and the most commonly injured vessel was the left iliac vein (Table 12.2) [4]. Intraoperative bleeding is more common than thrombosis and thromboembolism, though all may occur. While this chapter focuses on vascular injuries, for the

Table 12.2 Location and frequency of vascular injury in 269 anterior spine exposures

Location	*N* (269)	%
Left common iliac vein	21	7.8
Unnamed small vessel	7	2.6
Inferior vena cava	4	1.5
Iliolumbar vein	2	0.7
Lumbar artery	2	0.7
Left internal iliac artery	1	0.4
Left internal iliac vein	1	0.4
Aorta	1	0.4
Left common iliac artery	1	0.4

Reprinted with permission from Elsiever, *Annals of Surgery* 2013; 27:306–313 sake of completeness, other potential complications of anterior spine approach include blunt ureteral injury and retrograde ejaculation from pelvic plexus damage. Potential postoperative complications include skin or soft tissue infection, ileus, deep vein thrombosis, abdominal wall deformities/chronic pain, and seroma or hematoma of the dissection space.

Important risk factors that lead to complications include obesity and scar tissue. Obesity and scar tissue formation are similar themes due to the decreased visibility that both of these factors have in common. Small incisions are difficult in the obese due to the depth needed to achieve anterior lumbar spine exposure. There is a natural tendency toward a cone down view which leads to an even smaller operating field. Scar tissue may be present from previous surgery as discussed above; however, radiation and infection are two other entities that can lead to complete obliteration of the tissue planes that are essential to easily separate the vascular structures from the retroperitoneum. Inflammation or scar tissue from existing or previous infection can eliminate the ability to identify the veins in quite a daunting manner leading to their injury.

Additional factors that lead to increased risk for vascular injury include multi-level surgery, L4/5 exposure, and vascular anomalies. Multi-level surgery has increased risk for vessel injury primarily due to the extended dissection needed. In general, the incidence of multi-level ALIF is on the decline with the development and acceptance of lateral and oblique surgery (extreme lateral interbody fusion (XLIF) and oblique lateral interbody fusion (OLIF)). Exposure of L4/5 by these techniques can often be limited by the level of the iliac crest, favoring the option of ALIF at this level. L4/5 exposure is a separate factor for increased injury based on the variability of the level of the iliac vein bifurcation and the need for iliolumbar vein ligation with iliac artery and vein mobilization. Hamdan et al., in their single center series, found that 83% of the injuries occur at the L4/5 level, with injuries least frequent when L5/S1 was exposed as a single level [7]. Similarly, Chiriano et al. found venous injury to be three times greater in exposures involving L4/5 compared to other levels [8].

Vascular anomalies in the retroperitoneum primarily refer to venous anomalies. Larger vessels can be identified on preoperative imaging and include aberrant hypogastric vessels, left-sided inferior vena cava (IVC), and left renal vein variations. Several anomalies are difficult to identify on lumbar coned images. These include pelvic kidneys, accessory left renal arteries, and ureteral anomalies. In addition, the iliolumbar vein has two main variants which should be carefully dissected prior to ligation. One has a single main trunk from the iliac vein, and the second has two branches where one can be the ascending lumbar vein [9].

Most intraoperative vascular injuries can be divided into four categories: sharp, retraction, transection, or compression (Table 12.3). Sharp injuries are those related to direct vessel injury with scissors or some other sharp object. These are iatrogenic injuries performed during dissection. Some reasons why these occur include scar tissue, poor visualization as seen in obese patients, or compression of the vein and poor exposure of the vein wall. These more often occur on the anterior or leading lateral edges which can make them easier to repair. More difficult are the retraction

Table 12.3 Types of vascular injuries

Sharp	Retraction	Transection	Compression
Direct laceration	Avulsion	Loss of control	Vessel thrombosis
Dissection	Shearing	Inadvertent ligation	Intraluminal injury
Penetrating	Pseudoaneurysm		Thromboembolism

injuries that lead to avulsion or shear injury of the vessels. Retractors are key to all aspects of surgery; however, a slip or too much tension in a specific area can lead to an unintentional venotomy. In addition, manipulation of the retractors or other instruments during the spine discectomy and fusion can also lead to a retraction type injury. These injuries often are longitudinal or along the posterior aspect of vessels, making them much harder to repair. Some of these injuries are partial, not identified during surgery, and can lead to a weakening in the vessel wall and future pseudoaneurysm. The third type is a transection injury, for example when clips or ties fall off the iliolumbar vein with subsequent retraction of the branch vessel; this may create a larger defect than the original branch itself. On rare occasions, a major vessel may be inadvertently ligated. A combination of retraction or transection injury can be seen in injuries to the pelvic venous plexus, especially in circumstances where the dissection is too low. Compression injuries can occur with fixed retraction of a vessel leading to either distal outflow obstruction or intraluminal damage with plaque disturbance or dissection. Most often, these require a secondary procedure for repair.

Special Circumstances

Cancer operations in general tend to require larger exposures as resection (partial vs full corpectomy) requires a large field of view and an even more extensive reconstruction. Cancer cases, like fracture cases, can also be performed primarily for stabilization rather than resection, and while these require a smaller field of view than resection, they can have associated inflammation. It is fortunate that these cases encompass only a smaller percentage of exposures cases. Revision/redo operations and previous infection in the region of interest present similar difficulties. Each of these increases the complexity and thus the risk of vascular injury during surgery. The presence of scar tissue, inflammation, and phlegmon can make it very difficult to identify the retroperitoneal structures, especially the veins.

Proper preparation improves outcomes. Common among all is the communication between the surgeon performing the exposure and the spine surgeon. It is important to have a complete picture of the operative plan from the spine surgeon in regard to level, goals of operation, and planned reconstruction. Committing to the larger risk encompassed by these types of cases is made easier with better understanding of the patient needs, indications for surgery, and anticipated outcomes.

For redo operations, it is beneficial to review previous operative notes to identify the extent of previous dissection and laterality of the retroperitoneal approach. Utilizing a contralateral approach, most amenable for redo L5/S1 surgery, can often decrease the anterior abdominal scar tissue and provide a new window to approach the retroperitoneum. Reviewing the MRI or CT scan can also be helpful in identifying the location of the venous bifurcation, iliolumbar veins, and other major vessel anomalies. In cases of infection, the extent of the prevertebral phlegmon/edema can also be visualized. As previously suggested, all imaging including plain radiographs can help identify radiopaque markers or locations of previous surgery.

These larger cases also benefit from unique consideration of hospital capacity of additional services. Many routine spine access cases are safely performed in smaller facilities; however, consideration for availability of cell saver and blood bank may lead to a change in venue. Based upon level and concern for visualization, ureteral stents also may prove to be valuable. The availability of vascular surgeons or interventional radiologists with intraoperative endovascular capabilities has proven useful in additional control and reconstruction options that can decrease the morbidity of significant venous injuries. Some surgeons have anecdotally discussed their practice of early placement of venous sheaths for easy balloon occlusion in preparation for potential major venous bleeding.

"Dissect only where necessary" is an important maxim in these situations. Limiting the exposure solely to the space needed by the spine surgeon minimizes the risk of vascular injury. Within a phlegmon or scar tissue, vascular anatomy can be distorted or difficult to identify; however, awareness of three-dimensional anatomic location can minimize the extent of true vascular dissection needed for each level. Finding the plane for dissection can often lead one to use something nontraditional. For example, dissecting within the middle of the iliac veins down to the anterior lumbar ligament can allow dissection of the entire soft tissue phlegmon en bloc in an attempt to protect the iliac vein. In using this technique, intraoperative radiologic identification of the midline and correct level can help center the dissection. It also helps mentally to fuse the preoperative radiologic knowledge of the location of the iliac bifurcation with the actual surgery as this can be a point of injury.

Technical Considerations

A significant vascular problem can often be directly visualized at the time of injury if it is a sharp or transection type of injury. Any injury from retraction or compression may not be identified immediately at the time of injury. Retraction can provide control of venous injury given the low-pressure venous flow state. Thus, these injuries are often only identified once the retraction is removed. Compression leading to an intraluminal event may not be realized until the completion of surgery and after the drapes are removed, or even postoperatively. Utilization of toe digit pulse oximetry can assist in intraoperative identification of significant compression of or injury to an axial artery.

There are three key elements for management of all vascular injuries: recognition, hemostatic control, and repair. The first step once significant bleeding is encountered is application of direct manual pressure. Depending on the extent and location of bleeding, packing can be highly effective. At this point, taking a "bleeding time out" can help the team regroup, plan the next steps, and minimize blood loss while allowing for additional resuscitation if needed. Improper steps, such as blind clamping or en masse sutures, can be ineffective with ongoing bleeding and also can worsen the injury (especially venous injuries). After obtaining control, the surgeon should assess the next steps. Gauging the extent and location of injury will lead to specific decisions including requesting special instrumentation, need to extend the incision or exposure, and topical hemostatic use versus suture repair. Many such circumstances benefit from the hands of an additional surgeon.

Another important consideration at this point is whether the spine surgeon should continue with their portion of the operation. If good hemostatic control can be obtained with minimal additional risk, continuation of spinal fusion may be appropriate. Completing the spine portion prior to the venous repair may minimize reinjury as venous injuries are notorious for progression into more complex injuries due to the lack of muscular structure compared to their arterial counterparts. An injury to one aspect of the vein weakens the entire segment and limits the amount of further retraction that can be provided after repair. What may have started as a minor injury with seemingly minor delicate manipulation can rapidly become a large, rapidly bleeding defect.

Instrumentation

The right tools make a significant difference in repairing vessels effectively with minimal blood loss. Table 12.4 lists a collection of instruments that can be beneficial divide by category of use. Many of the instruments listed in the visualization column will already be available for the primary exposure. The sponge stick and

Table 12.4 Instrumentation often used during exposure and repair of vascular injuries

Visualization	Temporary hemorrhage control	Repair
Hands-free retractor Omni renal blades, ALIF designated retractor	Forceps 30 cm or longer	Needle driver Long Vascular: Castroviejo, Ryder
Headlight	Sponge sticks	Open laparoscopic knot pusher
Retractor based lighting	Kittners Laparoscopic	Monofilament polypropylene suture Half-circle needle
Renal vein retractors Wiley, spinal tech	Packing material Raytec, neurosurgery pattie/strip	Hemoclips Long, laparoscopic, or angled
Suction Cellsaver	Endovascular balloon	Topical hemostatic agents
	Allis, Babcock clamp	Endovascular stents or grafts

Kittners used for blunt dissection will find secondary use in pressure and hemorrhage control. Topical agents, especially those that come as sheets or strips, can also be used as packing material. Some instruments can be difficult to find during an emergency as they may be inside larger instrument trays for specialty surgery such as long thoracic, laparoscopic, or pelvic instruments (such as those used for gynecology or urology). Creation of an emergency spine tray can be invaluable. Specific instruments to include in this tray are long needle driver, Debakey forceps, open laparoscopic knot pusher, and angled medium clip applier. The open laparoscopic knot pusher is much easier to use than the closed knot pusher, especially with double armed suture. Sutures with half-circle needles, such as the RB1, RB2 (Ethicon; Bridgewater, NJ) or CV22 (Covidien; Minneapolis, MN), are quite versatile and provide additional maneuverability in deep, small exposure fields.

Exposure

Proper exposure is critical and is often determined by the extent of repair needed. Vascular surgery should be consulted as soon as a significant vascular injury is suspected. Focal injuries can often be repaired within the primary incision. The basic tenet of exposure remains true: more is better especially as the primary goal in these cases should be primary reconstruction/repair rather than ligation. The amount of exposure is also dictated by the technique used to obtain hemostatic control. The size of the instrumentation required for control (i.e., Debakey forceps vs. the larger sponge sticks) will affect the amount of remaining visual field in which to perform a repair. Whether proper exposure requires extending the incision, fascial release, rotation or additional dissection to formally control vessels, the goal is to establish a hand-free, well-lit exposure.

Similar to the need for additional exposure, the need for formal vessel control or clamping is dictated by the extent of injury and the type of repair. If identified early and carefully controlled without extensive manipulation, hemostasis can often be obtained quickly without extensive dissection. Control may require proximal and distal clamping to allow more precise repair. Venous injuries, given their propensity to enlarge with additional dissection, may need to be treated differently at the surgeon's discretion. Aortic, IVC, posterior venous wall, or bifurcation injuries often require a significant amount of vessel mobilization just to visualize the site of injury. In these cases, a balloon catheter sometimes inserted into the defect and gently inflated to achieve hemostasis while minimizing blood loss. Heparinization should be considered selectively after control has been obtained and is mostly reserved for prolonged arterial occlusion or management of thromboembolic complications or dissections.

Repair

Once the extent of injury is defined and adequate control has been obtained, repair can commence. Smaller punctate defects can often be controlled with hemostatic agents and packing. With the advancement of hemostatic products, the ability to manage even larger defects has been made possible especially if time and packing are possible. When considering hemostatic products, a surgeon must know the unique thrombogenic factors of each product for effective use. Nothing is more frustrating that watching the product get "washed away" or fail to stay in the desired location. It is important to consider the safety of continuing with further surgery after using hemostatic products. The lack of fixation can lead to theoretical dislodgement during the additional manual orthopedic manipulation required to complete the anterior or posterior fusion. Discussion with the spine surgeon may lead to a prudent decision to delay the posterior fusion to another day.

Suture repair can be very effective but often cumbersome in the small, deep spaces of the pelvis. Hemoclips can be a nice middle option for fixation. Given the depth of incision, appropriate length instrumentation is key for proper clip closure. Laparoscopic clip appliers, while offering options for directional rotation within the handle, come on a very long delivery handle. Deep in the pelvis, vessels tend not to run flat on surface but often dive deep into spaces. Angle clip appliers can be very precise without awkward hand contortions. They are also useful for placing side biting clips to control vessel injuries in a manner that is completely parallel to the vessel. At times clips, stacked side-to-side and perpendicular to the vessel, can be just as effective as parallel clips. Of course, the limitation of clips is that they can be dislodged leading to failure and recurrent bleeding. In some circumstances, additional suture control around the clip may be appropriate.

Monofilament suture repair is the gold standard for vessel repair and remains very effective. With the anatomical challenges presented by the vessels in these incisions, primary repair requires exposure, experience, and persistence. Patience in obtaining a sufficiently long needle driver and a needle of appropriate size and shape can help determine success. As previously mentioned, the half circle needles and knot pushers are very effective in deep spaces. The vein tends to be very accommodating in handling a variety of repairs from the traditional transverse closure to more longitudinal or purse-string repairs. Suture ligation of major vessels should generally be avoided and used primarily in cases of hemodynamic instability. Specifically, for arterial defects, additional attempts at improved vascular control and more formal repair should be undertaken if patient stability can be maintained.

Beyond using balloon occlusion to obtain vascular control, advanced endovascular techniques have also been used to repair major arterial and venous injuries. Covered stents and stent grafts have been used to reconstruct large defects such as in the IVC, the caval bifurcation, and the aorta and iliac arteries. Most often these patients are already positioned on a fluoroscopic table which facilitates the use of a C-arm for imaging. However, it can be difficult to maintain hands-free hemostasis while placing or exchanging devices. The larger sizes of the IVC and iliac veins require special attention to device sizing. Both endovascular infrarenal bifurcated and kissing limb stent graft options have all been described as technical options to reconstruct these vessels [2, 10–12]. The main considerations in choosing one of these approaches includes: goals of reconstruction, emergent availability of properly sized devices, options for access, and hemostatic control during device manipulation.

Intraluminal arterial injuries are most common in calcified vessels or when retraction has been prolonged. The latter is most common during a L4/5 exposure with manipulation and lateral compression of the left iliac artery. The injury can be thrombosis with risk of thromboembolism, dissection, or plaque rupture. The sequela of these injuries may not be recognized until the postoperative period and are best defined by contrast imaging. Conventional and CT angiography are equally diagnostic, and use of each is mostly determined by the location of the patient when the diagnosis is made and the severity of associated malperfusion. In general, thrombosis or thromboembolism is best managed by open thromboembolectomy. Dissection or plaque rupture with luminal compromise can often be more effectively treated by endovascular stenting.

Some postoperative vascular complications such as iliofemoral deep vein thrombosis or vessel stenosis can often also be treated by endovascular therapy in the post-operative setting. Some single center series show that patients with a vascular injury are more likely to have a postoperative deep vein thrombosis (DVT). In general, literature review suggests the DVT rate after ALIF to be 0–5% [4, 7, 8, 13]. Both mechanical and chemical thrombolytic techniques have been effective in treating these lesions and should be undertaken given the more central location of the thrombus and potential for underlying vessel stricture as well as future postphlebitic syndrome. Some of the newer mechanical thrombectomy devices are showing promise in the iliofemoral vessels and can be performed within the early postoperative period without use of thrombolytics. Any underlying lesion should be treated accordingly to prevent recurrence. Appropriate postoperative antiplatelet therapy should be in initiated in addition to anticoagulation according to current DVT guidelines [14]. Postoperative complications of arterial reconstruction or other complications such as arteriovenous fistulas or pseudoaneurysm are documented in single case reports. These should be treated as within vascular standards according to their presenting symptoms and lesion type.

Intraoperative vascular injuries can range from simple to complex. Unfortunately, they can be created by even the most capable of surgeons in seemingly ideal circumstances. Obsessively thorough preoperative evaluation can increase awareness of patient complexity and reduce these risks. When injuries occur, obtaining hemostasis can be accomplished by the proper exposure, a second pair of experienced hands, and the right tools. Topical hemostatics, suture and graft repair, and endovascular techniques can all be invaluable to providing successful outcomes. Good communication with both the spine surgeon and patient allows for transparency of risk and support during injury. Patients must be clearly informed about the nature of the complication, what was done to repair it, and what follow-up is necessary.

References

1. Linton RR, White PD. Arteriovenous fistula between the right common iliac artery and the inferior vena cava: report of a case and its occurrence following an operation for a rupture intervertebral disc with cure by operation. Arch Surg. 1945;50:6–13.
2. van Zitterer M, Fan B, Lohle PN, de Nie C, de Waal Malefijt, Vriens PW, et al. A shift toward endovascular repair for vascular complications in lumbar disc surgery during the last decade. Ann Vasc Surg. 2013;27:810–9.
3. Papdoulas S, Konstantinou D, Kourea HP, Kritikos N, Haftouras N, Tsolakis JA. Vascular injury complicating lumbar disc surgery. A systematic review. Eur J Vasc Endovasc Surg. 2002;24:189–95.
4. Zahradnik V, Lubelski D, Abdullah KG, Kelso R, Mroz T, Kashyap VS. Vascular injuries during anterior exposure of the thoracolumbar spine. Ann Vasc Surg. 2013;27:306–13.
5. Nguyen HV, Akbarnia BA, van Dam BE, Raiszadeh K, Bagheri R, Canale S, et al. Anterior exposure of the spine for removal of lumbar interbody devices and implants. Spine. 2006;31:2449–53.
6. Inamasu J, Guit BH. Vascular injury and complications in neurosurgical spine surgery. Acta Neurochir. 2006;148:375–87.
7. Hamdam AD, Malek JY, Schermerhorn ML, Aulivola B, Blattman SB, Pomposelli FB Jr. Vascular injury during anterior exposure of the spine. J Vasc Surg. 2008;48:650–4.
8. Chririano J, Abou-Zamzam AM Jr, Urayeneza O, Zhang WW, Cheng W. The role of the vascular surgeon in anterior retroperitoneal spine exposure: preservation of open surgical training. J Vasc Surg. 2009;50:148–51.
9. Jasani V, Jaffray D. The anatomy of the iliolumbar vein: a cadaver study. J Bone Joint Surg. 2002;84B:1046.
10. Zahradnik V, Kashyap VS. Alternative management of iliac vein injury during anterior lumbar spine exposure. Ann Vasc Surg. 2012;26:277.e15–8.
11. Bonasso PC, Lucke-Wold BP, d'Audiffret A, Pillai L. Primary endovascular repair of ilio-caval injury encountered during anterior exposure spine surgery Evolution of the paradigm. Ann Vasc Surg. 2017;43:316.e1–8.
12. Chou EL, Colvard BD, Lee JT. Use of aortic endograft for repair for intraoperative iliocaval injury during anterior spine exposure. Ann Vasc Surg. 2016;31:207.e5–8.
13. Brau SA, Delamarter RB, Schiffman ML, Williams LA, Watkins RG. Vascular injury during anterior lumbar surgery. Spine J. 2004;4:409–12.
14. Kearon C, Aki EA, Ornelas J, et al. Antithrombotic therapy for VTE disease: CHEST guideline and expert panel report. Chest. 2016;149(2):315–52.

Vascular Complications Associated with the Cardiac Patient

13

Juan E. Marcano, Mathew J. Wall Jr., and Ravi K. Ghanta

Introduction

Patients undergoing cardiac surgery are at risk for vascular complications and occasionally require vascular surgical intervention. Coronary artery disease, stenotic valvular disease, and thoracic aortic diseases share similar pathophysiologic pathways to peripheral atherosclerotic vascular disease. Consequently, it is not uncommon for patients presenting with severe cardiovascular disease to also have severe peripheral vascular disease, which may be unknown at the time of initial cardiac surgery evaluation. Furthermore, the advent of new devices and transcatheter technologies has enabled endovascular approaches to valvular heart disease and heart failure, which introduce possible peripheral vascular complications. In this chapter, we review common peripheral vascular complications associated with the cardiac surgery patient.

Preoperative Evaluation

Preoperative evaluation to document presence and extent of vascular disease is essential to avoid complications in the cardiac surgery patient. The Society of Thoracic Surgery (STS) has developed a widely utilized risk prediction model for coronary artery bypass grafting (CABG), aortic and mitral valve surgeries [1–3]. Presence of peripheral vascular disease, carotid stenosis, and cerebrovascular

J. E. Marcano · M. J. Wall Jr. · R. K. Ghanta (✉)
Division of Cardiothoracic Surgery, Michael E. DeBakey Department of Surgery, Baylor College of Medicine, Houston, TX, USA
e-mail: ravi.ghanta@bcm.edu

R. Gilani, J. L. Mills Sr. (eds.), *Vascular Complications of Surgery and Intervention*, https://doi.org/10.1007/978-3-030-86713-3_13

disease each increase predicted risk for cardiac surgery operations. Physical examination, including documentation of peripheral pulses, carotid auscultation, evaluation for venous stasis disease, and extremity tissue ischemia or loss, should be performed. Bilateral upper extremity blood pressure measurement is recommended for all patients undergoing coronary artery bypass grafting (CABG) to screen for potential left subclavian artery stenosis, which may compromise left internal mammary artery (LIMA) flow.

Concomitant carotid artery stenosis is present in 8% of patients who undergo CABG [4]. Most frequently patients are asymptomatic and incidence of carotid stenosis is greatest in patients greater than 65 years of age and with coronary artery disease, specifically left main coronary disease. Doppler carotid ultrasonography is recommended in patients with clinical symptoms of carotid artery stenosis, age greater than 65 years, left main coronary artery disease, and aortic stenosis [5]. Patients with a prior carotid operation, history of stroke, or positive findings on duplex ultrasonography may benefit from CT angiography of the head and neck to ascertain extent of cerebrovascular and carotid disease. The management of patients with concomitant cardiac disease and carotid stenosis is frequently debated and varies between surgical practices. Guidelines recommend combined carotid/CABG operation in patients with significant coronary artery disease and symptomatic carotid disease and/or bilateral severe carotid stenosis [5].

In patients with diminished pulses or claudication symptoms, vascular lab assessment of ankle-brachial index and pulse volume recordings should be considered, which may prompt additional imaging. Vein mapping to assess saphenous vein conduit is also frequently performed in patients undergoing CABG. Non-contrast chest CT to assess the amount and the pattern of calcification in the ascending aorta and arch vessels is helpful for preoperative planning of arterial cannulation strategy.

Patients with aneurysmal disease, reoperative sternotomy, or prior vascular events may benefit from additional preoperative imaging such as CT angiography of the chest, abdomen, and pelvis to assess for peripheral vessel diameter and suitability for peripheral cannulation for cardiopulmonary bypass and existence of concomitant intra-abdominal aortic or visceral vessel disease. With the advent of transcatheter approaches for valvular heart disease, CT angiography to gauge suitability for delivery devices is required, which may direct toward open femoral or iliac exposures for device delivery.

Postoperative Vascular Complications After Common Cardiac Operations

The etiology of vascular complications in the cardiac surgery patient can be broadly divided into iatrogenic injury, secondary to low cardiac output or vasodilation, cardioembolism, thrombotic state, or mechanical obstruction due to indwelling devices or catheters. The presence of peripheral vascular disease greatly increases the likelihood of these complications.

Vascular Complications Related to Vascular Access and Invasive Hemodynamic Monitoring

Cardiac surgery patients frequently require multiple intravascular lines for vascular access and hemodynamic monitoring. Large bore (9 French) catheters are placed in the internal jugular or subclavian vein for introduction of pulmonary artery catheters and central venous access. In patients with end-stage renal disease, who have often had multiple, previous indwelling vascular catheters, central vein stenosis or occlusion is a risk and venous access in these patients may result in iatrogenic injury. Careful review of preoperative imaging is helpful in these patients to obtain venous access and, in some cases, placement under fluoroscopy is indicated. Iatrogenic injury to carotid artery, subclavian vessels, innominate vein, or superior vena cava secondary to large bore venous access can occur and sometimes requires open surgical or endovascular repair.

Arterial access, usually via the radial artery, is routine in cardiac surgery patients. Furthermore, radial artery cannulation has now become a standard approach for diagnostic coronary catheterization. Consequently, evaluation of the hand should be a routine part of postoperative cardiac surgery care and recognition of vascular complication is critical to prevent loss of hand function. Other arterial access sites include the femoral artery, brachial artery, and axillary artery.

The femoral artery may be accessed for diagnostic cardiac catheterization, which may utilize closure devices of the access site. This, combined with systemic anticoagulation during cardiopulmonary bypass, introduces risks of pseudoaneurysm formation, hematoma formation, bleeding, or thrombosis. Therefore, evaluation of the groin and distal pulses should be a routine component of perioperative care. Presence of groin hematoma should warrant a duplex ultrasound study to rule out pseudoaneurysm.

In some cardiac operations, such as patients with prior sternotomy or minimally invasive cardiac surgery, peripheral arterial cannulation may be performed. For re-operative sternotomy, many surgeons percutaneously access the femoral artery and vein, which are then percutaneously cannulated for cardiopulmonary bypass if excessive mediastinal adhesions or cardiac injury is encountered during sternal re-entry. Some surgeons perform an open exposure of the femoral vessels for reoperative sternotomy. For minimally invasive sternal sparing cardiac operations the femoral vessels are cannulated for cardiopulmonary bypass. This may involve cannulation of the femoral vessel via Seldinger technique or placing an end-to-side 8 mm "chimney" graft to the femoral artery. The "chimney" graft allows bidirectional flow down the extremity and easier closure with less likelihood of stenosis of the femoral artery after de-cannulation.

Stroke

Stroke occurs in 1.8% of cardiac operations, with embolic stroke being the most common etiology [6]. Preoperative imaging (CT scan) and intraoperative imaging (epi-aortic ultrasound) helps guide cannulation strategy and may reduce risk of operative stroke [7]. Intraoperative measures such as maintaining adequate mean aortic pressure and hemoglobin during cardiopulmonary bypass are frequently utilized to reduce stroke risk [8]. Aortic arch surgery with deep hypothermic circulatory arrest (DHCA) is associated with a stroke risk as high as 19% [9]. To reduce the risk of stroke, most surgeons utilize cerebral perfusion during DHCA, either antegrade via the axillary artery and left carotid artery or retrograde via the superior vena cava [10]. New devices for use during open and transcatheter operations are in development to reduce embolic risk during surgery. As cardiac operations are lengthy and patients are sedated post-operatively, the timing of stroke may be unclear. Neuro-intervention should be considered in patients who have a perioperative stroke as favorable outcomes have been observed even in patients with longer times since potential stroke event [11].

Acute Mesenteric Ischemia

Mesenteric ischemia is rare (1%) post-cardiac surgery and is associated with high morbidity and mortality (87%) [12]. Risks factors for the occurrence of acute mesenteric ischemia include age >70 years, renal insufficiency, cardiogenic shock, peripheral vascular disease, atrial fibrillation, and need for prolonged inotropic support and need for IABP [13]. Tenderness on abdominal examination, blood in stools, or a rising lactate level should raise suspicion for mesenteric ischemia, particularly when other risk factors are present. Typically, CT angiography of the abdomen is diagnostic. Occlusion may be secondary to cardioembolism, particularly in the setting atrial fibrillation, ventricular aneurysms, or endocarditis. Usually, open surgical embolectomy and repair are required, although percutaneous options are also available. Non-occlusive mesenteric ischemia (NOMI) can be present in patients on vasopressors. Treatment may require initiation of mechanical circulatory support (MCS) to reduce vasopressor requirements and initiation of vasodilators. There have been case reports of successful outcomes with catheter directed continuous mesenteric infusion of vasodilators; however this condition is usually associated with a 90% mortality [14].

Lower Extremity Ischemia

Lower extremity ischemia can occur in patients with mechanical circulatory support, arterial lines and devices, low cardiac output, high vaso-pressor requirements, heparin-induced thrombocytopenia (HIT), or embolism. Risk is exacerbated in patients with peripheral vascular disease but limb ischemia can also occur in patients without peripheral vascular disease. Lower extremity ischemia can cause significant morbidity, extend length of stay, delay the return of the patient to the normal activities, and increased hospital cost. Figure 13.1 illustrates lower extremity ischemia/necrosis secondary to high vaso-pressor requirement. In patients with vaso-pressor-related limb necrosis, 70% require an amputation of the affected extremity [15].

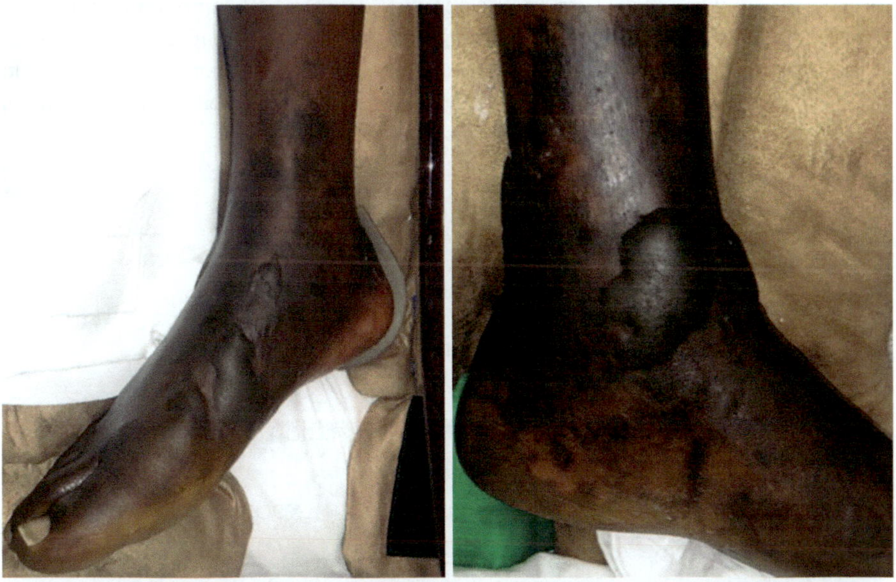

Fig. 13.1 Ischemic changes seen in the lower extremities of a critically ill patient with cardiogenic shock and multiorgan failure who required prolonged high-dose vasopressors

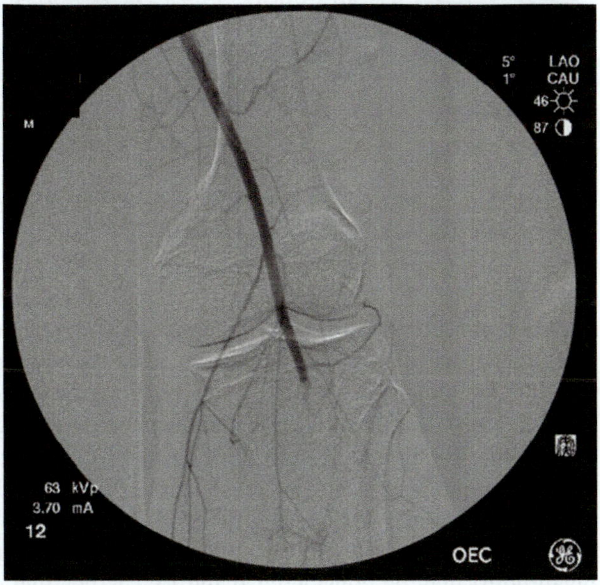

Fig. 13.2 This patient underwent aortic arch surgery and was found to have a cold leg and weak Doppler signals on POD#1. Angiogram showed embolization with popliteal artery occlusion

Limb ischemia may also result from cardioembolism, which may require open or endovascular intervention. Presentation can be early (within the same admission; Fig. 13.2) or late (usually weeks after the procedure; Fig. 13.3). Cardiac sources can be related to arrhythmias (atrial fibrillation). Heavy calcified vessels are prone to dissection and can easily develop flaps and release calcified debris that can embolize to a distal location.

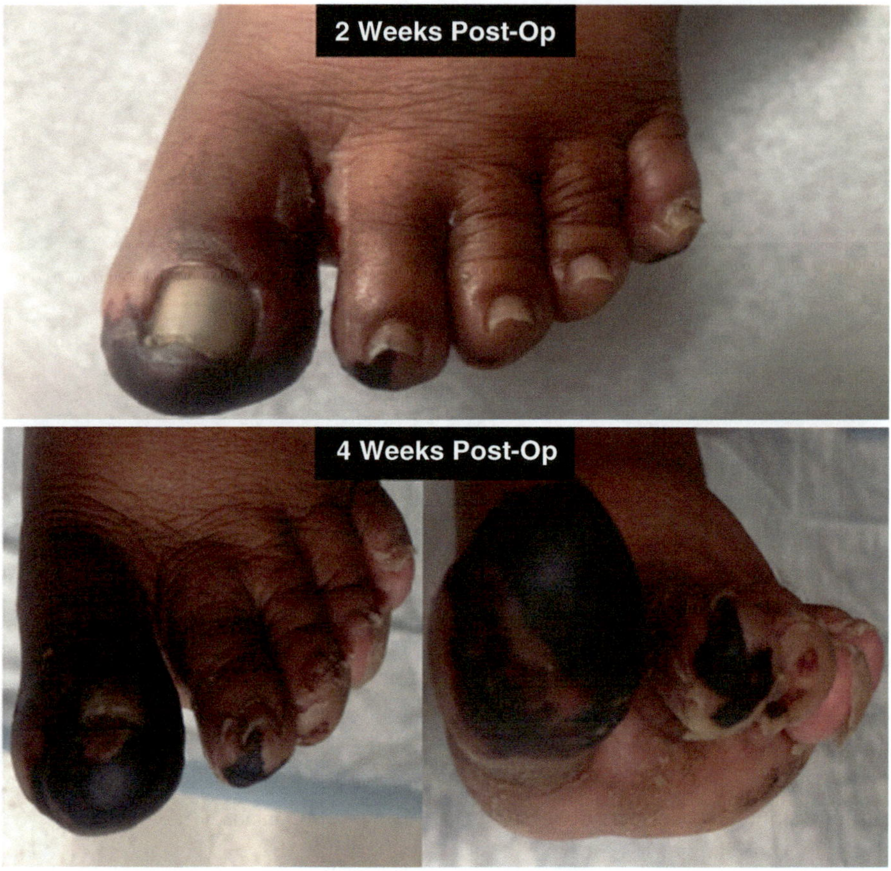

Fig. 13.3 Late distal extremity ischemia in patient 2 weeks after the index procedure. The lower pictures demonstrate the exam after 4 weeks

An estimated 3% of patients who undergo cardiac surgery develop HIT [16]. The presence of HIT results in a 50% increase in perioperative mortality. Patients with multiple heparin exposures and prolonged cardiopulmonary bypass are more at risk for HIT. The diagnosis of HIT can be challenging and clinical risk scores, such as the 4-T score do not take into account patients who go through cardiac surgery. Instead the timing and pattern may be more diagnostic [17]. Typically diagnosis requires serologic testing for anti-heparin-PF4 antibodies (sensitive, but not specific) and serotonin release assay (SRA; sensitive and specific). The SRA usually takes several days, and anti-coagulation with non-heparin anti-coagulants (such as bivalirudin) may be considered if the PF4 is positive or there is a strong clinical suspicion. If HIT is diagnosed, anti-coagulation is usually continued for 6 months post-operatively.

Vascular Complications Related to Mechanical Circulatory Support

Temporary mechanical cardiac support (MCS) in patients with low cardiac output can lead to lower extremity ischemia. A variety of MCS devices and configurations exist. The intra-aortic balloon pump (IABP) is the most common form of MCS and is a percutaneous, temporary, mechanical circulatory support device widely used for patients with cardiogenic shock. The IABP decreases afterload, increases coronary artery perfusion, and increases mean aortic pressure. The IABP is typically inserted percutaneously via the common femoral artery. This device may be inserted through an 8 French sheath or "sheathless" depending on operator preference and femoral vessel size [18, 19]. The main advantages of the IABP are related to overall low complication profile, ease of placement and removal, and low cost that makes it available in most of the centers. Complications rates of IABP vary between 12.9% and 29%, with leg ischemia the most common complication (9–25%) [20, 21]. However, contemporary data demonstrate an incidence between 1% and 3% with the use of low profile, sheath-less 8 Fr IABP devices [22]. IABP devices are removed percutaneously followed by manual pressure and bed rest. Complications of pseuodaneurysm or hematoma are possible, and patients require periodic examination. In cases with small femoral vessels and concerns for limb ischemia, open exposure and repair of the vessel may be required.

In patients with low cardiac output, shock, and/or respiratory failure, more advanced forms of MCS are required. Although a variety of devices exists, they share common traits. All devices have an inflow cannula that drains blood from the patient into an extra-corporeal pump that then returns blood to the patient via an outflow cannula. The location of the inflow and outflow cannula is dependent on the clinical requirements. Inflow and outflow cannulas may be positioned centrally for central veno-arterial extra-corporeal membrane oxygenation (ECMO) support or peripherally in the femoral or axillary vessels.

The most common configuration of MCS/ECMO is femoral arterial and femoral venous cannulation. The femoral arterial cannula is typically between 17 French and 21 French in size. The arterial cannula directs flow retrograde through the aorta (i.e., from the femoral artery towards the heart). As the cannula directs flow retrograde and occupies a portion of the femoral artery lumen, distal leg ischemia is possible. As these patients are in shock, high dose vasopressors further exacerbate this problem. In all patients who have indwelling femoral cannulae, periodic pulse examination is important. In most patients, pulsatile flow will be diminished, or non-existent and Doppler assessment is required. If the patient is stable, surgical exposure of the femoral artery and placement of a "chimney" 8 mm graft will provide bi-directional flow. This can be performed at the time of ECMO cannulation or can be performed in the contralateral groin once the patient is stabilized. Another option is to place the arterial cannula in the axillary artery if there is significant femoral atherosclerotic disease. An important and frequently utilized option to

Fig. 13.4 Patient status post cardiac surgery that required mechanical circulatory support. Femoral arterial cannula and the antegrade sheath can be seen. In the lower corner the CentriMag® Console is showing the speed and flow which for this patient is equivalent to full flow, so no or minimal pulsatility is expected

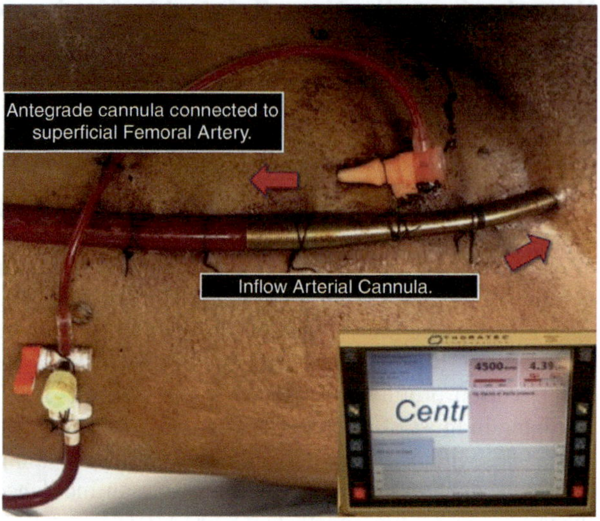

maintain distal limb perfusion during ECMO is to place an antegrade percutaneous sheath in the superficial femoral artery (SFA). Figure 13.4 depicts a patient on ECMO via a left femoral arterial cannula. An antegrade 7 French sheath is placed in the left SFA percutaneously. The sidearm of the sheath is then connected to the arterial limb of the ECMO circuit to provide additional flow to the extremity.

Vascular Complications Related to Transcatheter Valves

Transcatheter valves represent the newest innovation in structural heart disease [23, 24]. Transcatheter aortic valve replacement (TAVR) is currently being utilized in patients with aortic stenosis with appropriate anatomic criteria. TAVR can performed via a trans-femoral (TF-TAVR) or trans-apical approach through the left ventricle (TA-TAVR). Previously, TAVR devices were delivered through sheaths of 21 French or greater; however now devices can be delivered via 14 French systems. Thus TA-TAVR is rarely performed. The trans-apical approach however is utilized for transcatheter mitral valves (still in clinical trials in the United States in 2020) and remains a key technique for transcatheter valve delivery. Vascular complications related to transfemoral access occur in 4.2% of patients [25]. Risk factors for complications include advanced age, female gender (probably a surrogate marker for smaller vessel diameter), and sheath size greater than 19 French. Access site hematomas are the most common complication, followed by pseudoaneurysm. Retroperitoneal hemorrhage, arterial dissection, and femoral artery rupture are the most serious complications associated with TF-TAVR. Fortunately, with increased experience, smaller delivery systems, and improved pre-operative imaging, this complication is rare.

References

1. Shahian DM, et al. The Society of Thoracic Surgeons 2008 cardiac surgery risk models: part 1–coronary artery bypass grafting surgery. Ann Thorac Surg. 2009;88(1 Suppl):S2–22.
2. O'Brien SM, et al. The Society of Thoracic Surgeons 2008 cardiac surgery risk models: part 2–isolated valve surgery. Ann Thorac Surg. 2009;88(1 Suppl):S23–42.
3. Shahian DM, et al. The Society of Thoracic Surgeons 2008 cardiac surgery risk models: part 3–valve plus coronary artery bypass grafting surgery. Ann Thorac Surg. 2009;88(1 Suppl):S43–62.
4. Selnes OA, et al. Cognitive and neurologic outcomes after coronary-artery bypass surgery. N Engl J Med. 2012;366(3):250–7.
5. Hillis LD, et al. 2011 ACCF/AHA Guideline for Coronary Artery Bypass Graft Surgery: a report of the American College of Cardiology Foundation/American Heart Association Task Force on Practice Guidelines. Circulation. 2011;124(23):e652–735.
6. Fernandez FG, et al. The Society of Thoracic Surgeons National Database 2019 annual report. Ann Thorac Surg. 2019;108(6):1625–32.
7. Biancari F, et al. Epiaortic ultrasound to prevent stroke in coronary artery bypass grafting. Ann Thorac Surg. 2020;109(1):294–301.
8. Gold JP, et al. Improvement of outcomes after coronary artery bypass. A randomized trial comparing intraoperative high versus low mean arterial pressure. J Thorac Cardiovasc Surg. 1995;110(5):1302–11. discussion 1311–4
9. Ergin MA, et al. Hypothermic circulatory arrest in operations on the thoracic aorta. Determinants of operative mortality and neurologic outcome. J Thorac Cardiovasc Surg. 1994;107(3):788–97. discussion 797–9
10. Preventza O, et al. Unilateral versus bilateral cerebral perfusion for acute type A aortic dissection. Ann Thorac Surg. 2015;99(1):80–7.
11. Marcano J, Ghanta RK. Commentary: Tick, tock ... Time windows for intervention for stroke after cardiac surgery. J Thorac Cardiovasc Surg. 2019;158(1):199.
12. Warwick R, et al. Virchow's triad and intestinal ischemia post cardiac surgery. Asian Cardiovasc Thorac Ann. 2014;22(8):927–34.
13. Deng QW, et al. Risk factors for postoperative acute mesenteric ischemia among adult patients undergoing cardiac surgery: a systematic review and meta-analysis. J Crit Care. 2017;42:294–303.
14. Ogi K, et al. Successful treatment of nonocclusive mesenteric ischemia after aortic valve replacement with continuous arterial alprostadil infusion: a case report. Int J Surg Case Rep. 2017;35:8–11.
15. Kwon JW, Hong MK, Park BY. Risk factors of vasopressor-induced symmetrical peripheral gangrene. Ann Plast Surg. 2018;80(6):622–7.
16. Solanki J, et al. Heparin-induced thrombocytopenia and cardiac surgery. Semin Thorac Cardiovasc Surg. 2019;31(3):335–44.
17. Lillo-Le Louet A, et al. Diagnostic score for heparin-induced thrombocytopenia after cardiopulmonary bypass. J Thromb Haemost. 2004;2(11):1882–8.
18. Phillips SJ, et al. Sheathless insertion of the percutaneous intraaortic balloon pump: an alternate method. Ann Thorac Surg. 1992;53(1):162.
19. Erdogan HB, et al. In which patients should sheathless IABP be used? An analysis of vascular complications in 1211 cases. J Card Surg. 2006;21(4):342–6.
20. Patel JJ, et al. Prospective evaluation of complications associated with percutaneous intraaortic balloon counterpulsation. Am J Cardiol. 1995;76(16):1205–7.
21. Alle KM, et al. Iatrogenic vascular trauma associated with intra-aortic balloon pumping: identification of risk factors. Am Surg. 1993;59(12):813–7.
22. de Jong MM, et al. Vascular complications following intra-aortic balloon pump implantation: an updated review. Perfusion. 2018;33(2):96–104.

23. Smith CR, et al. Transcatheter versus surgical aortic-valve replacement in high-risk patients. N Engl J Med. 2011;364(23):2187–98.
24. Adams DH, Popma JJ, Reardon MJ. Transcatheter aortic-valve replacement with a self-expanding prosthesis. N Engl J Med. 2014;371(10):967–8.
25. Holmes DR Jr, et al. Annual outcomes with Transcatheter valve therapy: from the STS/ACC TVT registry. Ann Thorac Surg. 2016;101(2):789–800.

Vascular Insult of the Operated Extremity

14

Ahmed F. Khouqeer and Zachary S. Pallister

Patterns of Vascular Insults with Blunt Orthopedic Injuries

Introduction

> Hard signs are hard to miss. – Dr. Ramyar Gilani.

When a patient presents with "hard signs" of a vascular injury to the extremities, either associated with an operation or trauma, it is routine for the appropriate management to be carried out. However, these signs are not always present, and other confounding injuries such as orthopedic injuries can produce diagnostic uncertainty. We will discuss the most frequent presentations, etiologies, diagnostic modalities, and treatments required to appropriately manage patients presenting with vascular insults to the extremities associated with orthopedic procedures.

As a result of the proximity and similar axial course of both bony and vascular structures, certain patterns of blunt orthopedic injuries are highly associated with vascular injuries. Injuries caused by fractures, dislocations, contusions, crush, and traction account for 5–25% of traumatic vascular injuries that require treatment. Moreover, there is a spectrum of arterial injuries that includes spasm, intimal injuries, pseudoaneurysm, arteriovenous aneurysm formation, and partial or complete transection. Orthopedic injuries most frequently result in damage to the femoral, popliteal, or brachial arteries. Furthermore, long bone fractures causing vascular injuries are less likely in healthy individuals, with femur fractures being associated with 1–2% of superficial femoral artery injuries, and tibial fractures with 1.5–2.8%

A. F. Khouqeer (✉) · Z. S. Pallister
Michael E. DeBakey Department of Surgery, Baylor College of Medicine, Houston, TX, USA
e-mail: Ahmed.Khouqeer@bcm.edu

R. Gilani, J. L. Mills Sr. (eds.), *Vascular Complications of Surgery and Intervention*, https://doi.org/10.1007/978-3-030-86713-3_14

of popliteal, tibioperoneal trunk, and trifurcation injuries [1–5]. However, timely management of skeletal injuries by reduction can release the pressure from the externally compressed blood vessel and return distal blood flow. An arterial brachial index should be measured before and after reduction to assure no injury has been caused by the reduction itself. Additionally, all angiographic examinations, including CT angiography, should be performed following reduction if possible.

Injury Patterns

Axillary Artery Injury with Humeral Neck Fractures and Anterior Shoulder Dislocation

Approximately two thirds of patients with an axillary artery injury will have a vascular deficit on exam. Brachial plexus injuries are frequently associated with an axillary arterial injury due to their anatomic proximity. Therefore, brachial plexus neurologic deficits should increase suspicion of an axillary artery injury. Axillary artery injuries caused by orthopedic injuries are generally uncommon, occurring mostly with fractures [6, 7].

Traditionally, repair of the axillary artery injuries were performed with open exposure and primary repair or interposition graft reconstruction. Unfortunately, many obstacles are associated with open repair of this artery. The repair is inherently challenged by the location and fixation of the vessel proximally to the thoracic outlet. In addition, fracture of the humerus with disruption of the surrounding tissue caused both by the injury or by the orthopedic procedure itself makes open intervention difficult, as it is particularly challenging to achieve proximal control. Instead, an endovascular approach is increasingly being utilized, especially for subclavian and proximal axillary artery injuries. Endovascular repair has been described with good results in hemodynamically stable patients with retrograde femoral or antegrade brachial access [8, 9].

Brachial Artery Injury with Humeral Diaphysis Fracture and Elbow Dislocation

The association of humeral diaphysis fracture with brachial artery injury is common, especially in the pediatric age group. A neurovascular exam accompanied with a high index of suspicion for such patterns of skeletal injuries is useful. The brachial artery has a straight course, making proximal and distal control relatively easy. Repair is done primarily or with interposition grafting. Due to the young nature of this patient group, repair with autologous tissue, often with interrupted sutures that will accommodate future growth, is paramount, with endovascular stenting and prosthetic repair reserved only as a last resort.

Femoral Artery Injury with Femoral Neck Fracture and Hip Dislocation

Ninety percent of femoral artery injuries will present with distal ischemia or a pulse deficit. As with any other vascular injury however, clinical evidence of pulse deficits may not be apparent. Furthermore, normal distal pulses with profunda femoris injuries that may manifest with a non-expanding thigh hematoma could be overlooked or assumed to be from an accompanying orthopedic injury [10].

Femoral neck fractures and hip dislocation are commonly present in patients affected by high impact energy trauma situations, typically high-speed motor vehicle accidents. This injury is typically associated with multiple other extremity and torso injuries [11].

The treatment of femoral artery injuries depends on location. Common femoral injuries should be treated with open surgical repair whenever possible. Repair can be with either an interposition graft or a vein patch. The profunda femoris artery can be repaired in similar fashion. Superficial femoral artery injuries are more amenable to endovascular repair, but can similarly be repaired in an open fashion. In damage control situations or when the patient is in extremis, shunting is preferable to ligation whenever technically feasible.

Popliteal and Tibial Arterial Injuries with Supracondylar Femur Fractures, Proximal Tibial Fractures, and Posterior Knee Dislocations

Knee and proximal tibial injuries with close proximity to the knee joint have a high likelihood of a concomitant popliteal artery injury [12]. Popliteal artery injuries are associated with a high morbidity and should always be suspected in these types of trauma, as the arterial injury may not be as obvious or may present early only as a subclinical intimal injury. Moreover, preoperative planning, especially with popliteal artery injuries, is essential. Preoperative planning takes into account the best approach, positioning, and the possible need for vein harvest. These injuries have a high association with venous injury and arteriovenous fistula formation. Furthermore, imaging could prove to be beneficial with blunt injuries as well as fractures and dislocations, as the extent of the injury may vary.

Tibial artery injuries may not present with vascular exam changes, as all three vessels may be required to be compromised before ischemic signs and symptoms develop. Reconstruction is usually only required for injuries to multiple tibial vessels or the tibioperoneal trunk. Ligation of an injured tibial artery is frequently well tolerated with reported low amputation rates as long as there is adequate flow through the other arteries [13].

Who Should Operate First, Vascular or Orthopedic Surgery?

Who should intervene first has long been the subject of debate [14]. After establishing the diagnosis of combined orthopedic and vascular trauma, initial management often begins with bedside reduction. If possible, a discussion between both vascular and orthopedic surgeons should take place. The major concerns for the vascular service are ischemia time and the difficulty of either operating on an unstable leg or operating around fixed, orthopedic hardware. This is especially relevant when the patient requires placement of external fixation, which is often required in concurrent vascular and orthopedic injuries. Orthopedic surgeons are concerned about changes in length of the extremity after the orthopedic repair and the ability to manipulate the extremity without disruption of the arterial repair. Understanding those concerns makes it easier to reach the best decision and treatment plan for the patient. In our institution, we believe good communication between both services will often avoid issues for each team. Most importantly discussion should be centered in the following points:

1. Ischemia time: Will it pass the 6 hour mark? If so, arterial repair may be a priority for limb salvage.
2. Location of external hardware in relation to arterial exposure: Can placement be altered to allow the vascular repair to be done easily? Will the traction or manipulation required for orthopedic repair endanger vascular repairs? Affirmative answers would argue for orthopedic repair followed by vascular repair.
3. Extremity length change: Will the limb length be affected by the repair? Considering this will allow for operators to make the appropriate adjustments to the repair, especially when a bypass or interposition repair is required.

Common Elective Surgical Procedures with a Higher Risk for Vascular Insult

Injury to vascular structures during elective procedures is not uncommon, with the most frequent clinical scenarios being associated with orthopedic procedures. This can be attributed to the close proximity of the structures, manipulation of the joints and muscles around the vessels, and as a result of orthopedic instrumentation. Risk factors include pre-existing atherosclerosis and prior vascular procedures. Popliteal artery injuries during total knee arthroplasty are among the most common compared to other elective orthopedic procedures, with one retrospective review reporting a rate as high as 4% [15]. Recognition of the arterial injury is not uncommonly delayed until the post-operative period. This can be attributed to the increased blood loss during the procedure causing relative hypovolemia, relative hypothermia, and/or vascular spasm making an intra-operative accurate vascular exam difficult to obtain.

Although vascular injuries are uncommonly reported related to surgical procedures of extremities performed during general and plastic surgical operations, some exceptions exist. These include procedures in the axilla and groin (e.g., lymph node dissections). Mills et al. reported a single institution series of iatrogenic vascular injuries during elective procedures, with the majority occurring after cardiac catheterization (discussed in previous chapters). Only one injury (1.4%) occurred to the axillary artery during a wide local excision and lymph node dissection of a fibrous histiocytoma [16]. Injuries may also occur during excision of extremity sarcomas. However, with adequate preoperative planning, these are increasingly rare. Injury to the axillary vein occurs during axillary dissection for breast cancer. Vascular surgery should be consulted prior to oncologic or other types of surgery when involvement of major vascular structures is anticipated based on either clinical experience or preoperative imaging.

Resuscitative Endovascular Balloon Occlusion of Aorta

REBOA is a temporizing procedure in which a balloon is placed and inflated in the aorta in the setting of hemorrhagic shock in an attempt to exclude the injured portion of the aorta or iliac arterial systems to stabilize the patient until definitive operative intervention is possible. The most recent ER-REBOA system is a 7 French sheath system, downsized from the older 12 French models. Stannard et al. simplified the steps of this procedure into five steps [17], with each step posing different risks for extremity vascular insult (Table 14.1).

REBOA steps:

1. Arterial access.
2. Balloon selection and position.
3. Inflation.
4. Deflation.
5. Removal.

REBOA uses the basic endovascular retrograde access technique, most often through the CFA. It should be noted that in patients who are in shock and volume depleted, using an ultrasound to identify the artery and achieve safe access is of great importance. Secondly, balloon selection must be done carefully and positioning should be done under fluoroscopy, as the wire can injure the accessed vessel causing an intimal flap or dissection. Inflation of the balloon under direct fluoroscopic imaging is important as over inflation can cause dissection. Balloon deflation and sheath removal should be done slowly and after informing the whole team, noting the time of ischemia as many ischemic issues and electrolyte disturbances may arise afterwards.

Table 14.1 Summary of the steps of REBOA, with possible complications and measures to take to avoid them

Step	Possible complication	Preventive measures
Arterial access	High access (bleeding) or low access (thrombosis) Venous access	Ultrasound guidance
Balloon selection and positioning	Inadvertent wire movement (dissection, puncture)	Fluoroscopically guided. Assistant help with wire pinning.
Balloon inflation	Overinflation (dissection of aortic wall)	Fluoroscopically guided. Balloon to aortic wall profile
Deflation	Prolonged time to deflation. (prolonged ischemic time with risk of perfusion injury)	Conscious attention to time of inflation to deflation. Informing anesthesia while deflating
Removal	Loss of arterial control. Avulsion of the artery Ineffective closure	Closure device use with image guided removal. Adequate monitoring of limb perfusion afterwards

Recently, the use of REBOA has been discouraged after reports of complications including dissection, thrombosis, pseudoaneurysm, and limb ischemia in both the larger 12–14 and the 7–8 French systems [16]. Furthermore, the ACS TQIP data analysis showed a higher mortality and limb amputation rate associated with the REBOA group compared to the no-REBOA group [17]. The specific subset of trauma patients who might benefit from REBOA has yet to be determined.

Acute Compartment Syndrome (ACS)

ACS is defined as an increase in intra-compartmental pressures resulting in decreased perfusion to the tissue [18]. One of the most common vascular causes is the ischemia-reperfusion injury following acute limb ischemia [19]. Other non-vascular causes include extremity crush injuries, and orthopedic fractures. Risk factors include acute arterial ischemia, prolonged ischemia time greater than 6 hours, young age, hypotension, concomitant venous injuries, and popliteal artery injuries [20, 21]. Diagnosis of this condition is based on clinical findings, including severe pain, neurologic changes, tight compartments to palpation, and eventual loss of pulses with late presentations or delayed diagnosis. The diagnosis can be aided in case of uncertainty by obtaining objective measurements of individual compartment pressures.

Clinical suspicion should exist in all patients with a vascular injury and associated limb ischemia. Ischemia greater than 4 hours in duration prior to reperfusion increases the likelihood of ACS development. Patients who develop progressively painful extremities following reperfusion, tense compartments, and neurologic deficits despite adequate perfusion should raise suspicions of the diagnosis. Neurological (sensory and motor) deficits may point to the diagnosis although they are not always reliable in a recently operated extremity or are unable to be identified in an intubated or altered patient. Laboratory tests indicating muscle breakdown such as creatine kinase elevation are helpful to increase suspicion, but this is often a late finding and should not delay intervention. Measuring the delta pressure (ACS delta pressure = diastolic blood pressure – measured compartment pressure) is another tool to help direct management in patients with a difficult clinical exam. A delta pressure of greater than 30 mmHg serves as an objective finding in the diagnosis of ACS.

Compartment syndrome can occur in any location with enveloping fascia, with the most common locations being the lower leg and forearm. The diagnosis can be particularly challenging when the thigh, gluteal compartments, or upper extremity compartments are involved. The enveloping fascia is unyielding to increasing pressures, and this process will eventually compromise perfusion to the nerves within the compartments. This compartmental pressure will eventually compress micro- and macrovasculature and lead to distal ischemia. Appropriately timed fasciotomy

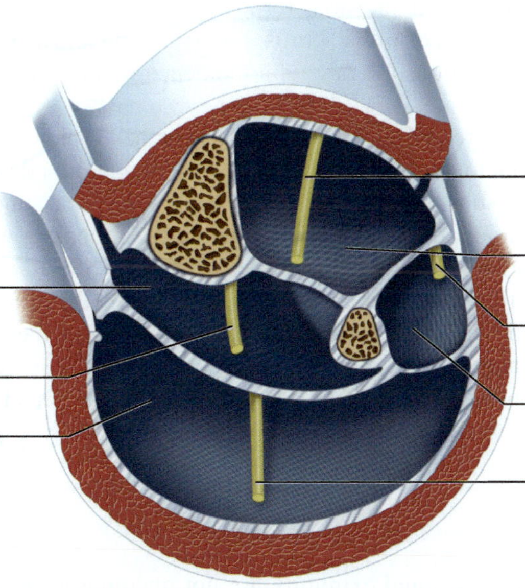

Fig. 14.1 Double incisions for lower extremity fasciotomy

is effective because it releases the enveloping fascia and decompresses the elevated compartment pressure, allowing muscle swelling and reversing compression of vessels allowing perfusion.

Lower Leg Compartment Syndrome

The lower leg consists of 4 compartments: anterior, lateral, superficial posterior, and deep posterior compartments. These compartments can be released through either a dual (medial and lateral) (Fig. 14.1) or single incision technique. The single incision is technically challenging to expose the deeper compartments but obviously has the advantage of a one lateral incision rather than two (medial and lateral).

Forearm Compartment Syndrome

The forearm, like the leg, consists of four distinct compartments. These include the dorsal, lateral, deep volar, and lateral volar compartments. Forearm fasciotomy is done by releasing volar compartment, dorsal compartment, and the mobile wad. The volar release is preferably done through an S-shaped incision on the volar aspect of the forearm starting about 1 cm from the medial condyle and may be extended down to the hand, taking care not to injure the palmar cutaneous branch of the median nerve (Fig. 14.2). It is also possible to decompress all 4 compartments with the volar incision, so evaluating the other compartments before making an extra incision is prudent.

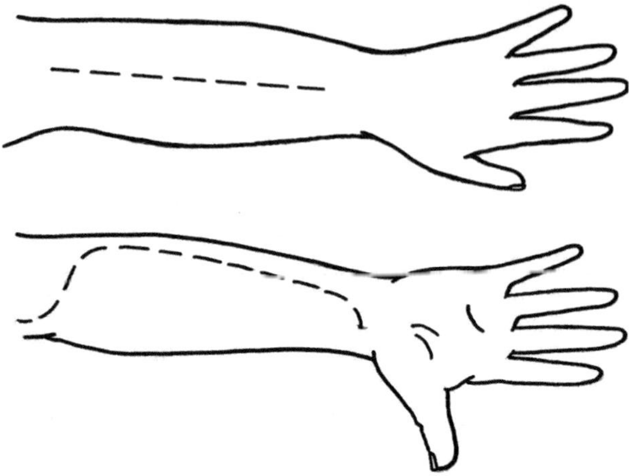

Fig. 14.2 Straight dorsal forearm incision and S-shaped volar incision

Conclusion

Vascular injuries of the operated extremity are not uncommon. Knowledge of the common patterns and presentations is helpful for early recognition and management. While associated most commonly with orthopedic procedures, an extremity vascular injury can occur during any extremity intervention. With new intravascular interventional technologies, complications will continue to arise. Being familiar and updated on these new technologies and the possible associated complications will help in early planning and mitigate any negative outcomes.

References

1. Mavrogenis AF, Panagopoulos GN, Kokkalis ZT, Koulouvaris P, Megaloikonomos PD, Igoumenou V, Mantas G, et al. Vascular injury in orthopedic trauma. Orthopedics. 2016;39(4):249–59. https://doi.org/10.3928/01477447-20160610-06.
2. Cooper C, Rodriguez A, Omert L. Blunt vascular trauma. Curr Probl Surg. 1992;29(5):281–357.
3. Rozycki GS, Tremblay LN, Feliciano DV, McClelland WB. Blunt vascular trauma in the extremity: diagnosis, management, and outcome. J Trauma. 2003;55(5):814–24. https://doi.org/10.1097/01.TA.0000087807.44105.AE.
4. Kootstra G, Schipper JJ, Boontje AH, Klasen HJ, Binnendijk B. Femoral shaft fracture with injury of the superficial femoral artery in civilian accidents. Surg Gynecol Obstet. 1976;142(3):399–403.
5. Feliciano DV, Moore FA, Moore EE, West MA, Davis JW, Cocanour CS, Kozar RA, McIntyre RC. Evaluation and management of peripheral vascular injury. Part 1. Western trauma association/critical decisions in trauma. J Trauma. 2011;70(6):1551–6. https://doi.org/10.1097/TA.0b013e31821b5bdd.
6. Graham JM, Mattox KL, Feliciano DV, DeBakey ME. Vascular injuries of the axilla. Ann Surg. 1982;195(2):232–8. https://doi.org/10.1097/00000658-198202000-00020.
7. Demetriades D, Chahwan S, Gomez H, Peng R, Velmahos G, Murray J, Asensio J, Bongard F. Penetrating injuries to the subclavian and axillary vessels. J Am Coll Surg. 1999;188(3):290–5. https://doi.org/10.1016/s1072-7515(98)00289-0.

8. Piffaretti G, Tozzi M, Lomazzi C, Rivolta N, Caronno R, Laganà D, Carrafiello G, Castelli P. Endovascular treatment for traumatic injuries of the peripheral arteries following blunt trauma. Injury. 2007;38(9):1091–7. https://doi.org/10.1016/j.injury.2007.02.044.
9. Ganapathy A, Khouqeer AF, Todd SR, Mills JL, Gilani R. Endovascular management for peripheral arterial trauma: the new norm? Injury. 2017;48(5):1025–30. https://doi.org/10.1016/j.injury.2017.02.002.
10. Asensio JA, Kuncir EJ, García-Núñez LM, Petrone P. Femoral vessel injuries: analysis of factors predictive of outcomes. J Am Coll Surg. 2006;203(4):512–20. https://doi.org/10.1016/j.jamcollsurg.2006.06.020.
11. Kaye J. A. Epidemiology of lower limb fractures in general practice in the United Kingdom. Injury Prevent. 2004;10(6):368–74. https://doi.org/10.1136/ip.2004.005843.
12. Halvorson JJ, Anz A, Langfitt M, Deonanan JK, Scott A, Teasdall RD, Carroll EA. Vascular injury associated with extremity trauma: initial diagnosis and management. J Am Acad Orthop Surg. 2011;19(8):495–504. https://doi.org/10.5435/00124635-201108000-00005.
13. Padberg FT, Rubelowsky JJ, Hernandez-Maldonado JJ, Milazzo V, Swan KG, Lee BC, Hobson RW. Infrapopliteal arterial injury: prompt revascularization affords optimal limb salvage. J Vasc Surg. 1992;16(6):877–85.; discussion 885–6. https://doi.org/10.1067/mva.1992.42019.
14. Allen MJ, Nash JR, Ioannidies TT, Bell PR. Major vascular injuries associated with orthopaedic injuries to the lower limb. Ann R Coll Surg Engl. 1984;66(2):101–4.
15. Wilson JS, Miranda A, Johnson BL, Shames ML, Back MR, Bandyk DF. Vascular injuries associated with elective orthopedic procedures. Ann Vasc Surg. 2003;17(6):641–4. https://doi.org/10.1007/s10016-003-0074-2.
16. Mills JL, Hallett JW. Minimizing mortality and morbidity from iatrogenic arterial injuries: the need for early recognition and prompt repair. J Vasc Surg. 1986;4(1):6.
17. Stannard A, Eliason JL, Rasmussen TE. Resuscitative Endovascular Balloon Occlusion of the Aorta (REBOA) as an adjunct for hemorrhagic shock. J Trauma. 2011;71(6):1869–72. https://doi.org/10.1097/TA.0b013e31823fe90c.
18. Joseph B, Zeeshan M, Sakran JV, Hamidi M, Kulvatunyou N, Khan M, O'Keeffe T, Rhee P. Nationwide analysis of resuscitative endovascular balloon occlusion of the aorta in civilian trauma. JAMA Surg. 2019;154(6):500. https://doi.org/10.1001/jamasurg.2019.0096.
19. Matsen FA. Compartmental syndrome. An unified concept. Clin Orthop Relat Res. 1975;113:8–14.
20. Papalambros EL, Panayiotopoulos YP, Bastounis E, Zavos G, Balas P. Prophylactic fasciotomy of the legs following acute arterial occlusion procedures. Int Angiol. 1989;8(3):120–4.
21. Abouezzi Z, Nassoura Z, Ivatury RR, Porter JM, Stahl WM. A critical reappraisal of indications for fasciotomy after extremity vascular trauma. Arch Surg (Chicago, Ill.: 1960). 1998;133(5):547–51. https://doi.org/10.1001/archsurg.133.5.547.

Interventional Alternatives for Vascular Injury

15

Ramyar Gilani

Introduction

Closed loop fluid circuits such as the cardiovascular system rely on structural integrity to maintain continuous fluid flow while harboring finite contents within a closed system. Vascular trauma often results in disruption of the structural architecture and leakage of contents requiring hemorrhage control and vessel repair. As with any fluid system, flow through the injured segment usually must be temporarily turned off to allow repair under direct vision. Only the most basic repair can be performed without interruption of flow through the segment to be repaired. As a result, the first order of business in vascular trauma is establishing flow interruption via proximal and distal control. Furthermore, given a finite volume of blood contained within the circulation, expeditious cessation of flow serves to maintain adequate system volume to allow for continued function within the remainder of the system while performing repair. Traditionally, vascular control has been established through open exposure and vessel clamping as well as tourniquet use in extreme conditions. Although very effective, these techniques can be suboptimal in circumstantial situations such as transition zones, re-operative fields, or patients in extremis (Fig. 15.1). Newer paradigms maintain principles of expeditious vessel control while overcoming such challenges by shifting focus from the immediate area of injury into a more controllable environment and utilizing the structural continuity of vessels to obtain access into proximity location and ultimately establishing flow control.

The pathophysiologic manifestations of vascular trauma, whether venous or arterial, often mandate acute surgical intervention. Furthermore, secondary sequelae can quickly spiral into multi-system derangements that call for a simple and expedient solution while mitigating impact to a patient with little remaining physiologic reserve. This characterization forms the impetus for application of endovascular

R. Gilani (✉)
Michael E. DeBakey Department of Surgery, Baylor College of Medicine, Houston, TX, USA
e-mail: rgilani@bcm.edu

R. Gilani, J. L. Mills Sr. (eds.), *Vascular Complications of Surgery and Intervention*, https://doi.org/10.1007/978-3-030-86713-3_15

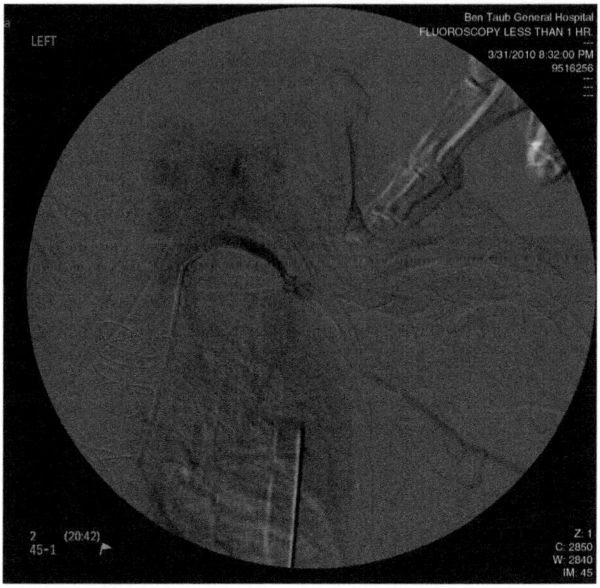

Fig. 15.1 Manual compression for hemorrhage control of left subclavian artery

surgery to acute care vascular surgery. Recent advances in technology have expanded application of intraluminal vascular solutions to an increasing variety of vascular conditions. Endovascular technologies allow for efficacious and safe interventions to occur at decreased overall impact to patients [1–5]. It should be no surprise that endovascular techniques are becoming increasingly utilized for acute care vascular dilemmas in patients who are often physiologically exhausted [6]. However, application of these technologies requires special skill sets to translate possibility into reality. Unfortunately, current trends in surgical practice demonstrate that few general or trauma surgeons possess adequate catheter-based skill sets. Furthermore, the number of open vascular operations performed during general surgical residency is steadily declining [7]. If these trends continue, the role for non-fellowship trained surgeons managing acute vascular conditions will be even further diminished.

The evolution of trauma care has fostered new requirements for operative, interventional, imaging and resuscitative capabilities. A “one-stop” for all patients is no longer possible as trauma patients often require resources throughout the geographic platform of most current institutions. The divergent locations of these resources exist in part because their increasing cost structure requires efficiency to maximize utilization, and therefore certain locational requirements are created. Often the local environments are developed under the conditions that occupy that resource for the greatest amount of time and therefore can be suboptimal to handle situations with additional stressors normally not present. The hospital power grid has not been designed to maximize efficiency during periods of maximal stress. Additionally, for circumstances in which patients require resources located in disparate locales and must be physically transported, significant logistical problems arise. The interface of patient, provider, and institution varies greatly among trauma centers, and no one solution is fit for overcoming all the possible challenges.

There is some feeling from critics that endovascular surgery is impractical and too costly from both a capital investment and inventory expenditure standpoint. In regard to capital, many endovascular procedures performed in the acute setting can be done so with existing equipment already present at most institutions (C-arm and fluoroscopy table). Although consumables in endovascular surgery can accrue significant expense, inventory required for acute care endovascular surgery need not be extravagant. As a testimony favoring endovascular technology, Rasmussen et al. reported their modern experience demonstrating the safety and efficacy of endovascular capability in the management of wartime injury [8]. Furthermore, they added that endovascular technology markedly expands capability in the management of the injured, and in certain circumstances is the preferred treatment. Having said this, endovascular surgery in its current state is not intended to replace traditional open surgical for acute care vascular surgery but rather be complementary as an alternative or as part of a hybrid procedure to the armamentarium of the modern-day acute care surgeon.

Technologies

The conduct of endovascular surgery is governed by general principles that are preserved regardless of procedure and ironically are in some ways comparable in concept to open vascular procedures. The foundation of endovascular surgery is built upon a platform consisting of over-the-wire techniques guided by live procedural imaging which is divergent from traditional surgery. However, parallels do exist in how endovascular and open surgical procedures are executed.

Access

All endovascular procedures by definition require the establishment of intravascular access much like open surgery requires an incision. Access sites are selected at points away from the location of intervention and where hemostasis can be ensured upon completion. Common points of arterial access are common femoral artery (CFA) (Fig. 15.2) and brachial artery because of underlying bony structures to ensure adequate compression for hemostasis. The need for manual compression against a bony landmark is less of a requirement for venous access. Once a site is selected and the vessel is cannulated, access is maintained by placing an access sheath which can be thought of as on on-ramp to the access vessel.

Catheters/Wires

After establishing access, the next step calls for dissection and visualization. In place of forceps and scissors for dissection and light for visualization, endovascular procedures use selective catheters and wires for dissection and most commonly

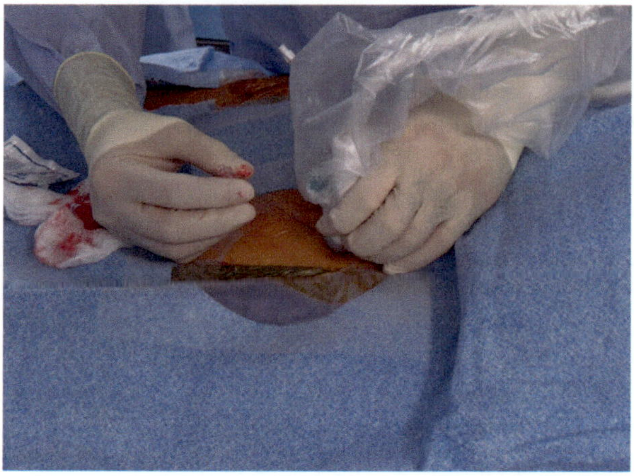

Fig. 15.2 Ultrasound guided access of left common femoral artery

fluoroscopy for visualization. Catheters are classified based on their shape, size, and length. There are many catheter shapes but all can be further classified into four categories: straight, single curved (gentle angles), double curved (acute angles), and reverse curved (reversing wire direction). Catheters are measured by the outer diameter (OD) in Fr which is different than sheaths and by the luminal diameter which indicates the corresponding wire diameter. Lengths and additional catheter properties are highly variable and are selected based on specific requirements.

Working through the lumen of the catheter is the guide wire. Angiographic wires can be characterized based on length, diameter, steerability, and stiffness. Various wire diameters exist, however most acute endovascular interventions can be performed with 0.035″ platforms and a few more with 0.014″ or 0.018″ wires. Among 0.035″ wires, there are varying degrees of steerability and support. Influencing the ability to steer a wire is the shape of the tip. Angle tip wires are able to engage branch vessel orifices, whereas straight or J-shaped tip wires are intended to follow the obtained lumen. Inversely related to steerability is stiffness. Stiffer wires are desired when increased wire support is required to maintain co-axial stability. Generally, a steerable wire is used to navigate and then exchanged for a stiffer wire to provide the stability needed to perform an intervention.

With the combination of wire and catheter working in unison, the vasculature is navigated from access point to site of intervention, all of this being performed under the watchful eye of fluoroscopy. Endovascular devices including catheters and wire have some radiopaque identification that allows for fluoroscopic visualization. At times during procedures, radiographic visualization of the vasculature for diagnosis and intervention planning is required and is achieved with contrast angiography.

Sheaths

During open surgical dissection, one would place and periodically re-adjust a fixed retractor to maintain the gained exposure. The endovascular corollary to a fixed retractor is a sheath. Sheaths are utilized to maintain established access into selected vessels and can be re-positioned as higher-order branch vessels are further selected. Sheaths are available in a multitude of lengths and sizes not to mention varied sheath properties. Sheath lengths are measured in cm. The diameter measurement is in Fr and refers to the inner diameter (ID). The reason for this difference in measuring of catheters and sheaths is to assist with catheter and sheath compatibility, i.e., a 5 Fr catheter will pass through a 5 Fr sheath.

Balloons/Stents/Coils

After making a diagnosis and obtaining access, it is time to perform an intervention. Rather than cut, sew, and tie, endovascular interventions can be thought of in terms of balloon, stent, and coil. Versatility of angiographic balloons goes beyond plaque dilation. The ability to obtain intraluminal vascular control especially in areas difficult to expose such as subclavian arteries (Fig. 15.3) or re-operative fields can't be overestimated. Furthermore, once control has been established, intervention can continue with endovascular techniques or can be converted to an open procedure as is the case for a ruptured aortic aneurysm, (Fig. 15.4) depending on case-related details.

In contrast to balloons, stents are almost always intended for therapeutic intervention. They are designed as balloon-expandable or self-expanding and constructed as bare-metal or covered with graft material and are available in any combination of those characteristics depending on intended use. Furthermore, stents are available in a wide array of sizes allowing for interventions ranging from coronary arteries to the aorta (Figs. 15.5 and 15.6). Covered stents are intended to quarantine blood flow

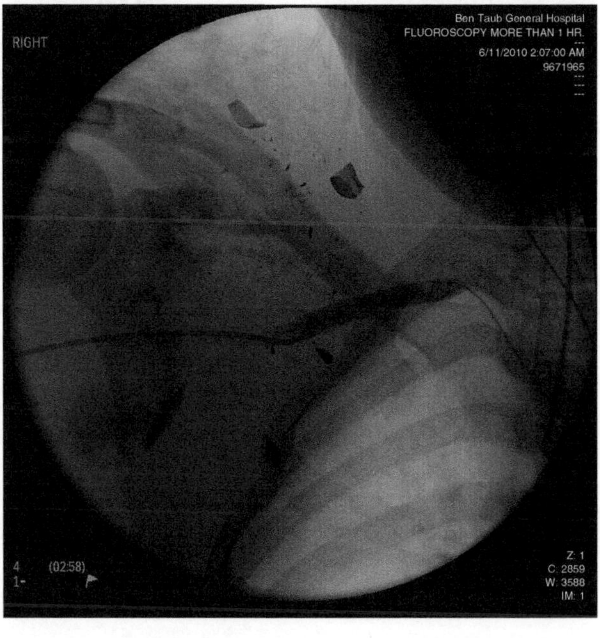

Fig. 15.3 Proximal balloon control for subclavian artery injury

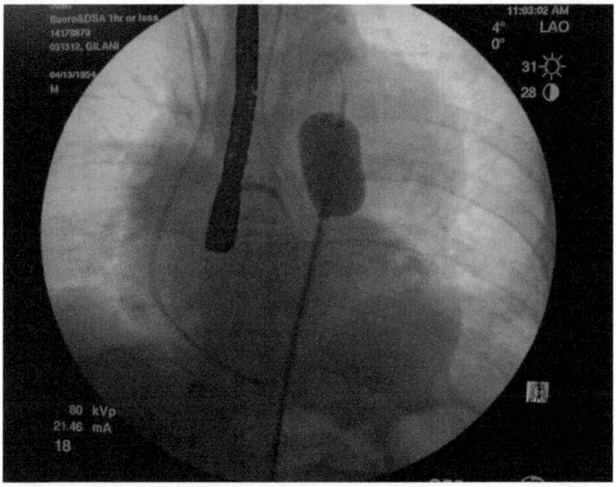

Fig. 15.4 Balloon deployment within the descending thoracic aorta

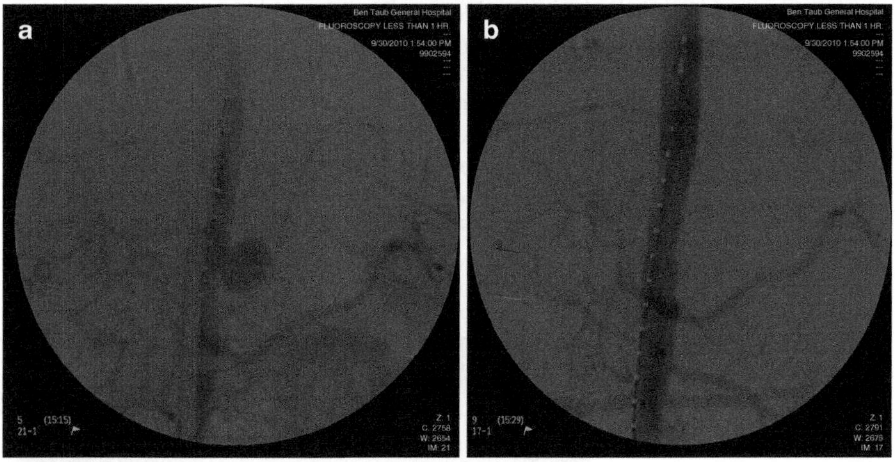

Fig. 15.5 Stent graft repair of descending aortic pseudoaneurysm. (**a**). Aortogram showing descending aortic pseudoaneurysm from penetrating wound (**b**). Completion angiogram of stent-graft graft repair for descending aortic pseudoaneurysm

away from an abnormal vessel such as an injury, an aneurysm, or an arteriovenous fistula, whereas bare-metal stents are designed to achieve or maintain luminal gain, as when treating a dissection or resistant plaque.

Surgical wisdom advises against "seek and destroy" methods for hemorrhage control from arteries of distribution such as hypogastric arteries (Fig. 15.7) and profunda femoris arteries. Uncontrolled bleeding from these vessels can create a difficult dilemma requiring directed hemorrhage control without causing additional collateral damage. A solution lies in the use of angiographic coils. These coils are

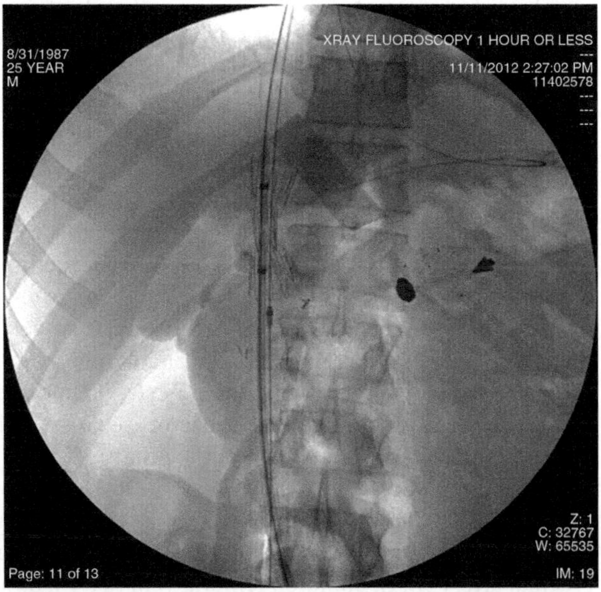

Fig. 15.6 Delivery and deployment of stent graft into inferior vena cava

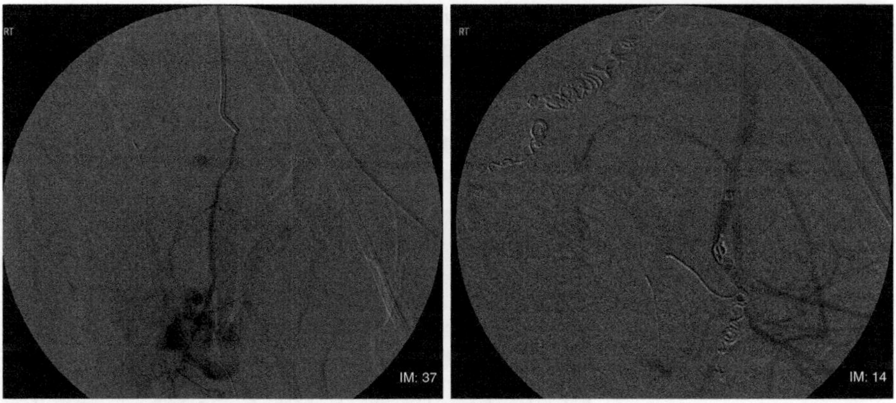

Fig. 15.7 Coil embolization for hypogastric artery hemorrhage control

constructed of various materials all of which are designed to stagnate blood flow and result in thrombosis. They can be directly delivered to the site of injury while minimizing damage and further thrombosis to adjacent structures and vessels.

Although very different in reality, conceptually endovascular surgery is guided by principles quite similar to those followed for open surgery, while offering different advantages as well as disadvantages. Despite potential for procedural complexity, endovascular basics are mostly conserved. These basics are purposefully kept simple and are intended to lay the groundwork of familiarity in an effort to bring awareness and possibility for endovascular application to acute vascular conditions.

Applications

Once it is determined that vessel control is required for hemorrhage or reconstruction, a decision must be made on how to proceed. While traditional open external vessel clamping remains a consideration, other methods exist and should be available to trauma surgeons. Although some of these techniques have been described for decades [9], the recent advent of endovascular surgery is creating a resurgence of interest in endoluminal control [10]. Endoluminal control is not synonymous with endovascular surgery; however there is significant interchangeability between the two terms. It is important to keep the terms separate as there are instances where one can be performed in the absence of the other.

Endoluminal control implies access to the lumen of a targeted vessel which is accomplished using a variety of techniques. Access can be established percutaneously using image guidance, for example, using the common femoral artery (CFA), brachial artery (BA), common femoral vein (CFV), or internal jugular vein (IJV), or it may be obtained open under direct vision using the iliac artery/vein, aorta, inferior vena cava (IVC). It is a preference of technique and skill set as well circumstantial as to what method to incorporate. As an example, a patient undergoing laparotomy with an IVC injury may be better suited for endoluminal control performed under direct vision where in the setting of a subclavian artery injury, a percutaneous image guided approach may be more feasible. Endoluminal control does not necessarily

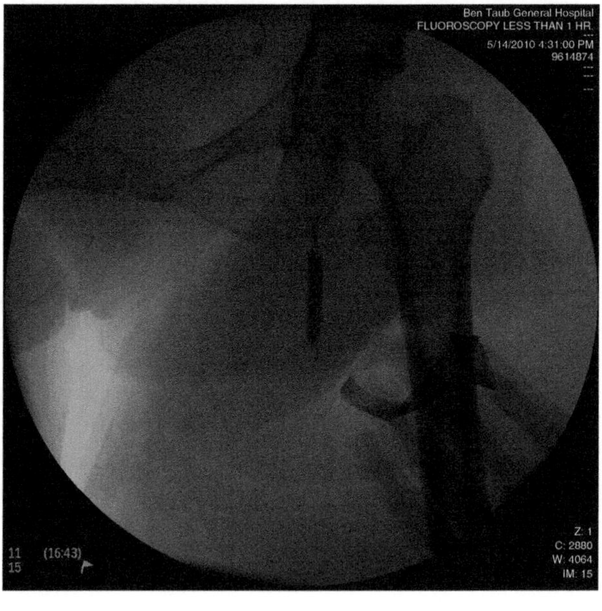

Fig. 15.8 Utilization of balloon control for superficial femoral artery injury while performing laparotomy

Table 15.1 Approximate artery sizes for balloon selection

Innominate – 10–14 mm
Carotid/subclavian/axillary – 8–10 mm
Common iliac – 8–10 mm
External iliac/common femoral – 6–8 mm
Superficial femoral/deep femoral – 5–7 mm
Aortic bifurcation – Bilateral common iliac balloons, Fogarty balloons or aortic occlusion balloon
Aorta – Aortic occlusion balloon

commit the operator to endovascular repair and can be effectively used in conjunction with open vessel reconstruction (Fig. 15.8).

Once appropriate access has been achieved, control is commonly obtained with the use of a balloon. A variety of balloons exist that are applicable in this setting such as angioplasty balloons, Foley catheters, Fogarty balloons, and aortic occlusion balloons. Balloons have a wide variety of properties that pertain not only to the balloon itself but also to its delivery and it is important to be facile with several in varying sizes (Table 15.1) so that any vessel in the body can be controlled either by an open or percutaneous approach. Vessel control can also be achieved via endoluminal delivery and deployment of a stent graft. A stent graft is comprised of traditional graft material supported by a stent exoskeleton. These devices function by quarantining blood within the fabric by proximal and distal seals opposing the vessel wall thereby sealing off the area of injury. These devices can also be introduced into position percutaneously with imaging or under direct vision and palpation. There use is increasing in vascular trauma [11] and their application is continuously expanding.

Temporary resuscitative occlusion in an effort to preserve systemic intravascular volume for continued perfusion of vital organs can also be performed via endoluminal techniques. Traditional open techniques such as emergency room thoracotomy often create additional incisions and are not without consequences [12]. Endoluminal control for resuscitation is not new in concept [13]; however its popularity has not been overwhelming despite theoretical advantages [14, 15]. Temporary occlusion of the thoracic or abdominal aorta is best performed utilizing imaging from a CFA approach either open through a cutdown or percutaneous. However in the setting of hemorrhage from a severe pelvic fracture, control of the distal aorta may be desirable [16] and can be readily performed without image guidance through bilateral CFA access and placement of appropriately sized Fogarty balloons through sheaths into the aorta and withdrawn to occlude the iliac orifice.

Techniques

It is difficult to imagine all the possibilities for endovascular solutions. However, understanding when traditional techniques may be challenging and being insightful in the pursuit of an endovascular approach is the first step to success. This begins the seemingly arbitrary but quite important process of preparation and mobilization before any intervention is initiated.

The first step is to obtain fluoroscopic capability along with a fluoroscopically compatible table. Furthermore, proper room configuration is dependent on access site and intervention site which then dictates position of the patient, table, and imaging assets. The patient is prepped and draped in anticipation of both an endovascular and open approach. Access is obtained through the selected access site, and navigation of the vasculature is performed. Obtaining diagnostic angiographic evidence further advances the status of intervention. The ability to achieve balloon control would mark a moment towards re-establishing control and correcting deranged physiology meanwhile recruiting more specialized personnel to proceed further.

These abilities would greatly facilitate expeditious progress towards an endovascular solution. It is not beyond the realm of ability for acute care surgeons to perform many of these tasks, especially obtaining access and temporary control of hemorrhage, but will require some experience in a step-wise approach. The goal should not be to become facile in endovascular surgery but rather to be willing and capable of performing definitive interventions in those crucial early moments in an effort to increase chances for successful clinical outcomes.

Summary

Endovascular (Open)

1. Access site (Incision)

↓

2. Catheter/Wire (Dissection)

↓

3. Fluoroscopy/Angiography (Exposure)

↓

4. Sheath (Self-retractor)

↓

5. Occlusion Balloon (Vascular clamps)

↓

6. Balloon/Stent/Coil (Cut/sew/tie)

Successful balloon occlusion can be thought of as a summation of a series of relatively simple, sequential maneuvers to perform that however do require some practice and attention to detail in order to avoid complications. Keep in mind that the procedure starts with patient positioning, requesting a C-arm and fluoroscopic bed and adequate prep to include the potential access sites. For most cases of balloon occlusion, the following sequence is followed at least in part until achieving control: access, vessel selection, sheath insertion, balloon delivery and inflation, and device removal.

Access

The most commonly used site for access is the CFA. Of course during the conduct of open surgery, any vessel large enough to accommodate the devices such as an iliac artery will suffice. The CFA can be accessed either percutaneously or via a cutdown. Ultrasound is very helpful here to find the CFA especially in a hypotensive patient and ensure that the CFA is cannulated rather than the iliac, deep femoral, or superficial femoral arteries. Problems with difficult access can be further mitigated with the use of a micropuncture set which uses a 0.018″ wire cannulation system which can be upsized to a 0.035″ wire system. The ultimate goal is to safely and accurately place at least a 5 Fr. sheath at the point of access. Completion of this step is similar to placing a fixed retractor for open surgery.

Vessel Selection

After placing the fixed retractor, it is now time to form some dissection. This is accomplished with a catheter and wire under image guidance. The aorta and virtually all of its first order branches can be selected with the use of single curve catheter (Bern) or a reverse curve catheter (VS1). Using the Bern catheter with a 0.035″ wire, repetitive motions of wire advancement and catheter advancement over the wire are performed under fluoroscopy until obtaining wire access into the descending thoracic aorta. At this point the dissection is complete and it is nearly time to insert the occlusion balloon.

Sheath Insertion

Aortic occlusion requires some special consideration and additional steps in comparison to other branch vessel occlusion. The hemostatic pressure within the aorta will exert a constant caudal force upon the inflated occlusion balloon. This can lead to caudal migration of the inflated balloon and loss of control. When attempting aortic balloon occlusion from below, additional axial columnar strength is necessary to provide support and prevent migration. This is accomplished by placing a sheath adequate in length to reach the zone of aortic occlusion and when properly performed the inflated balloon will rest upon the end of the sheath much like a sausage on a stick. The sheath must also be securely fixed to the skin to prevent the entire sheath-balloon combination from being dislodged. Also, balloons used for aortic occlusion have larger sheath requirements to accommodate larger aortic balloon profiles. Therefore, typical sheaths used for aortic occlusion from a CFA approach are 45–70 mm in length and range from 7 to 14 Fr. These sheaths are somewhat stiff and require additional wire support as they are introduced. Once the catheter is in place, a wire exchange is performed for a stiffer wire. The sheath can now be inserted into position and the dilator removed. When removing the dilator, it is important for someone to maintain the position of the sheath while another removes the dilator over the wire taking care to pin and pull so that the wire is not inadvertently removed.

Balloon Delivery and Inflation

With the lumen of the sheath now open, the next step is to introduce the balloon over the wire and bring it into the desired location. Under image guidance, one can see a radio-opaque marker on the end of most sheaths. The occlusion balloon will also have a pair of markers indicating the proximal and distal extents of the balloon. The proximal balloon marker should extend just beyond the marker on the sheath. Once this is accomplished, the balloon can be inflated. Balloon inflation is performed by attaching an appropriate size lure lock syringe filled with ½ contrast and ½ saline to the balloon port. The balloon is rapidly inflated to profile to occlude the target vessel and then the stopcock on the balloon port is closed. Once it appears the balloon is opposed to the vessel wall, further inflation of the balloon can lead to rupture and is not advised. Also, as the balloon is being inflated, some caudal migration may occur until the balloon engages the sheath and becomes supported. However, if too much migration occurs, the balloon must be deflated, the sheath and balloon advanced more cephalad and the balloon can be inflated once again. As a preventive maneuver, forward pressure should be applied to the sheath as the balloon is being inflated.

Device Removal

Once occlusion is no longer required, the final step is to remove the balloon, wire, and sheath. The balloon is completely deflated and removed over the wire. If wire access is longer needed, this can also be removed, and focus is turned towards sheath removal. For smaller sheaths (5–8 Fr.) used for branch vessel occlusion, the devices can often be simply removed and hemostasis achieved with manual pressure. However, the larger sheaths utilized for aortic occlusion will require more than manual pressure for successful hemostasis. If one has the ability and anticipates the use of a larger size sheath, a closure device can be placed prior to insertion of the larger sheath and used to control the arteriotomy upon completion. As an alternative for those not facile with closure devices, the large sheath is best removed after surgical exposure of the CFA. The sheath is removed only after the vessel is controlled proximally and distally. After sheath removal, the arteriotomy is repaired with interrupted 6–0 Prolene suture, taking care to perform appropriate flushing maneuvers prior to completing the repair.

Organizational Framework

Patient Needs

Severely injured trauma patients place great demand on providers and institutions; however, injuries occur in patterns and are somewhat constant and predictable. Trauma patients largely succumb to head injury and hemorrhage early on in their course. As a result, it is understood that trauma patients will need transfusion, imaging, surgery, critical care, etc. to manage such injuries. In addition care is expected to be provided expeditiously often without warning. Currently, the biggest drivers of conundrum for trauma patients and their movement are diagnostic and imaging requirements. In the era prior, it was generally accepted that injured patients were to be taken to operating theater for a "seek and destroy" mission. Then it became recognized that alternative diagnostic modalities could provide a more narrowed approach in a timely fashion and if allowable became preferred prior to operation. Moving beyond diagnosis, imaging could now help to decrease the undesirable impact of interventions, and, as a result, image-guided interventions are a big driver for trauma patient logistics. Given that the unpredictable is predictable, significant time should be utilized to evaluate trauma patient needs and generate a custom platform within a trauma center bringing together the combined strengths of providers and resources intended to meet the anticipated needs of trauma patients.

Provider Strengths

Provider capability varies greatly and is not indicative of skill level but rather is a function of training, practice pattern, interest, and needs of patients encountered. Because trauma patients have a predictably wide range of needs based on their injuries, often multiple providers with different capability are called into the care of patient. Generally speaking, providers prefer to practice in an environment that is familiar and designed to harness the impact of their efforts. Providers are a readily mobile and flexible resource and in comparison to fixed assets within a hospital are much more readily modified. Therefore inability to bring providers into interaction with patients because of geographic barriers should not be a limiting force to providing care. They should be willing to interact and provide a skill set to patient care regardless of where a patient is located. This may not be possible due to institutional resource limitations; however this should not be a provider issue. Also, providers are mostly willing and able to acquire additional skills necessary to care for patients through collaboration, especially when the need arises. On the contrary, providers are largely limited by their own perception and bias about new directions for trauma care. This is best countered through open objective dialogue among providers at local, national, and international forums.

Institutional Resources

The institutional resources that enter into the care of trauma resources are the largest and most variable component of the patient, provider, and institution formula. They are also often the most difficult to change but adequate care cannot be delivered without the most basic of resources. This is due to several important factors. First medical care has increasingly turned to sub-specialization and with it the increasingly narrowing focus within each unit. As each unit becomes increasingly specialized, the necessary resources have decreasing cross over into other specialties. This generates a conundrum of efficiency and possibility for hospitals. Although "anything is possible," in reality, not everything is achievable; therefore institutions must make decisions on resources that meet a certain threshold of need. However, by far the single biggest driver of institutional resource is cost. Within today's medical expenditure environment, this has become a make or break phenomenon. If utilization is not properly demonstrated and cost not justified assuming that funds are even available, resources will not make it to fruition. Imaging and interventional assets are a prime example of such a resource. They are incredibly costly. They may not always be maximally utilized. They create certain inefficiencies within hospital systems as they are incredibly specialized. They require dedicated teams, equipment, and support staff. Nonetheless, from a clinical perspective, they do offer incredible capability that in many ways provides improved care for trauma patients. Therefore, if the drawbacks can be mitigated through creative custom solutions for individual institutions then such resources become reality. The truth is that not all resources are possible but some are and it is imperative upon providers of care for trauma patients to be involved with such deliberations.

The Ideal

When discussing arenas for patient care two distinct terms surface: OR and IR, followed by a third more nebulous concept often referred to as Hybrid OR. The operating room (OR) has been the mainstay of trauma care basically since inception. Without a doubt, the OR provides tremendous capability in the care of trauma patients, particularly for head injury and hemorrhage. The OR as we know it in its true form does have certain limitations. It can be very sluggish to respond and react. Processes have to be thought out in great detail in advance before they can be implemented. This works well for planned elective operations, but in a time constrained situation, requesting even the most basic addition can be a real logistical mess. Second it is blind. This is to say that the ability to gather additional information during operation is basically limited by what one can see. This requires larger incisions, opening additional body cavities, etc. which can be harmful.

The antinode to the OR is the interventional suite. On the contrary, it is quick to react allowing for change in direction during procedures. It allows for gathering of additional information through alternative diagnostic modalities. However it is limited in scope and capability. Typically only one active issue is addressed at any given time. Secondly it is difficult to concurrently address ongoing needs for other problems.

The solution to each theater remains somewhere in between: a hybrid, meaning at times the ideal entity may be more like an OR and at other times more closely resemble an IR suite. It allows for angiography, endoscopy, intra-cranial imaging, and intra-vascular imaging. It would allow simultaneous operating, while resuscitation occurs. It must be flexible, such that when not in use for trauma care, it can be allocated for other uses. It would have crossover capability, meaning that it can function anywhere on the spectrum between operating room and interventional suite at any given time during operation. What does a Hybrid OR look like? It does not have to be what most would consider a hybrid OR but can be constructed out of the following elements at significantly reduced cost:

- Angiographic floating table.
- C-arm unit.
- Endovascular consumables.
- Vascular implants.
- Intravascular ultrasound.
- Laparoscopy.
- GI endoscopy.
- Aero endoscopy.
- Mobile ultrasound.
- General anesthesia capability.
- Massive transfusion.

Horizon Technologies

Imaging will continue to drive the evolution of the Hybrid OR in the near future. Currently, axial intra-cavitary imaging can be performed but remains cumbersome and sluggish. Furthermore, the cost of required machinery will likely be prohibitive for most centers. However, as has been true with most technologic advancements, cost decreases and capability increases over time. Therefore, a real practical solution for trauma care is likely on the horizon. This will markedly increase the information gathering ability in the OR especially for head trauma and additionally, open the door for alternative therapies for intra-cavitary injury. However solutions are only possible if providers can begin to imagine what is possible. Those who welcome technological advancement and place aside personal bias will benefit from what the future holds and those who fail to do so will continue to languish in what the past has offered.

Summary

- Hemorrhage and its subsequent sequelae are unintended but certain consequences of vascular injury.
- Obtaining control of vascular injury to stop hemorrhage and achieve repair is paramount and can be difficult with traditional techniques in certain settings such as infection, re-operative field, and anatomic transition zones.
- Endoluminal strategies offer an alternative spectrum of solutions for vascular control when traditional techniques are fraught with challenge.
- Anticipation and preparation for what is possible to be encountered and what will be required are essential to bring alternative strategies to fruition.

References

1. Barlow B, Rottenberg RW, Santulli TV. Angiographic diagnosis and treatment of bleeding by selective embolization following pelvic fracture in children. J Pediatr Surg. 1975;10:939–42.
2. Ouriel K, Veith FJ, Sasahara AA. A comparison of recombinant urokinase with vascular surgery as initial treatment for acute arterial occlusion of the legs. Thrombolysis or Peripheral Arterial Surgery (TOPAS) Investigators. N Engl J Med. 1998;338(16):1105–11.
3. Veith FJ, Ohki T, Lipsitz EC, Suggs WD, Cynamon J. Treatment of ruptured abdominal aneurysms with stent grafts: a new gold standard? Semin Vasc Surg. 2003;16(2):171–5.
4. White R, Krajcer Z, Johnson M, Williams D, Bacharach M, O'Malley E. Results of a multicenter trial for the treatment of traumatic vascular injury with a covered stent. J Trauma. 2006;60:1189–96.
5. Demetriades D, American Association for the Surgery of Trauma Thoracic Aortic Injury Study Group, et al. Operative repair or endovascular stent graft in blunt traumatic thoracic aortic injuries: results of an American Association for the Surgery of Trauma Multicenter study. J Trauma. 2008;64:561–70.
6. Reuben BC, Whitten MG, Sarfati M, Kraiss LW. Increasing use of endovascular therapy in acute arterial injuries: analysis of the National Trauma Data Bank. J Vasc Surg. 2007;46(6):1222–6.
7. Burkhardt GE, Rasmussen TE, Propper BW, Lopez PL, Gifford SM, Clouse WD. A national survey of evolving management patterns for vascular injury. J Surg Educ. 2009;66(5):239–47.

8. Rasmussen TE, Clouse WD, Peck MA, Bowser AN, Eliason JL, Cox MW, Woodward EB, Jones WT, Jenkins DH. Development and implementation of endovascular capabilities in wartime. J Trauma. 2008;64(5):1169–76. discussion 1176
9. Hughes CW. Use of an intra-aortic balloon catheter tamponade for controlling intraabdominal hemorrhage in man. Surgery. 1954;36:65–8.
10. Stannard A, Eliason JL, Rasmussen TE. Resuscitative Endovascular Balloon Occlusion of the Aorta (REBOA) as an adjunct for Hemorrhagic shock. J Trauma. 2011;71(6):1869–72.
11. White R, Krajcer Z, Johnson M, Williams D, Bacharach M, O'Malley E. Results of a multicenter trial for the treatment of traumatic vascular injury with a covered stent. J Trauma. 2006;60(6):1189–95. discussion 1195–6
12. Feliciano DV, Bitondo CG, Cruse PA, Mattox KL, Burch JM, Beall AC Jr, Jordan GL Jr. Liberal use of emergency center thoracotomy. Am J Surg. 1986;152(6):654–9.
13. Gupta BK, Khaneja SC, Flores L, Eastlick L, Longmore W, Shaftan GW. The role of intra-aortic balloon occlusion in penetrating abdominal trauma. J Trauma. 1989;29:861–5.
14. White JM, Cannon JW, Stannard A, Markov NP, Spencer JR, Rasmussen TE. Endovascular balloon occlusion of the aorta is superior to resuscitative thoracotomy with aortic clamping in a porcine model of hemorrhagic shock. Surgery. 2011;150:400–9.
15. Avaro JP, Mardelle V, Roch A, et al. Forty-minute endovascular aortic occlusion increases survival in an experimental model of uncontrolled hemorrhagic shock caused by abdominal trauma. J Trauma. 2011;71:720–5.
16. Martinelli T, Thony F, Declety P, et al. Intra-aortic balloon occlusion to salvage patients with life threatening hemorrhagic shock from pelvic fractures. J Trauma. 2010;68:942–8.

Part IV

Delayed

Dreaded Late Complications: Infection, Blowout, Pseudoaneurysm, Fistula

16

Zachary S. Pallister and Courtney Grant

Introduction

Late complications are an unfortunate but inevitable part of vascular surgery. These complications arise due to a number of complex pathophysiologic conditions. Infection plagues vascular reconstructions, especially with the use of prosthetic graft materials. Additionally, pseudoaneurysm, anastomotic aneurysms, and frank anastomotic blowout can occur at any time following vascular reconstruction. Aortoenteric fistula formation is also a dreaded complication of aortic reconstruction. Finally, lymphocele development and its associated complications can cause disastrous complications following open vascular surgery. All of these dreaded late complications require careful consideration, diagnosis, understanding of the disease process, and treatment. This chapter will discuss the etiology, diagnosis, pathophysiology, and treatment of these aforementioned complications.

Infection (Surgical Site Infection, Prosthetic Graft Infection)

A vascular surgical site infection (SSI) can range from a simple superficial wound infection to a deep wound or devastating prosthetic graft infection. Graft infections significantly increase the risks of graft failure, limb loss, and mortality. While standard treatment is graft excision and replacement via extra-anatomic bypass, methods such as in situ reconstruction and graft preservation have become increasingly accepted alternatives. Given the variety of treatment options available, the approach to managing graft infections must be individualized to each patient for an optimal

Z. S. Pallister (✉) · C. Grant
Division of Vascular and Endovascular Therapy, Michael E DeBakey Department of Surgery, Baylor College of Medicine, Houston, TX, USA
e-mail: zspallis@bcm.edu

R. Gilani, J. L. Mills Sr. (eds.), *Vascular Complications of Surgery and Intervention*, https://doi.org/10.1007/978-3-030-86713-3_16

outcome. This section reviews interventions for the management and prevention of prosthetic graft infection.

Incidence

The incidence of surgical site infection after vascular procedures ranges from 5% to 10% [1]. Peripheral artery bypass procedures have the highest reported rate of infection ranging widely between 3% and 44% with the groin being the most common site of infection [2–4]. Vascular SSI can range from superficial cellulitis, to subcutaneous tissue infection, to involvement of the vascular graft itself. These levels of infection are graded I–III respectively according to the Szilagyi classification [5]. The most dreaded SSI is graft infection which occurs in up to 15% of vascular reconstructions with incidence differing based on location [6]. This incidence is highest in the presence of groin incisions for lower extremity bypass procedures, up to 10.6%, and lowest for aortoiliac grafts ranging from 0.6% to 5% [2, 7–9]. Endovascular device infections are rare with incidence ranging from 0.1% to 1.2% [9, 10].

Vascular procedures are at greater risk of infection than typical clean procedures given a set of unique factors after arterial reconstruction that impede wound healing. These include edema, subsequent superficial wound separation, underlying hematoma or seroma formation, disrupted lymphatics, and non-healing wounds that can all lead to bacterial invasion [1]. Independent predictors of SSI after vascular lower extremity reconstructions include obesity, antiplatelet medication, and previous vascular surgery, particularly for aneurysmal disease and implantation of prosthetic conduits, dialysis dependence, hypertension, intraoperative thrombosis, prolonged operative time, high peak intraoperative glucose, and surgery performed at a larger hospitals or major teaching centers [2, 11].

Pathophysiology

Graft infections can be caused by intraoperative contamination via direct contamination by skin and soft tissue, extension of intra-abdominal infection, communication with the gastrointestinal or genitourinary tract, and graft seeding during episodes of bacteremia.

At the time of surgery, contamination can occur from poor handling of the graft and contamination with skin flora, the source of bacteria in most SSIs [12]. In addition, lymphatics and sweat glands in the groin and plaque and thrombus within vessels can all harbor bacteria. Direct communication with the gastrointestinal tract, such as aortoenteric erosions or fistulas, is uncommon, occurring in 1–2% after open aortic reconstruction. However, they account for up to 25% of endograft infections at time of presentation and will be discussed in further detail in a subsequent section [13, 14]. Extensions from intra-abdominal infections such as diverticulitis or appendicitis are limited to isolated case reports. Bacteremia or hematogenous spread of bacteria from distant sites of infection to grafts is rare, and it is often difficult to prove which infection came first. Transient bacteremia from colonoscopy or dental procedures may be a potential cause for late infection but evidence is also limited to case reports.

Microbiology

The most common isolated organisms in graft and endograft infections are gram-positive *Staphylococcus* species, including *S. aureus* and *S. epidermidis*, and the gram-negative organism *Pseudomonas aeruginosa* [1, 5, 15–17].

Early infections, occurring within the first 4–6 months, are most likely due to common gram-positive skin contaminants such as *S. aureus* and *Streptococcus* [11, 14, 17]. However, late graft infections are caused mostly by insidious, slow growing, low virulence organisms. The most commonly reported is *S. epidermidis*. These particular bacteria can be present in grafts for extended periods of time without overt evidence of gross infection or positive wound cultures due to production of a protective biofilm. Cultures of prosthetic graft infections may be negative in up to 40% of cases [9, 14–16]. Gram-negative bacteria are involved in approximately a quarter of vascular SSI and most commonly include *E. coli*, *Pseudomonas*, and *Proteus* species [18]. Gram-negative bacteremia in the presence of aortic graft infection should raise suspicion for aortoenteric erosion [1, 9].

Graft material does not appear to affect outcome of infection as much as the organism itself. In a study comparing inoculation of PTFE and vein grafts with low virulent *S. epidermidis* and high virulent *Pseudomonas*, Geary et al. found the virulent *P. aeruginosa* to cause anastomotic disruption in both graft types without discrimination [19].

Clinical Presentation

Diagnosis of infection begins with clinical presentation and physical examination, which varies depending on the graft location, organism, and timing of the infection. Early infections are defined as onset within the first 4–6 months postoperatively and are typically caused by more virulent, gram-negative bacteria [15]. Early peripheral infections tend to present with overt signs of high-grade infection such as drainage, dehiscence, or an abscess (Fig. 16.1), with or without systemic response [11], and have been associated with higher rates of bleeding from anastomotic disruption due to proteolytic characteristics of the more virulent bacteria [19]. Late, or delayed, infections typically present after the first year. Because they tend to be caused by more indolent organisms, they have a more insidious onset and may be more difficult to diagnose. Patients may lack systemic symptoms such as fever or sepsis, but rather may present with more nonspecific symptoms such as general malaise.

When there is concern for infection, wounds should be examined for surrounding cellulitis, drainage, and tenderness to palpation. These are signs of superficial

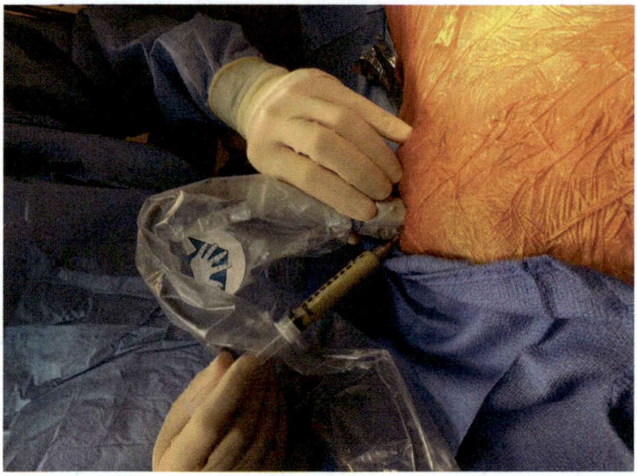

Fig. 16.1 Groin aspiration suggestive of underlying graft infection

wound infections but could also be signs of underlying graft infection. Pain and tenderness over a graft site with a sinus tract and drainage is the most common presentation for graft infection in the groin. Pseudoaneurysms and anastomotic bleeding should be assumed to be due to infection, as up to 60% of involved grafts are found to be culture positive [20]. Anastomotic pseudoaneurysm and blowout are discussed in detail in a subsequent section. Any exposed graft is considered infected.

Aortoiliac graft infections are not as clinically evident as lower extremity graft infections. Symptoms are less focal, and patients may complain of generalized malaise or dull abdominal or back pain. The most severe presentations consist of anastomotic bleeding, GI hemorrhage from aortoenteric erosion or fistula, and even septic emboli to the lower extremities [21]. Stent graft infections most commonly present with pain, fevers, and leukocytosis, with complaints of weight loss, fatigue, and generalized weakness in around 30% of cases [10, 17]. However, over a quarter have been found to present with aortic fistulas and endoleaks and 11% with rupture in a recent multi-institutional study [14]. A small number of aortoiliac graft infections are asymptomatic and found incidentally on routine follow-up imaging in a reported 5–10% of cases [10, 14].

Diagnosis

Diagnosis of prosthetic graft infection requires at least two of the following: (1) positive microbiological culture, (2) clinical or intraoperative signs of infection, (3) or radiologic evidence of graft infection with exclusion of other likely sources of infection [15].

Imaging can help establish the diagnosis and determine the extent of graft infection and involvement. Ultrasound is particularly useful in the extremity and often suggests infection with findings of perigraft fluid and pseudoaneurysms. Computed tomography (CT) is the most common initial study to evaluate for graft infection

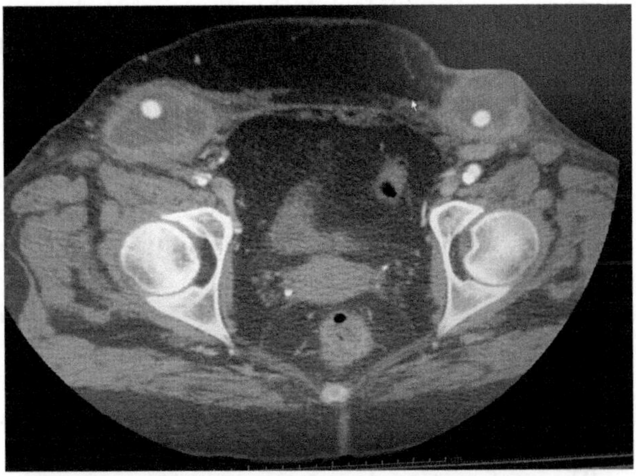

Fig. 16.2 CT scan showing infected femoral-femoral prosthetic bypass

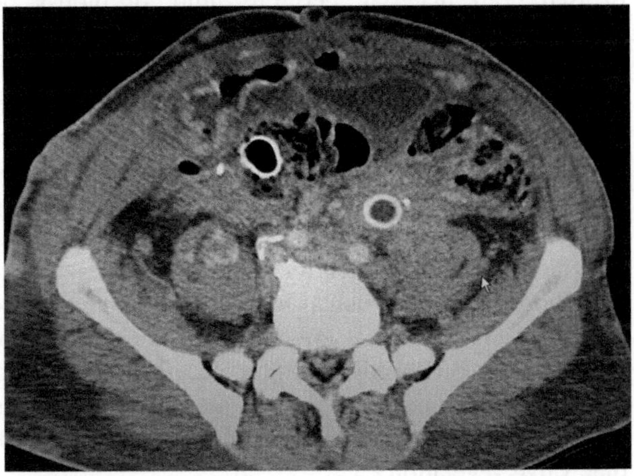

Fig. 16.3 CT scan showing graft limb within the colon lumen and surrounding inflammatory changes

with a reported sensitivity of 67–92% in published studies [7, 17]. Signs of graft infection on CT include perigraft fluid, gas, surrounding soft tissue stranding or inflammation, and pseudoaneurysm development (Figs. 16.2 and 16.3). However, one must keep in mind that perigraft air may persist for up to 2 months and fluid up to 3 months after surgery and thus should not be considered pathognomonic within this time frame [20]. Nuclear medicine studies can suggest the presence of infection, especially when there is clinical uncertainty. Leukocyte scintigraphy, or tagged white blood cell scan (TWBCS), uses a radioisotope to detect leukocytes involved in infection or inflammation and can identify 90% of graft infections. With a lower specificity of 82% there is some risk of false negatives, but fewer than CT scan alone [7]. 18-fluorine-fluorodeoxyglucose positron emission tomography (18F-FDG PET) uses a radioactive glucose isotope to detect the high glucose utilization of activated leukocytes in areas of infection and inflammation. Meta-analyses show focal uptake of glucose to have a sensitivity and specificity up to 97% and 89% [6,

7]. One concern with both leukocyte scintigraphy and PET is detection of inflammation which may or may not be associated with infection. Thus, performing these studies within the first 2–3 months after surgery may lead to false positives due to normal postoperative inflammation or uninvolved infections in the vicinity of the graft. Combining PET and TWBCS with CT, however, reportedly increases diagnostic accuracy by enabling differentiation between graft and soft tissue infection, making PET/CT and WBC SPECT/CT more favorable than CT imaging alone [6, 7]. The disadvantage is limited accessibility to these types of imaging in many institutions. MRI findings of graft infection include a high intensity signal surrounding the graft in T2-weighted imaging and have been described as being more accurate in detecting small fluid collections from staphylococcal epidermidis infections [20]. Angiography is not typically useful unless delineating unclear anatomy. When acute GI bleeding is involved or there is suspicion for aortoenteric fistula, endoscopy is recommended.

The confirmatory diagnostic study for graft infection is a direct culture from excised graft material, perigraft fluid, or biopsy of surrounding deep tissue. Superficial wound swabs are discouraged due to high risk of skin flora contamination. Intraoperative cultures during exploration and graft assessment are imperative, especially in cases of vague presentations or negative imaging studies with high clinical suspicion. Intraoperative findings of graft infection include the presence of perigraft fluid, gross purulence, and lack of graft incorporation. It is important to note that despite these findings, cultures can still be negative in the case of biofilm producing organisms such as *S. epidermidis*, which requires culture in chocolate agar media to reliably identify.

Laboratory values such as leukocytosis and increased inflammatory markers can raise suspicion for graft infection, but are not diagnostic and may be normal in occult cases. CRP, ESR, and procalcitonin are all studies used as adjunctive evidence of infection, although they are notoriously nonspecific. Blood cultures are commonly negative; however, when positive, they should prompt evaluation for cardiac valve vegetation.

Treatment

The primary principle for surgical infection treatment is source control and culture-based antibiotic therapy. With the exception of superficial skin infections, antibiotic therapy alone is largely inadequate. Deep wound infections and large lymphoceles at risk of infection require exploration, with cultures obtained from surrounding tissue, fluid, or graft material itself, followed by extensive lavage and debridement. For prosthetic graft infection, the gold standard treatment is complete graft or endograft excision. When graft removal is determined to be likely to result in limb or life-threatening ischemia, then reconstruction must be performed either by extra-anatomic bypass followed by graft excision or alternatively in situ reconstruction. In appropriately selected peripheral cases, wound exploration with graft preservation and wound sterilization is feasible. Overall, the approach to the management of infected prosthetic grafts is largely patient specific and depends on the location, extent, and timing of infection, as well as the type of graft and organism involved.

When there is extensive contamination of the graft with gross purulence and revascularization is required, extra-anatomic bypass to avoid reconstruction in an infected field is generally recommended. In peripheral bypasses, commonly described routes include lateral bypass of the groin and obturator bypass. Aortoiliac routes include most commonly the axillobifemoral bypass to the common femoral artery. In the case of groin infection, alternative distal anastomosis sites such as the profunda femoris or superficial femoral arteries via a lateral approach are considered. Obturator canal aorta to femoral artery bypasses serve as an alternative extra-anatomic bypass with improved patency compared to axillofemoral bypass [22]. If immediate revascularization is required, reconstruction can be performed simultaneously or staged with bypass construction followed by excision of the infected graft in stable patients. This occurs ideally 2–3 days later but depends on the patient's condition and the urgency of graft removal [23]. In cases of hemorrhage or gastroenteric communication, simultaneous reconstruction is necessary. It is imperative that the wound bed is aggressively debrided and, for aortic stumps, that the closure be doubly oversewn and covered with an omental flap to prevent subsequent infection and rupture. Overall, extra-anatomic bypasses, particularly in aortic infections, have been shown to have significant morbidity with rates of aortic stump rupture up to 20%, reinfection up to 15%, and poor primary patency rates as low as 64% at 5 years [9, 17, 21, 23, 24]. For this reason, in situ reconstruction has become increasingly utilized and preferred when possible.

In situ replacement of infected grafts has superior outcomes with patency rates as high as 97% at 5 years and lower rates of limb loss and reinfection depending on the chosen conduit [8]. This technique is mostly recommended in complex reconstruction cases associated with minimal contamination and lower virulence organisms. If pursued, the graft must be totally excised, including anastomotic sites and the wound bed aggressively debrided. Partial graft excision can be considered when the infection is confined to a focal segment not involving the anastomoses, leaving uninvolved graft left behind; however, outcomes tend to be inferior [25]. The optimal conduit for in situ graft replacement is debated. Options include autologous vein, cryopreserved allografts, and antibiotic bonded prosthetic grafts. In peripheral reconstruction, including hemodialysis access, bioprosthetic conduits have excellent patency with low reinfection risk [26].

Autologous saphenous, femoropopliteal, and less commonly iliac veins are used for reconstruction. Vein conduits have the lowest rate of reinfection (1–2%) and late mortality (30–50%). They also have the highest primary patency, up to 91% in aortic reconstructions [8, 20]. This makes them ideal in stable patients with excessive gross contamination and more virulent organisms [21]. Use of femoral vein (Fig. 16.4) for NeoaortoIliac System (NAIS) reconstruction has been described by some as the standard of care for aortic graft infections and is the recommended reconstruction in stable patients [20, 27]. Venous reconstructions do however have disadvantages. Harvesting lengthens operative time, limiting use to stable patients. Rates of reintervention are high with reported rupture risk of 5%, and femoral vein

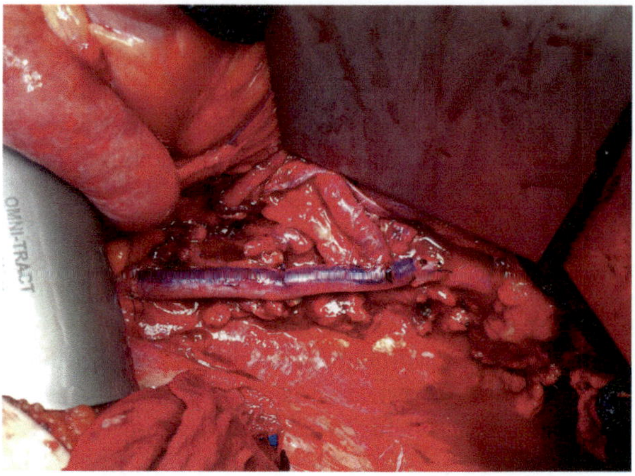

Fig. 16.4 Femoral vein conduit for infected aorta-femoral bypass reconstruction

harvesting includes risk of postoperative fasciotomy (12%) and chronic venous insufficiency (15%) [20, 21, 24].

Cryopreserved allografts have emerged as a frequently used option, with positive outcomes close to those using autologous vein grafts, specifically low reinfection (3–4%), similar rupture and mortality rates, and high primary patency of 93–97% at 5 years [8, 9, 25]. They are recommended in cases of minimal contamination and have the benefit of avoiding the morbidity of vein harvesting and decreasing operative time, each of which is advantageous in unstable patients. Disadvantages, however, include high rates of degeneration, cost, and limited availability [9, 25].

Antibiotic-bonded grafts have been studied with mixed results and most have been performed in animals. When studied in vivo, patency rates of rifampin bonded Dacron grafts rival both autologous and cryopreserved grafts with primary patency of 93% at 5 years and late mortality of 40–50% [21]. Reinfection rates have been reported to be as high as 4–11.5%, associated mostly with highly virulent and antibiotic-resistant organisms [8, 18, 21]. Reinfection risk is decreased when combined with tissue coverage of the graft [17]. Antibiotic-impregnated grafts have been described most successfully in elective cases with minimal to no gross contamination, and low virulence organisms [18, 21], especially in localized peripheral infections. Silver-coated grafts have also been described but reports are limited. While primary patency rates were 93% at 32 months with the benefit of not contributing to increasing antibiotic resistance, these grafts were associated with the highest reinfection rate up to 15.7% [8, 9]. Current guidelines only recommend the use of antibiotic or silver impregnated grafts in unstable patients needing immediate reconstruction [27].

Irrespective of conduit type, meta-analyses have shown overall graft failure and morbidity to be lower for in-situ graft replacement than extra-anatomic bypass [8]. The types of reconstruction for aortoiliac graft and endograft infections have not been shown to affect mortality [17]. Mortality is higher if grafts are not removed and treated non-operatively rather than surgically, with low survival rate of 33% versus 58%, respectively [16].

After graft removal, there is no standard recommendation for the duration of antibiotic treatment. Most studies describe continuation of tailored antibiotics for 4–6 weeks postoperatively. Some cases will require indefinite antibiotic suppression, especially with retained prosthetic material or in an immunosuppressed patient [14, 17, 24]. Antimycotic agents should be considered for patients with aortoenteric associated infection [9].

Finally, graft preservation with wound sterilization has been reported with success in appropriately selected cases. Graft preservation is most suitable for patent femoral or distal grafts with infection limited to the bed of the graft and not involving suture lines, in patients not presenting with sepsis or hemorrhage. Graft preservation should not be considered in the presence of high virulence organisms such as *Pseudomonas* [5, 11, 28]. Wound sterilization begins with thorough operative debridement and copious irrigation, with or without adjuncts such as betadine, hydrogen peroxide, or bacitracin. Sterilization with povidone-iodine-soaked dressing changes over exposed grafts was the original method described with successful graft preservation around 71% [28]. More recently, sterilization using antibiotic beads to deliver highly concentrated doses to a local wound has been reported. The technique consists of creating antibiotic beads intraoperatively by mixing polymethyl methacrylate powder with vancomycin and either tobramycin or gentamicin, rolling the mixture into small beads, linking them on a suture while solidifying, and once the thermal reaction has cooled they are inserted into the wound which is then sutured closed. Serial washouts and antibiotic bead exchanges are continued every 3–5 days until negative cultures are obtained, requiring a range of 1–3 explorations after initial bead placement [4, 11]. At the time of final closure, muscle flap coverage should be considered in the case of significant graft exposure or large soft tissue defects. Postoperative antibiotic course consists of at least 4–6 weeks of parenteral culture-specific antibiotics. Wound sterilization rates of 87–94% with reinfection rates of 11–12.5% are reported [4, 29]. Higher reinfection rates up to 20% were seen using therapy guided by the clinical appearance of the wound instead of culture results [4]. An association with late pseudoaneurysm formation seen in 4–5% of graft preservation patients highlights the need for long-term surveillance [4, 11].

Prevention

The ultimate treatment for infection is prevention. Giving prophylactic antibiotics prior to vascular arterial reconstruction reduces risk of wound infection by three quarters and early graft infection by two thirds [30]. Thus, prophylaxis against common gram-positive and gram-negative skin contaminants with first- or second-generation cephalosporin is recommended. Alternatively, clindamycin or vancomycin can be utilized in the case of a beta-lactam allergy. It is important to redose in the case of lengthy operations. Given that SSIs rates are doubled with operative time greater than 250 minutes, efficiency during procedures is essential [2].

Reference A

Skin preparation with chlorhexidine instead of povidone-iodine has been shown to reduce SSI in vascular surgical procedures. [Ref: Factors associated with surgical site infection after lower extremity bypass in the SVS VQI. Kalish JA, Farber A, Homa K, Trinidad M, Beck A, Davies M et al. J Vasc Surg 2014;60:11238–46}.

Intraoperatively, when handling graft material, one should avoid unnecessary contact with the skin. The use of iodine containing adhesive drapes to act as a microbial barrier has been shown to have no effect on SSI rate when compared to no drapes [12]. Optimizing patient factors such as maintaining blood sugar level below 180 mg/dL and avoiding hypothermia have shown association with lower SSI rates [2, 18]. Simultaneous gastrointestinal operations with aortic grafting should be avoided.

At closure, aortic grafts should be covered by reapproximating the posterior peritoneum, and if this is not possible, an omental flap is recommended. Groins should be closed in layers with soft tissue coverage to protect grafts from contact with skin. Placing vancomycin powder into groin wounds at the time of closure showed a small but statistically significant decrease of 7.9% in superficial infections alone, within the first 30 days [31]. Closed incision negative pressure therapy for the first 5–7 days after surgery has been suggested as an effective strategy to maintain approximation of skin edges, protect the wound from bacteria, and remove proinflammatory fluid and edema. Studies have reported reduced wound infections from 25–30% to 6–8.5% in high-risk femoral incisions [3, 32].

Postoperatively, antibiotics are not indicated for prevention. However, after a patient has undergone graft or endograft placement, prophylactic coverage is recommended when undergoing certain procedures such as dental work, colonoscopy, or cystoscopy [27].

Conclusion

Surgical site and graft infections are a frequent and dreaded complication of both open and increasingly endovascular vascular surgery. A diverse microbiological pathophysiology drives the clinical presentation and treatment algorithms. An understanding of diagnosis, microbiology, treatment, and prevention is paramount to performing safe and high-quality vascular surgery.

Late Anastomotic Complication: Pseudoaneurysm, Anastomotic Aneurysm, and Blowout

Late anastomotic failure presents in a variety of ways. The first form of anastomotic failure would be the formation of a true anastomotic aneurysm. This presents late as a dilation of the native artery at the site of the anastomosis and includes all walls of the vessel with containment of blood flow. The next, and more common entity, is the pseudoaneurysm or false aneurysm, with blood flow outside of the artery contained within a pseudocapsule with continuous flow and arterial pressure within the pseudoaneurysm. Finally, frank rupture of the anastomosis or "blowout" can occur.

Early anastomotic failure typically occurs due to a technical problem or virulent infection. Following the initial postoperative period, the etiology of late failure is more complex. This section will focus on late anastomotic complication.

Pathophysiology

Anastomotic complications can occur due to several underlying pathophysiologic causes. The majority of episodes will involve native artery to prosthetic anastomoses, though these can all occur in relation to autogenous tissue anastomoses in rare circumstances [33]. Failure can occur at multiple sites in patients who undergo arterial reconstruction that have multiple anastomoses. Additionally, while anastomotic aneurysms and blowout can occur at any location, late manifestation is most frequently seen with aortoiliac and aortofemoral reconstruction and for reconstructions performed for occlusive rather than aneurysmal disease.

The anastomosis is initially dependent only on suture material for integrity. However, with time fibrous scarring will contribute to building integrity along with the suture material, and this must also be affected in order to have anastomotic failure [34]. Therefore, these late complications require failure of the suture line, the fibrous scar tissue, and/or prosthetic conduit at the anastomosis. This can occur due to primary suture failure, technical failure, arterial or prosthetic degeneration, or infection.

If arterial or autogenous graft dilation is the underlying cause, a true aneurysm involving all walls of the vessel can develop. Additionally, prosthetic conduit itself can dilate with time. Often this can be attributed to aneurysmal degeneration of the anastomosis proximal or distal to the conduit. This can be seen after aortic aneurysm repair with proximal degeneration involving the juxtarenal aorta or distally involving the iliac arteries when a tube graft was performed. This is also frequently seen at the femoral anastomosis in aortobifemoral reconstructions. Poor control of blood pressure, atherosclerotic disease progression, and excessively deep endarterectomy can attribute to full thickness dilation of the blood vessel creating a true aneurysm. Finally, compliance mismatch between graft and autologous tissue has been implicated as a cause of native artery true aneurysm formation [35].

Occurring more frequently than dilation and true aneurysm formation, a break in the vessel wall or anastomosis may allow blood to exit the lumen into the surrounding tissues to form a pseudoaneurysm. Suture line fracture, conduit, or native artery full thickness tears, infection, or technical errors such as poor graft sizing, excessive tension, or redundancy can contribute to anastomotic failure and manifest late as a pseudoaneurysm (Fig. 16.5). Graft failure or defect can also lead to this complication, though this is very rare. Pseudoaneurysms can erode through the skin causing external hemorrhage (Fig. 16.6) or into adjacent bowel which can contribute to aortoenteric fistula formation [36].

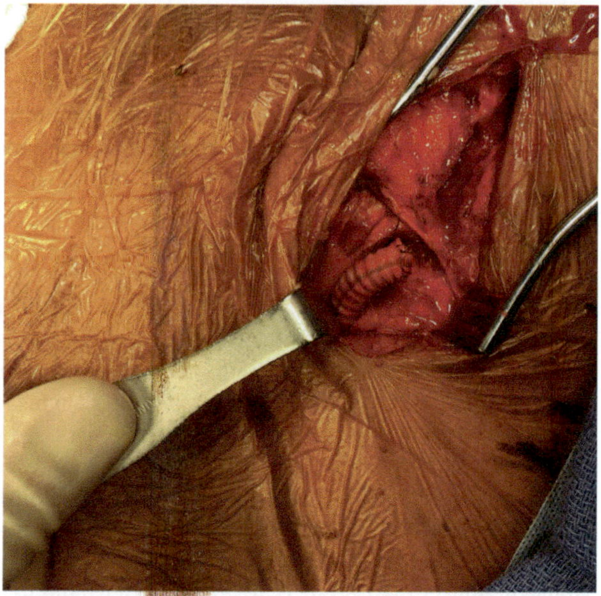

Fig. 16.5 Late graft anastomotic disruption

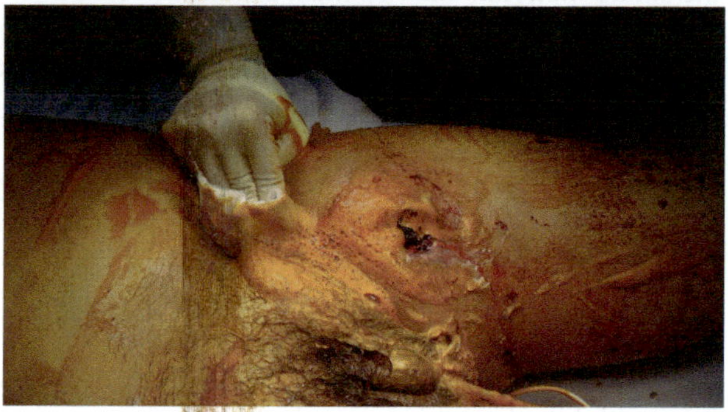

Fig. 16.6 Pseudoaneurysm of femoral artery eroding through the skin

The development of a late anastomotic failure is also associated with systemic disorders. Vasculitides and connective tissue disorders increase the risk of anastomotic failure [37]. Smoking is also a known risk factor for anastomotic failure. Poor control of hypertension can also contribute to this complication. Finally, the need for systemic anticoagulation and/or antiplatelet agents can contribute to persistent flow in pseudoaneurysms.

Diagnosis

Presentation of anastomotic complications varies based on the etiology of the underlying complication. In a series of 142 femoral anastomotic aneurysms, 64% presented with a painless pulsatile mass, 19% presented with acute limb ischemia,

8% presented with a painful mass, and 7% presented with hemorrhage [38]. Early presentation, within the first 6 weeks following intervention, is more likely to include pain, signs of infection, bleeding, and acute ischemia. Late presentations typically appear as painless pulsatile masses.

The most common site of late anastomotic complication is the femoral artery following reconstruction, with 3% of all patients developing aneurysms. The incidence is higher when patients are undergoing aortofemoral reconstruction, with 6–8% of patients developing anastomotic complications following aortobifemoral bypass [39].

A physical examination will often suggest the presence of a femoral aneurysm or pseudoaneurysm. Oftentimes, pseudoaneurysm development will be accompanied by pain, local tissue inflammation, and edema. Aortic anastomotic complication would more likely present as an incidental imaging finding, retroperitoneal rupture, or with development of an aortoenteric fistula [40]. Duplex ultrasonography can be suggestive of anastomotic complication and is particularly helpful when identifying a pseudoaneurysm with classic "to and fro" flow within an extravascular space. Cross-sectional imaging, most commonly CT scan, would definitively diagnose the lesion and allow evaluation of the entire reconstruction for asymptomatic involvement of other sites. Pseudoaneurysms at multiple sites (e.g., after aortobifemoral reconstruction) should raise the question of an underlying infection. If there is concern for infection at the site of anastomotic complication, some advocate for the use of PET CT scanning, though this will often not change the course of management. Additionally, some advocate for routine surveillance CT to assess for asymptomatic anastomotic aneurysms at 5 years post reconstruction. MRA can also be a useful adjunct in these patients when radiation exposure is a concern.

Treatment

Management of anastomotic complications is based on the underlying cause and location of the lesion.

Overt hemorrhage requires immediate operative intervention to control the source of bleeding, regardless of the presence of infection. Late blowout generally involves infection or graft failure. One should plan for massive transfusion and consider both open and endovascular treatment to address the cause of bleeding. Often endovascular exclusion can be used as temporizing measure prior to definitive, planned reconstruction.

All retroperitoneal aortic anastomotic aneurysms and pseudoaneurysms should be treated urgently when diagnosed to avoid rupture and erosion. In the presence of infection, excision and extra-anatomic bypass or in-line repair should be considered. However, when infection is unlikely, endovascular exclusion is becoming increasingly used as a safe and effective definitive treatment. Aortoenteric fistula treatment is discussed in a later section of this chapter.

All femoral anastomotic pseudoaneurysms should be considered for immediate treatment. Due to the high frequency of infection or graft failure as the cause of late lesions, these generally require open revision. Some advocate for converting all end-to side aortofemoral anastomoses to an end-to-end configuration unless retrograde flow is required to perfuse the ipsilateral hypogastric artery. When infection is not suspected, primary repair is possible by repairing the site of graft or suture line failure. However, if infection is suspected, resection of the graft and extraanatomic bypass reconstruction should be considered. Conversion to an aortopopliteal or iliopopliteal bypass via the obturator canal is an option for infected femoral artery anastomoses [33]. If in-line reconstruction is performed, autologous tissue coverage is imperative. The use of muscle flap coverage has been extensively reported and is a very useful adjunct when local autologous tissue is insufficient for coverage [41].

True femoral anastomotic aneurysms should be fixed when they exceed 2 cm in greatest diameter [42]. Repair can often be performed with simple resection of the aneurysmal segment and interposition reconstruction. Again, conversion to an end-to-end configuration is often required when the aneurysmal segment of the native artery is involved and excised. A growing body of literature has suggested that endovascular exclusion has acceptable results, though long-term data is lacking.

Conclusion

Late anastomotic blowout, pseudoaneurysm and true aneurysm formation are complicated clinical problems. They require a high index of suspicion on symptom and examination findings. Additionally, infection must always be considered as the underlying cause. These unique clinical situations require urgent recognition and repair to prevent disastrous outcomes.

Aortoenteric Fistula

Aortoenteric fistula (AEF) occurs in both primary and secondary forms. Primary AEF is a rare entity which is associated with aneurysmal degeneration of the aorta. This chapter will focus on secondary AEF as a late complication of open and endovascular aortic intervention. This complication is uncommon, but carries a high mortality rate and requires prompt identification and treatment.

Incidence

Secondary AEF (SAEF) has a relatively low incidence. In a series of 307 patients by Hallett et al., 1.6% of patients developed a secondary AEF following aortic intervention [43]. In a selective review of patients presenting with SAEF, Pipinos et al. demonstrated 98% of patients had undergone reconstruction with prosthetic graft material [44]. Of these patients, they were nearly equally weighted between abdominal aortic aneurysm repair and aortobifemoral bypass performed for aortoiliac occlusive disease. These findings counter previous reports of increased occurrence of SAEF following AAA repair. A proximal end-to-side configuration has been associated with increased risk of SAEF formation. Of note, there is minimal evidence to support increased occurrence of SAEF with a retroperitoneal exposure. These fistulas occur either at the anastomosis (graft enteric fistula) or along the graft material (graft enteric erosion). Additionally, aortoenteric fistula formation has been demonstrated following endovascular exclusion of AAAs [45]; however it remains rare, with an incidence of 0.01% following EVAR in the MAEFISTO study reviewing 3932 patients [46].

The most common presentation of secondary AEF is gastrointestinal hemorrhage. Classically, a small volume herald bleed will occur, though massive hemorrhage can certainly occur without herald bleeding. SAEFs can also present with chronic findings of weight loss, malaise, fevers, sepsis, and graft thrombosis. It is important to appreciate that many patients with SAEF will not present with clinical bleeding. The most frequent presentations of SAEF include one or more of the following clinical signs and symptoms: gastrointestinal bleeding (80%), sepsis (44%), abdominal pain (30%), back pain (15%), groin mass (12%), and abdominal pulsatile mass (6%) [47].

Even with treatment, morbidity and mortality with secondary AEF remains very high. Untreated SAEF are uniformly fatal and postoperative mortality of those who undergo all forms of repair still approaches 50%.

Pathophysiology

Aortoenteric fistula formation most frequently occurs between the duodenum and the proximal aortic graft [48] due to the close proximity of the bowel to the anastomosis on infrarenal aortic reconstructions (Fig. 16.7). The duodenum is a retroperitoneal structure at this location and minimal intervening tissue is present between the bowel and the graft. The most common site of secondary AEF formation is also

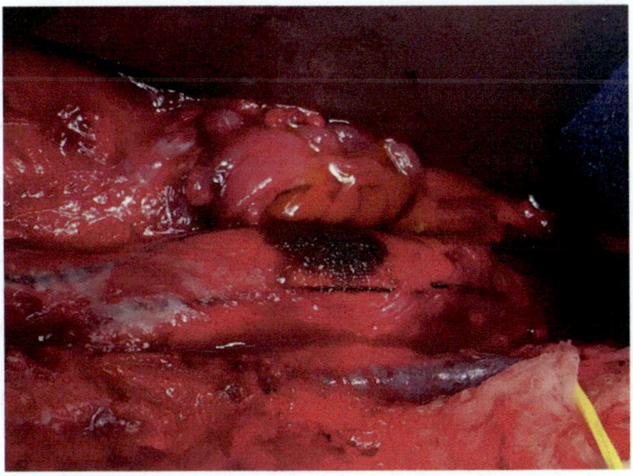

Fig. 16.7 Aortic graft erosion into duodenum

the duodenum (62%) followed by the jejunum and ileum (12%) and then colon (5%). Fistulous tracts have been reported to occur at any level of the graft, with approximately 4–6% occurring away from the anastomosis [49]. Careful approximation of tissue between the structures, use of an omental pedicle flap, and a retroperitoneal approach to the aorta for reconstruction are thought to decrease the risk of SAEF.

Secondary AEF occur due to several possible underlying mechanisms [50]. Infection of the aortic graft can contribute to local inflammation and tissue destruction. Virulent bacteria, especially *S. aureus*, are most often attributed to formation in animal models [51]. However, two thirds of operative cultures are generally polymicrobial, owing to the contamination with enteric contents. An additional component seen is the high frequency of *Candida* species growing in operative cultures [52]. This organism is thought to contribute to development of the fistulous connection. This is often difficult to distinguish however, as the infection may have been the underlying cause or the result of graft exposure to the enteric contents. The pulsatile nature of the aortic graft also is thought to contribute to graft erosion and fistula formation. This pulsatility produces constant friction as well as pressure and potential ischemia to the bowel tissue. Technical errors during the procedure may also contribute to SAEF development. Bowel injury, graft contamination, and inadequate separation of graft and bowel can all potentially occur during the operation.

SAEF following EVAR occur due to unique problems associated with endovascular aortic exclusion. One mechanism is sac enlargement due to persistent endoleak and direct erosion of the aneurysmal aorta into bowel. Infection can contribute to development of SAEF following EVAR as well as graft endotension and migration. Importantly, more than 30% of EVAR-related AEF were related to a defect in the aortic stents themselves such as fracture, erosion, or angulation of the stent [53].

Diagnosis

Diagnosis of SAEF is driven primarily by the presentation of the patient. Unfortunately, a high index of suspicion must be maintained in order to promptly make the correct diagnosis, and AEF should thus always be a consideration in patients with previous aortic intervention and GI bleeding. When a patient presents with hemodynamic instability and massive gastrointestinal hemorrhage, AEF will most often be diagnosed at the time of exploratory laparotomy. A subset of these patients will be diagnosed by aortography or endoscopy. If the patient is stable, they often first undergo endoscopy. This is insensitive for the diagnosis of AEF, with a sensitivity of only 50% [54]. Ideally, these patients should undergo CT angiography for full evaluation of the aortic graft and surrounding tissues. This imaging is also useful in operative planning for treatment of the condition. The sensitivity of CTA for diagnosis is still not ideal, with only 61% of patients being diagnosed correctly [55]. Findings associated with AEF include loss of fat planes around the aorta, perigraft fluid and gas, tethering of adjacent bowel loops to the graft, and extravasation of contrast from the aorta into the involved segment of bowel. Angiography has not been found to be useful in stable patients, as active bleeding is rarely seen at the time of the procedure.

In patients who present with constitutional symptoms without gastrointestinal bleeding, additional tools often aid in diagnosis. CT angiography will often have the aforementioned findings around the aortic graft. PET scanning and tagged WBC scanning can be used as an adjunctive measure to diagnose AEF when aortic graft infection is present [56]. Finally, if communication exists between the colon and aortic graft, colonoscopy can be diagnostic.

Treatment

Treatment for secondary AEF should be catered to the presentation of the patient. Patients with massive hemorrhage, instability, or ongoing severe sepsis require specialized, emergent therapy to try to stave off an extremely high mortality condition. A stable, non-toxic patient presenting with a classic herald bleed has time for preoperative planning, diagnostics, and resuscitation prior to treatment. However, even they should be treated in an urgent manner, that is, during the index hospitalization.

Hemodynamically unstable patients must be urgently resuscitated, transfused, started on broad spectrum antibiotics, and brought to the operating room for emergent exploration. The preferred approach is midline laparotomy, and the first step is rapid proximal aortic clamping for control. Balloon control is also a reasonable option for obtaining proximal control given the potentially hostile nature of a reoperative abdomen. Distal control should similarly be obtained with iliac clamping or balloon occlusion. Some have advocated for the use of Resuscitative Endovascular Balloon Occlusion of the Aorta (REBOA) for temporary control by inflating a compliant balloon to bridge the aortic defect, while the aorta is exposed and controlled [57]. The affected bowel should be controlled with bowel clamps, the fistula excised, and bowel closed primarily or resected with primary anastomosis. The aortic stump should be oversewn and covered with omentum, and the retroperitoneum should be drained widely. Traditionally, aortic reconstruction necessitates complete graft excision and extraanatomic bypass, often with axillobifemoral bypass. However, immediate in situ reconstruction can also be performed with Cryoartery, antibiotic-soaked Dacron, or creation of a Neo-Aortoiliac system with autogenous femoral vein (Fig. 16.8). There is not a superior conduit, and much of the conduit choice reflects individual surgeon and institutional practices [58]. Specific descriptions of these procedures are beyond the scope of this chapter.

Some have advocated for endograft exclusion of the AEF, typically used as a temporizing step or as a palliative option for patients would not physiologically tolerate excision and reconstruction [59]. However, long-term data is needed to fully evaluate the viability of endograft exclusion of SAEF as a destination therapy.

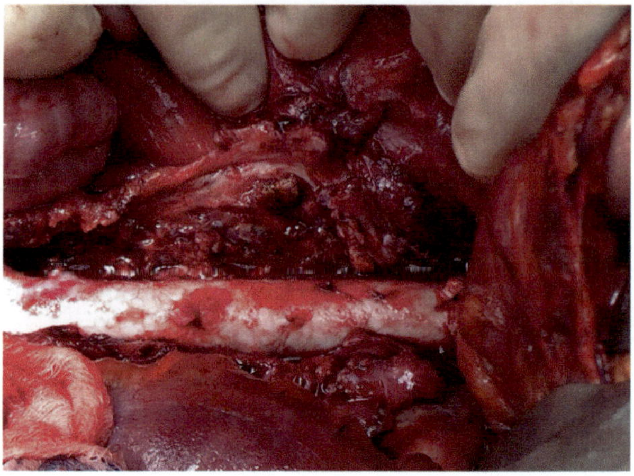

Fig. 16.8 Aortoenteric fistula repair with cadaveric aorta

Conclusions

Secondary AEF is a dreaded complication of open and endovascular aortic aneurysm repair as well as reconstructions for aortoiliac occlusive disease. Complex pathophysiologic mechanisms appear to lead to the development of these fistulas. While this diagnosis portends high morbidity and mortality, prompt diagnosis and treatment can improve outcomes.

Lymphocele/Lymphatic Fistula/Chylous Ascites

Lymphatic complications following vascular surgery are complex and irksome complications. Their presentation varies from early postoperative developments to late clinical findings. A spectrum of outcomes can be expected. Lymphoceles can be incidentally found and behave in benign fashion or may present as massive lymphatic leaks with infection which require operative intervention and can lead to significant morbidity and mortality. An understanding of the clinical findings and treatments are imperative for vascular surgeons.

Etiology

Damage to the lymphatic channels is a known complication of open surgical procedures, leading to lymphorrhea. If the lymph fluid is contained within the surrounding tissues, it is known as a lymphocele. If there is external communication, it is termed a lymphocutaneous fistula. This complication most frequently occurs during kidney transplantation, lymphadenectomies, and pelvic oncologic resections. For vascular surgery, the most common site of lymphatic injury is the groin during open reconstruction of the femoral vessels, and in the retroperitoneum following aortoiliac reconstruction [60, 61] because of the dense concentration of lymphatic tissue within the femoral triangle and the retroperitoneum. Risks for lymphorrhea include failure to ligate lymphatic channels, reoperative surgical fields, infection, and placement prosthetic graft material [62]. These complications potentially delay wound healing, increase risk of infection, and increase fluid losses contributing to dehydration and increased length of stay. Additionally, the high triglyceride concentration within chyle can lead to nutritional deficiency, especially with high volume cutaneous loss or ascites. The change from lymph to chyle occurs in the retroperitoneal and intraabdominal lymphatic tissue when emulsified fats are added to the lymph fluid by the small intestine.

Incidence

The incidence of lymphoceles after groin arterial reconstruction is relatively common, with a large series demonstrating 4% [63]. In order for a lymphocele to develop, a persistent communication with a lymphatic channel is required. Lymphoceles develop pseudocapsules which contain the lymph fluid within a discrete space. The accumulation typically occurs in the first postoperative month, though lymphocele and lymphatic fistula can occur at any time following intervention [64]. Lymphocutaneous fistula is diagnosed when there is continuous drainage of clear to straw colored fluid from the incision site. These have occurred in fewer patients compared to contained lymphocele. Kalman et al. demonstrated a frequency of only 0.1% in a surgical series of 4000 patients undergoing femoral artery reconstruction [62]. Fistulas require more aggressive management when compared to lymphoceles due to the increased fluid losses, wound complications, and infection risk. Lymphatic complications can also occur with open aortoiliac surgery, demonstrated by both development of retroperitoneal lymphocele or chylous ascites [61]. This complication is noted to be rare and only sparingly reported in literature.

Diagnosis

Lymphocele is typically diagnosed with ultrasonography. If lymphocele develops further than 1 month following the operation, contrast-enhanced CT is helpful to distinguish the collection from pseudoaneurysm or abscess. Lymphocutaneous fistula is typically diagnosed with the aforementioned findings, though CT scan and ultrasound are useful adjuncts to rule out concomitant retroperitoneal involvement. The gold standard to diagnose a lymphocele, lymphatic fistula, or chylous ascites is lymphoscintigraphy [65]. This technique is also useful to distinguish contained collections from simple seromas during the early postoperative period.

Treatment

Treatment of lymphoceles should be considered in the presence of compressive symptoms, clinical signs of infection, or increase in size. Small lymphoceles are more appropriately observed as they often resolve spontaneously. When a lymphocele develops in proximity to prosthetic graft reconstruction, many advocate for prophylactic intervention to prevent graft infection. Some symptomatic lymphoceles will resolve with percutaneous drainage, often augmented by the use of sclerosing agents. Ethanol, povidone-iodine, tetracycline, doxycycline, bleomycin, talc, and fibrin glue have been used as sclerosing agents. There is a reported 50% recurrence rate for retroperitoneal lymphocele with drainage alone [66]. Wounds with refractory lymphorrhea should be explored with direct ligation of the lymphatic pedicle and resection of the pseudocapsule. Lymphocutaneous fistulas typically require intervention to aid in wound healing and avoid superinfection. However, conservative management with bed rest, local wound care, and empiric antibiotics has been advocated by some [67]. Increasing utilization of negative pressure wound vacuum closure has also been used to treat fistulae with excellent results, including a series by Haman et al. describing 100% closure of the fistulae [68]. Wound exploration with ligation of the damaged lymphatic channel is again advocated for lesions failing conservative therapy. Chylous ascites often requires treatment due to severe symptoms and nutritional losses and is mostly driven by dietary modifications. The use of total parenteral nutrition or restriction to a medium chain triglyceride only diet leads to decreased chyle production and resolution of chyle accumulation [69]. Percutaneous and operative interventions have been performed rarely for refractory cases of chylous ascites. In a series of patients who developed chylous ascites following open aortic surgery by Pabst et al., patients requiring operative management had high surgical success of lymphatic channel ligation; however the team recommends utilizing this approach only as a last resort [70]. In their series, chyle leak associated mortality following aortic intervention was reported at 11.5% regardless of treatment approach.

Conclusion

Lymphatic complications are diverse and complicated. These complications can present early in the postoperative course, but late presentation or superimposed infection can often lead to serious adverse patient morbidity. An understanding of the pathophysiology and clinical presentations drives prevention and treatment.

Conclusion

Dreaded late complications in vascular surgery encompass a broad clinical presentation and pathophysiology. Infection, anastomotic complications, aortoenteric fistula, and lymphatic complications can create devastating clinical morbidity and mortality. Vascular surgeons should be aware of modern diagnostic modalities and treatments to address each of these late complications.

References

1. Bandyk DF. Vascular surgical site infection: risk factors and preventive measures. Semin Vasc Surg. 2008;21(3):119–23. https://doi.org/10.1053/j.semvascsurg.2008.05.008.
2. Davis FM, Sutzko DC, Grey SF, Mansour MA, Jain KM, Nypaver TJ, Gaborek G, Henke PKJ. Predictors of surgical site infection after open lower extremity revascularization. Vasc Surg. 2017;65(6):1769–1778.e3. https://doi.org/10.1016/j.jvs.2016.11.053. PMID: 28527931.
3. Matatov T, Reddy KN, Doucet LD, Zhao CX, Zhang WW. Experience with a new negative pressure incision management system in prevention of groin wound infection in vascular surgery patients. J Vasc Surg. 2013;57(3):791–5. https://doi.org/10.1016/j.jvs.2012.09.037. Epub 2013 Jan 9.
4. Stone PA, Mousa AY, Hass SM, Dearing DD, Campbell JR 2nd, Parker A, Thompson S, AbuRahma AF. Antibiotic-loaded polymethylmethacrylate beads for the treatment of extracavitary vascular surgical site infection. J Vasc Surg. 2012;55(6):1706–11. https://doi.org/10.1016/j.jvs.2011.12.037. Epub 2012 Mar.
5. Szilagyi DE, Smith RF, Elliott JP, Vrandecic MP. Infection in arterial reconstruction with synthetic grafts. Ann Surg. 1972;176(3):321–33.
6. Rojoa D, Kontopodis N, Antoniou SA, Ioannou CV, Antoniou GA. 18F-FDG PET in the diagnosis of vascular prosthetic graft infection: a diagnostic test accuracy meta-analysis. Eur J Vasc Endovasc Surg. 2019;57(2):292–301. https://doi.org/10.1016/j.ejvs.2018.08.040. Epub 2018 Sep 18. Review. PMID: 30241981.
7. Reinders Folmer EI, Von Meijenfeldt GCI, Van der Laan MJ, Glaudemans AWJM, Slart RHJA, Saleem BR, Zeebregts CJ. Diagnostic imaging in vascular graft infection: a systematic review and meta-analysis. Eur J Vasc Endovasc Surg. 2018;56(5):719–29. https://doi.org/10.1016/j.ejvs.2018.07.010. Epub 2018 Aug 16.
8. O'Connor S, Andrew P, Batt M, Becquemin JP. A systematic review and meta-analysis of treatments for aortic graft infection. J Vasc Surg. 2006;44(1):38–45. Review.
9. Ben Ahmed S, Louvancourt A, Daniel G, Combe P, Duprey A, Albertini JN, Favre JP, Rosset E. Cryopreserved arterial allografts for in situ reconstruction of abdominal aortic native or secondary graft infection. J Vasc Surg. 2018;67(2):468–77. https://doi.org/10.1016/j.jvs.2017.06.088. Epub 2017 Aug 18.
10. Argyriou C, Georgiadis GS, Lazarides MK, Georgakarakos E, Antoniou GA. Endograft infection after endovascular abdominal aortic aneurysm repair: a systematic review and meta-analysis. J Endovasc Ther. 2017;24(5):688–97. https://doi.org/10.1177/1526602817722018. Epub 2017 Jul 31.
11. Zamani N, Sharath SE, Barshes NR, Braun JD, Kougias P. Long-term outcomes of lower extremity graft preservation using antibiotic beads in patients with early deep wound infections after major arterial reconstructions. J Vasc Surg. 2019. pii: S0741-5214(19)31786-0.; https://doi.org/10.1016/j.jvs.2019.06.192.
12. Webster J, Alghamdi A. Use of plastic adhesive drapes during surgery for preventing surgical site infection. Cochrane Database Syst Rev. 2015;4:CD006353. https://doi.org/10.1002/14651858.CD006353.pub4.
13. Hallett JW Jr, Marshall DM, Petterson TM, Gray DT, Bower TC, Cherry KJ Jr, Gloviczki P, Pairolero PC. Graft-related complications after abdominal aortic aneurysm repair: reassurance from a 36-year population-based experience. J Vasc Surg. 1997;25(2):277–84; discussion 285–6.
14. Smeds, Duncan, Harlander-Locke. Treatment and outcomes of aortic endograft infection. J Vasc Surg. 2016;63:332–40.

15. Rawson TM, Lee MJ, Khanna P, Gopal Rao G, Renton S, Buckley J. Microbiological characterisation of prosthetic vascular graft infection. J Infect. 2015;71(3):400–2. https://doi.org/10.1016/j.jinf.2015.04.008. Epub 2015 Apr 23.
16. Li H, Chan YC, Cheng SW. Current evidence on management of aortic stent-graft infection: a systematic review and meta-analysis. Ann Vasc Surg. 2018;51:306–13. https://doi.org/10.1016/j.avsg.2018.02.038. Epub 2018 Jun 11.
17. Davila, Stone, Duncan, et al. A multicenter experience with the surgical treatment of infected abdominal aortic endografts. J Vasc Surg. 2015;63:877–83.
18. Bandyk DF, Novotney ML, Johnson BL, Back MR, Roth SR. Use of rifampin-soaked gelatin-sealed polyester grafts for in situ treatment of primary aortic and vascular prosthetic infections. J Surg Res. 2001;95(1):44–9.
19. Geary KJ, Tomkiewicz ZM, Harrison HN, Fiore WM, Geary JE, Green RM, DeWeese JA, Ouriel K. Differential effects of a gram-negative and a gram-positive infection on autogenous and prosthetic grafts. J Vasc Surg. 1990;11(2):339–45; discussion 346–7.
20. Chung J, Clagett GP. Neoaortoiliac System (NAIS) procedure for the treatment of the infected aortic graft. Semin Vasc Surg. 2011;24(4):220–6. https://doi.org/10.1053/j.semvascsurg.2011.10.012.
21. Oderich GS, Bower TC, Hofer J, Kalra M, Duncan AA, Wilson JW, Cha S, Gloviczki P. In situ rifampin-soaked grafts with omental coverage and antibiotic suppression are durable with low reinfection rates in patients with aortic graft enteric erosion or fistula. J Vasc Surg. 2011;53(1):99–106, 107.e1–7; discussion 106–7. https://doi.org/10.1016/j.jvs.2010.08.018.
22. Masaki H, Tabuchi A, Yunoki Y, et al. Long-term results of obturator bypass. Ann Vasc Dis. 2016;9(2):80–4.
23. Seeger JM, Pretus HA, Welborn MB, Ozaki CK, Flynn TC, Huber TS. Long-term outcome after treatment of aortic graft infection with staged extra-anatomic bypass grafting and aortic graft removal. J Vasc Surg. 2000;32(3):451–9; discussion 460–1.
24. Heinola I, Kantonen I, Jaroma M, Albäck A, Vikatmaa P, Aho P, Venermo M. Treatment of aortic prosthesis infections by graft removal and in situ replacement with autologous femoral veins and fascial strengthening. Eur J Vasc Endovasc Surg. 2016;51(2):232–9. https://doi.org/10.1016/j.ejvs.2015.09.015. Epub 2015 Nov 2.
25. Harlander-Locke MP, Harmon LK, Lawrence PF, Oderich GS, McCready RA, Morasch MD, Feezor RJ, Vascular Low-Frequency Disease Consortium, Zhou W, Bismuth J, Pevec WC, Correa MP, Jim J, Ladowski JS, Kougias P, Bove PG, Wittgen CM, White JV. The use of cryopreserved aortoiliac allograft for aortic reconstruction in the United States. J Vasc Surg. 2014;59(3):669–74. https://doi.org/10.1016/j.jvs.2013.09.009. Epub 2013 Nov 14.
26. Lindsey P, Echeverria A, Lin PH. Lower extremity bypass using bovine carotid artery graft (artegraft): an analysis of 124 cases with long-term results. World J Surg. 2017. PMID: 28819879.
27. Chaikof EL, Dalman RL, Eskandari MK, Jackson BM, Lee WA, Mansour MA, Mastracci TM, Mell M, Murad MH, Nguyen LL, Oderich GS, Patel MS, Schermerhorn ML, Starnes BW. The Society for Vascular Surgery practice guidelines on the care of patients with an abdominal aortic aneurysm. J Vasc Surg. 2018;67(1):2–77.e2. https://doi.org/10.1016/j.jvs.2017.10.044.
28. Calligaro KD, Veith FJ, Schwartz ML, Goldsmith J, Savarese RP, Dougherty MJ, DeLaurentis DA. Selective preservation of infected prosthetic arterial grafts. Analysis of a 20-year experience with 120 extracavitary-infected grafts. Ann Surg. 1994;220(4):461–9; discussion 469–71.
29. Poi MJ, Pisimisis G, Barshes NR, Darouiche RO, Lin PH, Kougias P, Bechara CF. Evaluating effectiveness of antibiotic polymethylmethacrylate beads in achieving wound sterilization and graft preservation in patients with early and late vascular graft infections. Surgery. 2013;153(5):673–82. https://doi.org/10.1016/j.surg.2012.10.011. Epub 2012 Dec 24.
30. Stewart A, Eyers PS, Earnshaw JJ. Prevention of infection in arterial reconstruction. Cochrane Database Syst Rev. 2006;3:CD003073. Review. PMID: 16855996.
31. Mohammed S, Pisimisis GT, Daram SP, Bechara CF, Barshes NR, Lin PH, Kougias P. Impact of intraoperative administration of local vancomycin on inguinal wound complications. J Vasc Surg. 2013;57(4):1079–83. https://doi.org/10.1016/j.jvs.2012.09.073. Epub 2013 Jan 11.

32. Kwon J, Staley C, McCullough M, Goss S, Arosemena M, Abai B, Salvatore D, Reiter D, DiMuzio P. A randomized clinical trial evaluating negative pressure therapy to decrease vascular groin incision complications. J Vasc Surg. 2018;68(6):1744–52. https://doi.org/10.1016/j.jvs.2018.05.224. Epub 2018 Aug 17. PMID: 30126781.
33. Gaylis H, Dewar G. Anastomotic aneurysms: facts and fancy. Surg Annu. 1990;22:317–41.
34. Evans WE. Anastomotic femoral false aneurysms. In: Complications in vascular surgery. New York: Grune & Stratton; 1985. p. 205–12.
35. Mehigan DG, Fitzpatrick B, Browne HI. Is compliance mismatch the major cause of anastomotic arterial aneurysms? Analysis of 42 cases. J Cardiovasc Surg (Torino). 1985;26:147–50. PMID: 3156861.
36. Satiani B. False aneurysms following arterial reconstruction. Surg Gynecol Obstet. 1981;152:357–63. PMID: 7466589.
37. Alpagut U, Ugurlucan M, Dayioglu E. Major arterial involvement and review of Behcet's disease. Ann Vasc Surg. 2007;21(2):232–9. PMID: 17349371.
38. Demarche M, Waltregny D, van Damme H, Limet R. Femoral anastomotic aneurysms: pathogenic factors, clinical presentations and treatment. A study of 142 cases. Cardiovasc Surg. 1999;7(3):315–22.
39. Chavez CM. False aneurysms of the femoral artery: a challenge in management. Ann Surg. 1976;183:694–700. PMID: 135534.
40. Perdue GD, Smith RB, Ansley JD. Impending aortoenteric hemorrhage: the effect of early recognition on improved outcome. Ann Surg. 1980;192:237–43. PMID: 6967716.
41. Meland NB, Arnold PG, Pairolero PC, Lovich SF. Muscle-flap coverage for infected peripheral vascular prostheses. Plast Reconstr Surg. 1994;93(5):1005–11.
42. Demarche M, van Damme H, Limet R. Femoral anastomotic aneurysms: pathogenic factors, clinical presentations and treatment. A study of 142 cases. Cardiovasc Surg. 1999;7(3):315–22.
43. Hallett JW Jr, Marshall DM, Pettterson TM, Pairolero PC. Graft-related complications after abdominal aortic aneurysm repair: reassurance from a 36-year population-based experience. J Vasc Surg. 1997;25:277. PMID: 9052562.
44. Pipinos II, Carr JA, Haithcock BE, et al. Secondary aortoenteric fistula. Ann Vasc Surg. 2000;14:688. PMID: 11128470.
45. Riera del Moral L, Fernández Alonso S, Stefanov Kiuri S. Aortoenteric fistula arising as a complication of endovascular treatment of abdominal aortic aneurysm. Ann Vasc Surg. 2009;23(2):255.e13–7. Epub 2008 May 22. PMID: 18513484.
46. Kahlberg A, Rinaldi E, Piffaretti G. Results from the Multicenter Study on Aortoenteric Fistulization After Stent Grafting of the Abdominal Aorta (MAEFISTO). J Vasc Surg. 2016;64(2):313–20. PMID: 27289529.
47. Reynolds JY, Galloway JMD. Primary aortoduodenal fistula: a case report and review of the literature. Ir J Med Sci. 1991;160:381–4.
48. O'Mara C, Imbembo AL. Paraprosthetic-enteric fistula. Surgery. 1977;81(5):556–66. PMID: 300510.
49. Bergqvist D. Arterioenteric fistula. Review of a vascular emergency. Acta Chir Scand. 1987;153(2):81–6. PMID: 3303777.
50. Elliott JP Jr, Smith RF, Szilagyi DE. Proceedings: aortoenteric and paraprosthetic-enteric fistulas. Problems of diagnosis and management. Arch Surg. 1974;108(4):479–90. PMID: 4815922.
51. Bussuttil RW, Rees W, Baker JD. Pathogenesis of aortoduodenal fistula: experimental and clinical correlates. Surgery. 1979;85:1–13. PMID: 153003.
52. Chopra A, Cieciura L, Modrall JG, et al. Twenty-year experience with aorto-enteric fistula repair: gastro-intestinal complications predict outcome. J Am Coll Surg. 2017;225:9–18. PMID: 28161484.
53. Bergqvist D, Bjork M, Byman R. Secondary aortoenteric fistula after endovascular aortic interventions: a systemic literature review. J Vasc Interv Radiol. 2008;19:163–5. PMID: 18341942.
54. Deijen CL, Smulders YM, Coveliers HME. The importance of early diagnosis and treatment of patients with aortoenteric fistulas presenting with herald bleeds. Ann Vasc Surg. 2016;36. PMID: 27423720.

55. Raman SP, Kamaya A, Federle M. Aortoenteric fistulas: spectrum of CT findings. Abdom Imaging. 2013;38:367. PMID: 22366854.
56. Krupnick AS, Lombardi JV, Engels FH. 18-fluorodeoxyglucose positron emission tomography as a novel imaging tool for the diagnosis of aortoenteric fistula and aortic graft infection–a case report. Vasc Endovasc Surg. 2003;37(5):363–6. PMID: 14528383.
57. Miyamoto K, Inaba M, Kojima T, et al. Intra-Aortic Balloon Occlusion (IABO) may be useful for the management of secondary aortoduodenal fistula (SADF): a case report. Int J Surg Case Rep. 2016;25:234–7. PMID: 27414993.
58. Saers SJF, Scheltinga MRM. Primary aortoenteric fistula. Br J Surg. 2005;92:143–52. PMID: 15685700
59. Kakkos S, Christeas N, Lampropoulos G, Papadoulas S, Makri R, Zampakis P, et al. Endovascular management of aortoenteric fistulas with aortic cuff extenders: report of two cases. Int Angiol. 2011;30(3):290–4.
60. Croft RJ. Lymphatic fistula: a complication of arterial surgery [letter]. BMJ. 1978;2:205. PMID: 678862.
61. Savrin RA, High R. Chylous ascites after abdominal aortic surgery. Surgery. 1985;98:866. PMID: 3933135.
62. Kalman PG, Walker PM, Johnston KW. Consequences of groin lymphatic fistulae after vascular reconstruction. Vasc Endo Surg. 1991;25:210.
63. Roberts JR, Walters GK, Zenilman ME, Jones CE. Groin lymphorrhea complicating revascularization involving the femoral vessels. Am J Surg. 1993;165:341–4. PMID: 8447539.
64. Sidaway AN, Perler BA. Local complications: lymphatic. In: Rutherford's vascular surgery and endovascular therapy, vol. 52; 2018. p. 647.
65. Stolzenberg J. Detection of lymphaticocutaneous fistula by radionuclide lymphangiography. Arch Surg. 1978;113:306. PMID: 637696.
66. Karcaaltincaba M, Akhan O. Radiologic imaging and percutaneous treatment of pelvic lymphocele. Eur J Radiol. 2005;55:340–54. PMID: 15885959.
67. Obara A, Dziekiewicz MA, Maruszynski M. Lymphatic complications after vascular interventions. Wideochir Inne Tech Maloinwazy. 2014;9:420. PMID: 25337168.
68. Hamed O, Muck PE, Smith JM, Krallman K, Griffith NM. Use of vacuum-assisted closure (VAC) therapy in treating lymphatic complications after vascular procedures: new approach for lymphoceles. J Vasc Surg. 2008;48:1520. PMID: 19118737.
69. Weninger M, D'Haese JG, Angele MK, Kleepies A. Treatment options for chylous ascites after major abdominal surgery: a systematic review. Am J Surg. 2016;211:206. PMID: 26117431.
70. Pabst TS, McIntyre KE, Schilling JD, et al. Management of chyloperitoneum after abdominal aortic surgery. Am J Surg. 1993;166:194–8. PMID: 8352415.

Reference A

Skin preparation with chlorhexidine instead of povidone-iodine has been shown to reduce SSI in vascular surgical procedures. [Ref: Factors associated with surgical site infection after lower extremity bypass in the SVS VQI. Kalish JA, Farber A, Homa K, Trinidad M, Beck A, Davies M et al. J Vasc Surg 2014;60:1 1238–46].

Considerations for Surgery in Hostile Zones

17

Jessica M. Mayor and Joseph L. Mills Sr.

Introduction

Re-operative surgery poses additional considerations and may benefit from the consultation of a vascular surgeon. Primary reasons for preoperative vascular surgery consultation include anticipation of the potential need for vascular reconstruction, hemorrhage, and assistance with difficult dissections [1–4]. These consults take place preoperatively, as part of surgical planning, or intraoperatively when unanticipated vascular issues arise. In this chapter, we aim to describe general concepts that can potentially improve patient outcomes during re-operative surgery.

Case Example

The following case illustrates several potential considerations that could have improved this patient's perioperative course. A highly functional, middle-aged woman presented with hypothyroidism, prior pulmonary embolus, and left renal cell carcinoma (RCC) status post left nephrectomy several years earlier. She was found to have a local recurrence 2 years later, which was resected. Surveillance imaging subsequently showed a 2.5 cm left periaortic mass and a 1.5 cm right lung nodule (Fig. 17.1). Both were biopsied, with pathology positive for metastatic RCC. She underwent wedge resection of the lung nodule and, after recovering, was scheduled for elective resection of the left periaortic nodule.

J. M. Mayor · J. L. Mills Sr. (✉)
Division of Vascular Surgery and Endovascular Therapy, Michael E DeBakey Department of Surgery, Baylor College of Medicine, Houston, TX, USA
e-mail: Joseph.Mills@bcm.edu

R. Gilani, J. L. Mills Sr. (eds.), *Vascular Complications of Surgery and Intervention*, https://doi.org/10.1007/978-3-030-86713-3_17

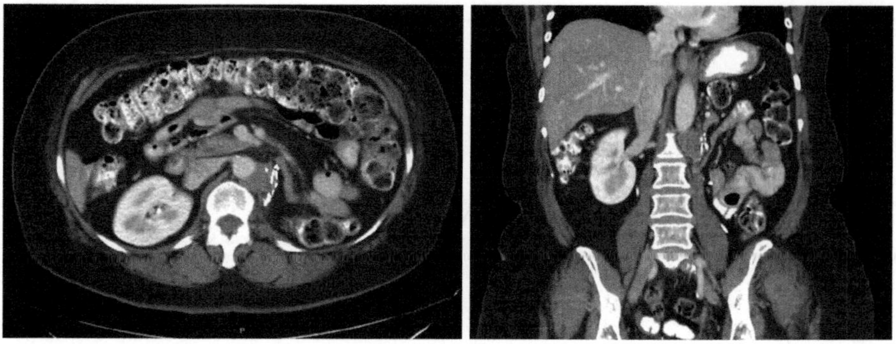

Fig. 17.1 Computed tomography imaging of a patient with recurrent renal cell carcinoma at previous resection bed abutting the abdominal aorta

Using a left subcostal incision (through her previous scar), the urology service exposed the left retroperitoneum. During attempted resection of the mass, significant bleeding was encountered, and the urology team was concerned for adventitial aortic injury. Vascular surgery was consulted emergently during the operation for assistance and repair. While not initially evident, the aortic injury was sufficiently extensive such that primary repair was not possible. At this point there was massive hemorrhage, which could not be controlled with manual compression. The incision was extended superiorly to allow for supraceliac aortic clamp placement. A segment of the juxtarenal aorta was resected, en bloc with the cancerous mass, while visualizing and preserving the right renal artery ostium. A beveled Dacron interposition tube graft was used to replace the abdominal aortic segment. The clamp was moved onto the graft after the proximal anastomosis was performed to restore visceral and right renal perfusion.

Intraoperatively, the patient lost 2.5 L of blood and required massive transfusion and the administration of vasopressors. Her hypovolemic shock was so severe that she required close to 30 minutes of abdominal aortic compression during resuscitation. Her subsequent postoperative course was smooth, and she was discharged home on post-operative day 7.

General Considerations

This case highlights several potential preoperative considerations that could have been anticipated during the preoperative planning stage and subsequently improved this patient's peri-operative course. Preoperative cross-sectional imaging is important to determine the proximity to major vascular structures.

While minimally invasive surgery generally results in decreased peri-operative pain and length of stay, often these incisions do not facilitate obtaining proximal and distal control. In re-operative fields, in which one can anticipate dense adhesions and obliterated tissue planes, wide exposure of the operative field can be beneficial. Especially when operating in the retroperitoneum, in fields that have been previously explored or irradiated, anticipation of the need for proximal and distal arterial control of any major vessels involved with or abutting the tumor should be a priority.

If vascular reconstruction is a possibility based on review of cross-sectional imaging, the vascular surgeon must consider conduit options. During a history and physical examination, one must ascertain the patient's history of previous surgery, varicose veins/venous insufficiency, and central venous access. Personal and family history of hypercoagulable disorders and deep vein thromboses may also be relevant in maintaining patency of the vascular reconstruction.

Oncologic Considerations

Oncologic surgery, among the various surgical subspecialties, is a common source of vascular surgeon operative consults. As surgical technique and neoadjuvant therapy have advanced, oncologic surgeons are operating on patients who may not have been offered an operation in the past. Vascular resection and reconstruction are often required to safely complete these operations.

Substantial benefits for preoperative vascular surgery consults for oncologic cases have been described. Preoperative consults have been associated with increased use of autologous grafts and fewer vascular injuries than urgent intraoperative consults [5, 6].

Sarcoma

Sarcoma resections are also a common vascular surgery operative consult. Current systemic therapies are often ineffective. Therefore, complete surgical resection remains the primary therapy for many of these tumors. Due to the nature of sarcomas, these patients can require reoperations for tumor recurrence and, depending on their histology, may even have previously received radiation therapy. Some centers routinely consult vascular surgery preoperatively as part of a multidisciplinary team, including surgical and medical specialists, as well as radiation oncologists. All of these patients should receive preoperative computed-tomography angiography and routine lower extremity vein mapping of the femoral and great saphenous vein, and they all should ideally meet with the vascular surgeon preoperatively [7, 8]. Fig. 17.2a shows preoperative imaging of a child with a sarcoma in the left neck. Vascular surgery was preoperatively consulted and was available to assist with left carotid resection and interposition graft using internal jugular vein conduit (Fig. 17.2b).

When compared to sarcoma cases that did not have vascular involvement requiring reconstruction, cases with vascular reconstruction had significantly higher complication rates (74% vs. 44%, $p = 0.002$) and increased transfusion requirements (66% vs. 33%, $p < 0.001$); however, 30-day mortality, 90-day mortality, local recurrence, and overall survival were not significantly different between groups [8]. As cases with vascular involvement tend to be more advanced, this study matched the

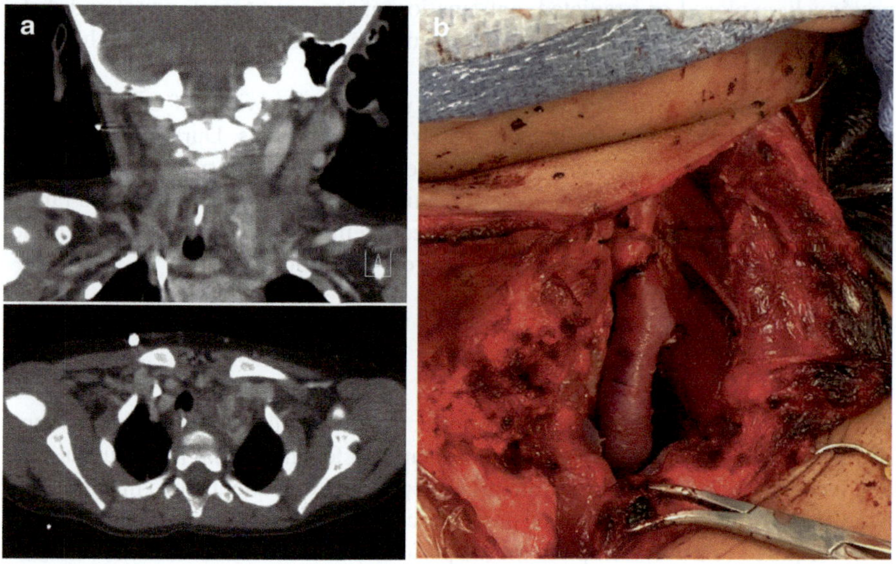

Fig. 17.2 (**a**) Preoperative computed tomography of a child with a sarcoma in the left neck abutting the common carotid artery. (**b**) Left carotid artery replacement with internal jugular vein interposition graft

patients in the two groups based on oncologic variables, such as anatomic size, tumor grade, and primary vs. recurrent disease [8]. This information may be useful during preoperative discussions with the patient and family.

A classification system has been proposed to differentiate the vascular involvement of soft tissue sarcomas in order to aid in surgical planning and to standardize reporting (Fig. 17.3). Type I tumors have both arterial and venous involvement; type II tumors have only arterial involvement; type III tumors have only venous involvement; and type IV tumors have no vascular involvement. In these two series, 9.9% of patients with lower extremity soft tissue sarcomas and 17.7% of patients with retroperitoneal soft tissue sarcomas had some vascular involvement (types I, II, and III) [9, 10].

RCC

Renal cell carcinoma (RCC) is unique in that it is one of the few tumor types that can form tumor thrombus in a renal vein that may extend into the inferior vena cava (IVC) and even reach the right atrium. Depending on the thrombus extent, thrombectomy and primary repair, patch angioplasty, and interposition grafting may be used to reconstruct the IVC. The Mayo Clinic determined that the following preoperative imaging findings are associated with an increased risk for IVC resection: right-sided tumors, an anterior-posterior diameter of the IVC at the renal vein orifice of >24 mm, and complete occlusion of the IVC at the renal vein orifice [11].

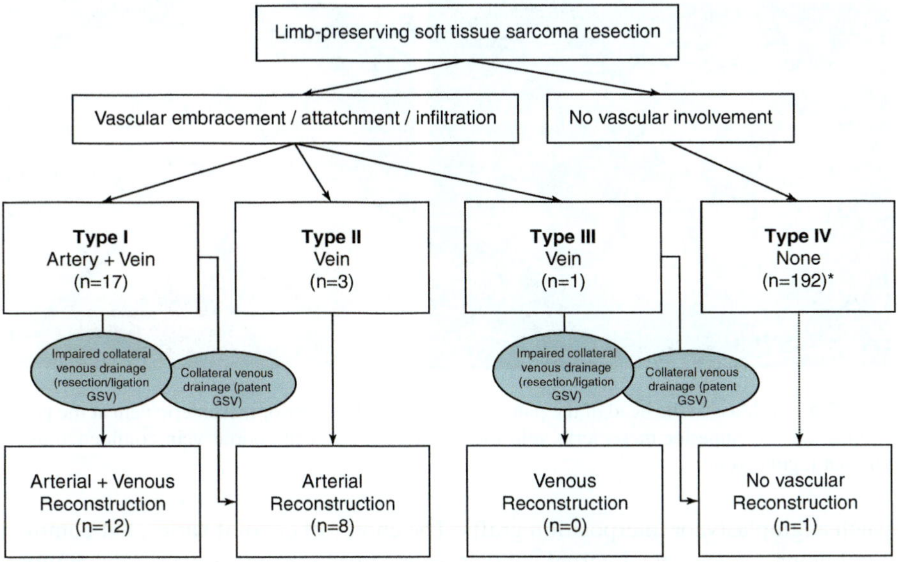

Fig. 17.3 Type of vascular involvement and algorithm for vascular reconstruction in patients with extremity soft tissue sarcoma. *Number of patients with type IV soft tissue sarcomas treated during the study period (excluded from further analysis). GSV greater saphenous vein

However, others have not found these factors to be significantly associated with risk for IVC reconstruction, although there were higher crude rates of IVC reconstruction with more Mayo Clinic risk factors [12]. More rarely, IVC tumor thrombus can be seen with adrenal cortical tumors, leiomyosarcomas, and pheochromocytomas [13].

Pancreatic Adenocarcinoma

Whether or not masses in the head of the pancreas are resectable is often dependent on regional vascular involvement. Masses of borderline resectability demonstrate some involvement of the portal vein, superior mesenteric vein, superior mesenteric artery, and/or celiac axis vessels, and complete resection of these masses requires vascular reconstruction. Despite increased blood loss and operative time, when vascular reconstructions are required during pancreaticoduodenectomy, there is no difference in short-term survival between traditional pancreaticoduodenectomy and pancreaticoduodenectomy with vascular reconstruction [14–17]. Computed tomography (CT) scan is the modality of choice to examine the relationship of the tumor to the vessels with review by a multidisciplinary care team [18]. This process facilitates surgical planning and, if needed, preoperative vascular surgery consultation. Despite CT imaging, many patients who do not appear to have tumor invasion on imaging are found intraoperatively to have vascular invasion [17]. Depending on extent of tumor invasion, reconstruction can be performed with primary repair,

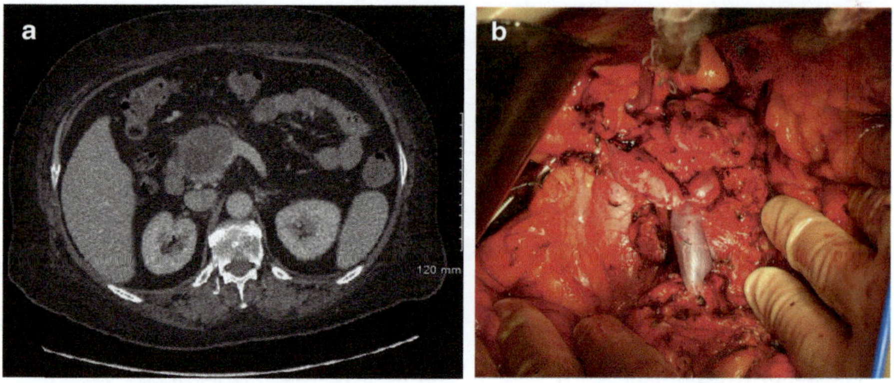

Fig. 17.4 (**a**) Mass in the head of the pancreas involving the superior mesenteric vein at the portal confluence. (**b**) Superior mesenteric vein interposition graft at the portal vein confluence using internal jugular vein

patch angioplasty, or interposition grafts. The choice of conduit varies, but common autologous choices are internal jugular vein, great saphenous vein, and femoral vein; use of allogeneic conduits, such as CryoVein, has also been reported [15–18].

The most common vascular structure requiring vascular reconstruction during resection of pancreatic head masses is the portal vein, often at the confluence of the superior mesenteric and splenic veins. Figure 17.4 shows an example of a case in which preoperative imaging showed a tumor in the head of the pancreas involving the superior mesenteric vein at the portal venous confluence. Vascular surgery was consulted preoperatively, and the left internal jugular vein was used to create an interposition graft. Postoperative abdominal duplex imaging showed patency of the graft. The patient recovered uneventfully. Risk factors for portal vein thrombosis include use of prosthetic graft conduit and prolonged operative time [19].

Arterial reconstructions during pancreatic surgery are more rare, and usually only performed if the tumor has responded to systemic therapy. The superior mesenteric artery margin is the most likely surgical margin to be positive following pancreaticoduodenectomy [18]. Resection of this vessel remains controversial, as it is associated with significant morbidity due to injury to autonomic nerves to the small intestine. Tumors of the pancreatic body or tail may involve the celiac axis, which can be resected without reconstruction because the proper hepatic artery usually receives supply from the gastroduodenal artery [18, 20]. The common hepatic artery (CHA) can be involved in pancreatic head or body masses. CHA resection mandates reconstruction, as it provides blood supply to the bile ducts and biliary anastomosis [18, 20].

Other Considerations/Benefits

In addition to the direct patient care benefit, there are other potential benefits of vascular surgeon involvement as co-surgeons, including financial and educational. In cases with the involvement of a vascular surgeon as a co-surgeon, there is evidence of financial benefit to the hospital system. Vascular surgeon consult cases significantly increase the contribution margin compared to non-consult cases (\$14,406 vs. \$5491, $p = 0.002$). This difference did not depend on whether the consult was planned or unplanned [21]. These cases resulted in an average of approximately 20–30 additional work relative value units (wRVUs) per case for the vascular surgery portion [1–3]. At one academic medical center, these cases provided an additional 1371.46 wRVUs per year and accounted for almost 7% of the case volume for the division of vascular surgery [2]. However, while these cases generate additional financial benefit, these data fail to account for the detrimental effect on the vascular surgeon's scheduled cases or clinic appointments, especially when these consults are unplanned [3].

From an educational point of view, as fewer open vascular cases are being performed, intraoperative vascular consults for cases such as these, which very often require open bypass, patch angioplasty, or primary repair of major vessels, provide a major educational opportunity for trainees. As there is a wide variation in the anatomic location for which these consults arise, knowledge of a breadth of vascular exposures is mandated, particularly in the abdomen, but also the pelvis, the neck, and the extremities [2, 3, 5, 6].

The availability of vascular surgeons for consultation is another topic worthy of consideration. Intraoperative vascular surgery consults often require significant time and effort and can often disrupt the vascular surgeon's other clinical and administrative duties [1]. One way for hospitals and healthcare systems to resolve this problem is to form vascular surgery teams who can cover for each other in the event of emergent intraoperative consultations. To facilitate this approach, healthcare systems may need to provide additional resources, such as advance practice providers, to vascular surgery groups. Smaller hospitals with limited vascular surgeon availability may need to make arrangements for patient transfer to tertiary care centers with established multidisciplinary teams.

References

1. Danczyk RC, Coleman J, Allensworth J, Azarbal AF, Mitchell EL, Liem TK, et al. Incidence and outcomes of intraoperative vascular surgery consultations. J Vasc Surg. 2015;62(1):177–82.
2. Tomita TM, Rodriguez HE, Hoel AW, Ho KJ, Pearce WH, Eskandari MK. Implications of intraoperative vascular surgery assistance for hospitals and vascular surgery trainees. JAMA Surg. 2016;151(11):1032.
3. Manzur MF, Ham SW, Elsayed R, Abdoli S, Simcox T, Han S, et al. Vascular surgery: an essential hospital resource in modern health care. J Vasc Surg. 2017;65(6):1786–92.
4. Kalipatnapu S, Agarwal S. IPC23. Vascular Surgery in a Tertiary Care Center—Profile and outcomes of intraoperative consultations. J Vasc Surg. 2019;69(6):e94.
5. Smith MC, Connolly P, Meltzer AJ. PC114. The role of the vascular surgeon in open oncologic resection: benefiting everyone involved. J Vasc Surg. 2019;69(6):e237.
6. Mogannam AC, Chavez de Paz C, Sheng N, Patel S, Bianchi C, Chiriano J, et al. Early vascular consultation in the setting of oncologic resections: benefit for patients and a continuing source of open vascular surgical training. Ann Vasc Surg. 2015;29(4):810–5.
7. Song TK. Major blood vessel reconstruction during sarcoma surgery. Arch Surg. 2009;144(9):817.

8. Poultsides GA, Tran TB, Zambrano E. Sarcoma resection with and without vascular reconstruction: a matched case-control study. J Vasc Surg. 2015;62(6):1677.
9. Schwarzbach MHM, Hormann Y, Hinz U, Bernd L, Willeke F, Mechtersheimer G, et al. Results of limb-sparing surgery with vascular replacement for soft tissue sarcoma in the lower extremity. J Vasc Surg. 2005;42(1):88–97.
10. Schwarzbach MHM, Hormann Y, Hinz U, Leowardi C, Böckler D, Mechtersheimer G, et al. Clinical results of surgery for retroperitoneal sarcoma with major blood vessel involvement. J Vasc Surg. 2006;44(1):46–55.
11. Psutka SP, Boorjian SA, Thompson RH, Schmit GD, Schmitz JJ, Bower TC, et al. Clinical and radiographic predictors of the need for inferior vena cava resection during nephrectomy for patients with renal cell carcinoma and caval tumour thrombus. BJU Int. 2015;116(3):388–96.
12. Overholser S, Raheem O, Zapata D, Kaushik D, Rodriguez R, Derweesh IH, et al. Radiologic indicators prior to renal cell cancer thrombectomy: implications for vascular reconstruction and mortality. Urol Ann. 2016;8(3):312–6.
13. Boneschi M, Miani S, Erba M, Giuffrida GF, Giordanengo F. Malignant neoplasms invading into the inferior vena cava. Surgical indications. Minerva Cardioangiol. 1995;43(3):91–5.
14. Zhang X, Zhang J, Fan H, He Q, Lang R. Feasibility of portal or superior mesenteric vein resection and reconstruction by allogeneic vein for pancreatic head cancer—a case-control study. BMC Gastroenterol. 2018;18(1):49.
15. Cheung TT, Poon RTP, Chok KSH, Chan ACY, Tsang SHY, Dai WC, et al. Pancreaticoduodenectomy with vascular reconstruction for adenocarcinoma of the pancreas with borderline resectability. World J Gastroenterol. 2014;20(46):17448–55.
16. Sgroi MD, Narayan RR, Lane JS, Demirjian A, Kabutey N-K, Fujitani RM, et al. Vascular reconstruction plays an important role in the treatment of pancreatic adenocarcinoma. J Vasc Surg. 2015;61(2):475–80.
17. Lee DY, Mitchell EL, Jones MA, Landry GJ, Liem TK, Sheppard BC, et al. Techniques and results of portal vein/superior mesenteric vein reconstruction using femoral and saphenous vein during pancreaticoduodenectomy. J Vasc Surg. 2010;51(3):662–6.
18. Younan G, Tsai S, Evans DB, Christians KK. Techniques of vascular resection and reconstruction in pancreatic cancer. Surg Clin N Am. 2016;96(6):1351–70.
19. Glebova NO, Hicks CW, Orion KC, Abularrage CJ, Weiss MJ, Cameron AM, et al. Portal vein reconstruction in pancreatic resection: technical risk factors for portal vein thrombosis◊. J Vasc Surg. 2014;60(3):831–2.
20. Christians KK, Pilgrim CHC, Tsai S, Ritch P, George B, Erickson B, et al. Arterial resection at the time of pancreatectomy for cancer. Surgery. 2014;155(5):919–26.
21. Johnson CE, Manzur MF, Wilson TA, Brown Wadé N, Weaver FA. The financial value of vascular surgeons as operative consultants to other surgical specialties. J Vasc Surg. 2019;69(4):1314–21.

Medical and Legal Implications of Failure to Rescue

18

George E. Anton and Robbin S. Sabo

In 2000, the Institute of Medicine published the report *To Err is Human: Building a Safer Health System* which was intended to inspire national efforts to improve patient safety. The Institute of Medicine recommended that medicine adopt a safety and error-free framework similar to aviation. Prior to that initiative, experts agreed that too many people have been harmed by unintentional medical errors. Historically, professional training has focused on technical, rather than on interpersonal skills.

As early as 1924, W. Wayne Babcock, M.D., FACS, raised a critical question: "How efficient a lifesaving station have you in your operating room?" [14]. Lipshy and Loporta observed that this answer remains elusive over nine decades later.

In 1990, James Reason identified that errors occur due to two types of failure: either the correct action does not proceed as intended (failure of execution) or the original intended action is not correct (errors of planning). As most surgeons know, a tragic ending to a patient's life is not always abrupt or unexpected. In the late 1980s, leaders in patient safety including Gaba and Runciman identified that small errors and system failures interact to produce serious complications. Gaba noted that there are often multiple opportunities to interrupt the evolutionary cascade of events [20]. Instead, these failures are often accompanied by a steady cascade of clinical cues [7].

In his Presidential Address to The Society for Vascular Surgery's in 1995, Dr. Norman Hertzer recognized that good surgeons acted decisively when the best interests of their patients were at stake. Dr. Hertzer recommended that surgeons need to stand for results and concluded that "results mean everything" [9].

G. E. Anton (✉)
Cleveland Clinic, Department of Vascular Surgery, Heart, Vascular and Thoracic Institute, Mayfield Heights, OH, USA
e-mail: ANTONG@ccf.org

R. S. Sabo
Cleveland Clinic, Heart & Vascular Institute Regional Vascular Lab, Mayfield Heights, OH, USA

R. Gilani, J. L. Mills Sr. (eds.), *Vascular Complications of Surgery and Intervention*, https://doi.org/10.1007/978-3-030-86713-3_18

Failure to rescue was defined by Silber, Williams, Krakauer and Schwartz in 1992 as hospital deaths which occurred from adverse conditions [24]. The theory of failure to rescue initiates the idea that healthcare systems should be able to rapidly identify and treat complications as they occur. Ghaferi further categorized factors of failure to rescue into two classifications, timely response and appropriate response, including correct management and treatment [26].

According to Rosero et al. [22], failure to rescue is a measure of how proficient a hospital is at recognizing and treating serious complications and is more strongly associated with hospital characteristics than patient variables. In fact, high-performing hospitals may be identified and characterized by how well they are able to rescue patients from major complications. There is a growing body of evidence suggesting complications and mortality are not related. Ghaferi et al. [6] identified that high mortality hospitals had nearly two times the likelihood of dying after development of major complications as did their counterparts in very low mortality hospitals. McEwan et al. [16] reported that approximately 70% of adverse events in medical settings are not due to individual errors but, as a result of breakdown in teamwork.

In 1990, James Reason introduced the model commonly known as the "Swiss cheese model of accident causation." This theory focuses on creating safe work habits. James Reason reflected that "Accidents do not occur because people gamble and lose, they occur because people believe that the accident that is about to occur is not at all possible" (Reason 2003). The Swiss cheese model is comprised of long-standing, preexisting latent conditions that ultimately contribute to *active failures*. There are many latent conditions in the operating room. The lack of communication between surgeon and staff can be detrimental. If the staff is informed of the surgical plan in advance, it allows the staff autonomy in checking for supplies and potential equipment that could possibly be needed. Such a process empowers the staff to be able to improvise and adapt during a procedure if necessary. It is often too late, once the patient has been anesthetized, to recognize that special needs of the patient have not been met. For instance, one example would be not having nickel free appliances available for a patient with nickel allergies. Situational awareness will help to identify latent conditions so that the system's defenses can be improved. Constant vigilance, surveillance, and keeping your head in the game will dramatically improve preparation and responsiveness.

Crew Resource Management

Healthcare is often compared to the aviation industry as both have highly trained professionals interacting with technology in high risk situations. In both professions, errors can impact safety and public trust. Agha et al. [1] reported that the application of aviation based strategies to surgical disciplines has focused on improving both technical and non-technical skills.

Safety culture encompasses all attitudes and perceptions that contribute to an organization's commitment to safety. Teamwork is paramount to ensure safety in both aviation and healthcare [13] reported based on confidential interviews with surgeons that approximately 43% errors were a result of poor communication.

Crew resource management (CRM) is a set of training procedures for use in environments in which human error can have devastating effect. Used primarily for improving air safety, CRM focuses on non-technical skills such as leadership, interpersonal communication, teamwork, situational awareness, decision-making, workload management, stress management, and fatigue management [15]. Support of all team members without traditional hierarchies is meant to promote effective communication and thus improve the safety culture.

Crew resource management (CRM) was developed at a conference focusing on the contribution of human factors to airplane crashes. This conference was convened in response to the National Transportation Safety Board (NTSD) investigation of the United Airline Flight 173 crash and the 1977 Tenerife airport disaster. Flight 173 crashed when they ran out of fuel over Portland, Oregon, while troubleshooting a landing gear malfunction [11]. The Tenerife airport disaster occurred when two Boeing 747 aircraft collided on the runway killing 583 people. The crash was a result of environmental conditions and organizational influences. The KLM captain was a strong autocratic leader that did not allow his team to act as a team [25]. In 1981, United Airlines became the first airline to provide CRM training for its cockpit crews. By the 1990s, CRM training had become a global standard and continues to be required in ground school for pilots and staff.

The term "cockpit resource management" was coined in 1979 by NASA psychologist John Lauber who had studied communication processes in cockpits for several years. While retaining a command hierarchy, the concept was intended to foster a less authoritarian cockpit culture, one in which co-pilots were encouraged to question captains if they observed them making mistakes.

Airline statistics have shown that human error produced far more accidents than mechanical malfunction. The most common human error was the failure of the crew members to communicate effectively and failure to utilize available resources.

CRM in the operating room requires a surgeon to become a designated leader in their specialty and to establish a group climate that encourages participation and exchange of information without fear of retribution. CRM emphasizes consistent performance in pre-operative, intra-operative, and post- operative phases [32]. Preparation, planning, and vigilance (situational awareness) will determine the extent to which an operating room crew will recognize new threats and develop contingencies and *ACT* accordingly. One must always be thinking ahead of the airplane! This concept is a long-term cultural change in surgical suites and hospitals and requires consistent reinforcement and practice.

In 2000, the Institute of Medicine advised health care organizations to implement crew resource management (CRM) to enhance safety and improve outcomes where human error can have devastating effects. CRM is an operating philosophy that promotes team member input and is proactive in accident prevention. CRM is an effective use of all available resources to assure a safe and efficient operation, reducing error and avoiding stress. CRM is accepted by other "high-reliability" industries dealing with the combination of advanced technology and complex risk.

In 2010, the National Center for patient safety of the Veteran's Health Administration initiated a multisite pilot program in CRM. The outline included building a safety culture, leadership building, and situational awareness, countering fatigue, briefings-debriefings, and checklists and reducing distractions. Young-Xu et al. [31] observed a significant decrease in failure to rescue events from 25% prior to the training to 12% ($P = 0.03$).

The ultimate success of CRM training in medicine is quite variable and complex. Bacon et al. [2] postulated that a strong organization safety culture complimented by comprehensive CRM training would improve failure to rescue and reduce in-hospital mortality. They found that the reduction in failure to rescue and in-hospital mortality was not realized after implementation of CRM, but the study did not include refresher CRM training. The authors advocated for periodic or refresher staff training to reinforce and strengthen the desired safety behavior.

Salas et al. [23] endorsed that CRM training should be provided and practiced continuously. Training should not be a one-time event. If safety is the main concern, then recurrent training is a must.

Weller and Boyd [30] found that briefing protocols, checklists, team training, and organizational change have a positive impact in teamwork in the operating room. However, the positive effects initially realized decayed over the following 4 years, reinforcing the need for ongoing monitoring and evaluation. The educational process must be sustained.

Musson and Helmreich [18] advocated that hospital, medical organizations, nursing schools, and medical schools should play an important role in developing team training and CRM programs. Physicians must take a leadership role and provide long-term commitment to fostering and sustaining such training programs. To improve relevance, these programs need to be established and tailored to medicine and not necessarily taken directly from aviation.

Resilience

During a commencement speech at Williams College in 2012, Atul Gawande noted that he observed the critical skills of the best surgeons and recognized their ability to handle complexity and unpredictability. He noted that the surgeons had developed judgment and understanding of teamwork and were willing to accept accountability for their decisions. Gawande further identified that the best hospitals were not better at controlling and minimizing risks but rather better at preventing things from going wrong [5].

Weick and Sutcliffe [28] determined resilience to be a defining characteristic of high-reliability organizations (HRO). Resilience is defined as the ability to adapt successfully in the face of stressful circumstances. Resilience consists of three components: the ability to absorb stress and continue to function, the ability to bounce back, and the capability to learn from errors. Resilient teams manage what they consider inherently uncertain conditions by scanning for potential problems and working quickly to mitigate these problems as they arise. Resilient teams consistently update their understanding of a situation using interpersonal trust and respectful interaction to inquire about characteristics of the situation and consider new data to inform their situational awareness, a process known as sensemaking. During this period of sense making, where new information is being processed and integrated, the surgeon is vulnerable to loss of situational awareness and impaired decision-making. Team resilience developed from sound crew resource management skills will compensate for less resilient individuals resulting in a safe outcome. Resilience can be developed through effective communication, attention to recovery, and continual learning opportunities and reinforcement. Commitment, competence, and cognizance are essential components of a resilient team. The collective mindfulness of risks is one of the defining characteristics of a HRO.

Multiple studies reveal that surgical mistakes escalate with simple increase in disruptions such as information breakdown, equipment, or technology complications, interruptions, or fatigue. Lipshy and LaPorta [14] determined that the loss of situational awareness occurs when the team is overstressed, distracted, or trapped in confirmation biases. As a result, the team has lost touch with reality. [19] identified when people are focused on a task, they often fail to notice an unexpected but fully visible object. This phenomenon is known as inattentional blindness. The more distracted we are the less likely we are to be aware of our surroundings. Under conditions of distractions, we tend to develop tunnel vision. The concept of inattentional blindness underscores the importance of preparation, education, and situational awareness [8].

Lipshy and Laporta advocate that once maladaptive responses are under control, then competent leadership, decisive communication, risk assessment, planning, and implementation create a route for successful outcome. Just as the leader must be selected before a crisis develops, guidelines pertaining to team cooperation must be planned in advance. The authors further emphasized the importance of debriefing after any crisis.

High Reliable Organizations (HRO)

The concept of high reliability is appealing for healthcare due to the complexity of operations and the potential for catastrophic consequences when failures occur. HROs cultivate resilience by prioritizing safety over other performance pressures. Highly reliable organizations tend to have pre-occupation with failure, reluctance to simplify, sensitivity to operations (situational awareness), and commitment to resilience. People in HROs know that the people closest to the work are generally the most knowledgeable about that work. Commitment to resilience is entrenched in the fundamental understanding of the frequently unpredictable nature of system failures. The local leaders drive a culture of safety and create an atmosphere that provides for psychological safety. High reliability is an ongoing process, an organizational frame of mind. The Joint Commission suggests that healthcare organizations need to work to create a strong foundation which includes developing a leadership commitment to mitigate harm and establish a positive safety culture. Patient safety is one aspect of the culture of safety, but it is more of an aspirational goal. A culture of safety also includes psychological safety, accountability, teamwork, communication, and negotiation [6].

Healthcare has often been compared to the aviation industry. Both involve highly trained personnel interacting with advanced technology in high risk situations. Wachter [27] proposed that surgery has always had the two most important ingredients for a safety program: passionate commitment and a sense of accountability. The author further suggested that a safe culture is one in which trainees (and others) should understand that calling for help when one is in over one's head is a sign of strength and not a weakness.

[13] identified that teamwork is imperative to establish safety in both aviation and healthcare. The similarities between aviation and healthcare include a primary goal of safety. Both domains have become safer as a result of technology, but teamwork is essential to mitigate or treat errors. Both have multiple sources of threat to safety: technological, human and environmental factors.

What does a safe culture look like? Ghaferi and Dimick [7] referred to the shared, often unconscious, attitudes that govern behavior. The authors proposed that forces shaped by an organization's values, beliefs and traditions impact its culture. Ghaferi stressed that the understanding of culture is imperative to change it. The signature of a highly reliable organization (HRO) is not that it is error-free, but that errors don't disable it.

Weller et al. [29] recognized that failures in interpersonal teamwork and communication lead directly to compromised patient care as well as staff stress, distress, tension, and inefficiency. These factors contribute to >60% of sentinel events. HROs view of near misses is that they are an opportunity for learning and improvement. When people see a near miss as success, this reinforces their acceptance that current performance is satisfactory to forestall inadvertent sequelae. The application of Band-Aids is not a resilient process.

Success generates confidence. The obstacle is that if people assume success establishes competence, they are more likely to drift into complacency. A near miss needs to be interpreted as danger in the pretense of safety rather than safety in the guise of danger. Successful rescue hinges on early recognition and timely management of complications once they occur. The ultimate goal is to provide a high quality response to an initial complication and thereby avoid a progressive cascade of adverse events that may lead to "failure to rescue." A resilient team is continually scanning the patient and environmental horizon for major changes in condition so as to be able to act quickly to mitigate additional harm.

Implementation of the OODA Loop

A process that improves an organization's ability to act quickly and decisively is to employ the OODA Loop (Fig. 18.1). OODA Loop was originated by a fighter pilot and instructor for the US Air Force, Colonel John Boyd. Boyd was dubbed "forty-second Boyd" for his standing bet as an instructor pilot that beginning from a position of disadvantage; he could defeat any opposing pilot in air combat maneuvering in less than forty seconds. Boyd advocated that decision-making occurs in a recurring cycle of observe-orient-decide-act. The observations are raw data in which decisions and actions are based. Boyd advocated that OODA loops are time sensitive and a series of OODA loops are necessary for decision-making in complex procedures [17].

According to Boyd, OODA loop is a recurring cycle of making rapid, accurate, and critical decisions under stress.

OBSERVE: Gather information
ORIENT: Decipher information (sense making)
DECIDE: Based on previous knowledge and experience
ACT: Implement the plan without impulsive behavior

Integrating the OODA loop with sound CRM skills, sound leadership and teamwork, effective communication skills, sound situational awareness, decision-making, and task assignment will offer the best opportunity for preventing, identifying, and managing adverse events.

Closing the Loop

It has been my anecdotal observation that during a crisis, 90% of people will be stunned or paralyzed leading to indecision, and the other 10% are doing the wrong thing. As strong leaders, we must demonstrate an ability to compensate for less resilient team members, so as to facilitate recovery. Clarity and focus enhance problem-solving abilities during crisis management. State your intention in a calm and definitive fashion. Under these circumstances, it is important to exhibit good judgment, sound decision-making, and competence based on experience and knowledge. Contemporaneous and accurate medical chart documentation provides the

Fig. 18.1 OODA loop

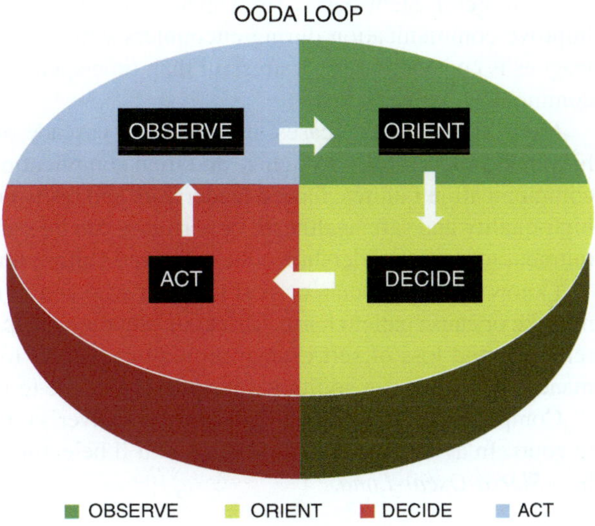

most powerful evidence to either avoid or defend a lawsuit. Timely and accurate documentation leaves little uncertainty and doubt about your testimony and credibility during legal investigation. Malpractice claims take many months or years to sort out. One cannot simply rely on memory alone. Having a permanent record of the rapid response, strong teamwork, and technical expertise will provide objective evidence of team confidence and resilience.

Conclusion

Hospital safety has been a target of initiatives since the 1990s. Despite the safety initiatives and plethora of safety information, failure to rescue remains a timely topic. Hospital errors are multifactorial and complex. The successful rescue of a patient who develops an unexpected complication relies on the hospital system and their teamwork.

Physicians have the opportunity to impact lives and safety at the local level. Patients entrust their lives and well-being to the providers of their care and that is a sacred trust. The essential role of leadership in developing a safe culture should be a first priority to physicians and hospital systems according to the Joint Commission [12].

Successful rescue hinges on early recognition and timely management of serious complications. Striving to create a high reliable organization (HRO) and a culture of safety that mitigates mistakes is paramount. The critical portion of creating a true culture of safety requires a leader/physician champion committed to prioritizing and creating a culture of safety as important as the time and resources devoted to revenue, system integration, and productivity. It is my opinion, that physician leadership in this endeavor is imperative for both eventual acceptance and maximum relevance.

Weick and Sutcliffe (2001) advocated that culture is a product of that which is done on a consistent basis. Time spent developing the techniques and habits that improve communication during encounters with patients and exchanges with colleagues is considerably less stressful than time spent defending care resulting from communication breakdown.

Medical malpractice cases often reveal a cascade of missed opportunities for a hospital to successfully recognize and treat complications. Frequently identified are communication failures, flawed leadership, and decision-making skills. Providing a high-quality and safe healthcare opportunity can be realized with unwavering commitment to strong leadership, education, and culture improvement.

I know of no physician or staff member who comes to work intending to make a mistake or cause patient harm. Threat of litigation, hospital sanctions, loss of patient referrals, and loss of self-esteem provide incentives to elevate a surgeon's performance. Pilots have an additional incentive, a desire to live.

Complications in medicine will cause caregiver's remorse, and they may car pool to court. In aviation, if you land long, you'll be eating alfalfa. Either way you will be – *Sierra-Oscar-Lima.*

References

1. Agha R, Fowler A, Sevalis N. The role of non-technical skills in surgery. Ann Med Surg. 2015;4:422–7.
2. Bacon C, McCoy T, Henshaw D. Failure to rescue and 30-day in-hospital mortality with and without crew-resource-management safety training. Res Nurs Health/Early View. 2019. Retrieved from: https://onlinelibrary.wiley.com/doi/10.1002/nur.22007.
3. Bickell W, Wall M Jr, Pepe P, Martin R, Ginger V, Allen M, Mattox K. Immediate versus delayed fluid resuscitation for hypotensive patients with penetrating torso injuries. N Engl J Med. 1993;331:1105–9.
4. Crico Strategies. Malpractice risks in communication failures. 2015 annual benchmarking report. 2015.
5. Gawande A. Failure to rescue. The New Yorker. 2010, June 2. Retrieved from https://www.newyorker.com/new/news-desk/failure-and-rescue
6. Ghaferi AA, Birkmeyer JD, Dimick JB. Variation in hospital mortality associated with inpatient surgery. N Engl J Med. 2009;361(14):1368–75.
7. Ghaferi AA, Dimick JB. Understanding failure to rescue and improving safety culture. Ann Surg. 2015;261(5):839.
8. Hatchimonji JS, Kaufman EJ, Sharoky CE, Ma L, Whitlock AEG, Holena DN. Failure to rescue in surgical patients: a review for acute surgeons. J Trauma Acute Care Surg. 2010;87(3):699–706.
9. Hertzer N. Presidential address: outcome assessment in vascular surgery-results mean everything. J Vasc Surg. 1995;1995(21):6–15.
10. Institute of Medicine. To error is human: building a safer health system. 2000. Retrieved from http://www.nap.edu/books/030906837/html/.
11. Jedick RA. United Airlines 173- the need for CRM. 2014. Retrieved from https://goflightmedicine.com/united-airlines-173.
12. Joint Commission. The essential role of leadership in developing a safety culture. Sentinel Event Alert. 2017;(57):1.
13. Kao L, Thomas E. Navigating towards improved surgical safety using aviation-based strategies. J Surg Res. 2008;145(2):327–35.
14. Lipshy KA, LaPorta A. Operating room crisis management leadership training: guidance for surgical team education. Bull Am Coll Surg. 2013;98(10):24–33.
15. Martin W. Crew resource management and individual resilience crew resource management. 3rd ed. San Diego: Academic Press; 2019. p. 218.
16. McEwan D, Ruissen GR, Eys MA, Zumbo BD, Beauchamp MR. The effectiveness of teamwork training on teamwork behaviors and team performance: a systematic review and meta-analysis of controlled interventions. PLoS One. 2017;12(1):e0169604.
17. Mulder P. OODA loop. 2017. Retrieved 17 Oct 2019 from Tools Hero: https://www.toolshero.com/decision-making/ooda-loop/.
18. Musson D, Helmreich R. Team training and resource management in healthcare: current issues and future Musson and Helmreich team training and resource management. Harvard Health Policy Rev. 2004;5:25–35.
19. Neisser R. Becklan R. Selective looking: Attending to visually specified events. Cogn Psychol. 1975;7(4):480–94.
20. Reason J. Understanding adverse events: human factors. BMJ Qual Saf. 1995;4(2):80–9.
21. Reason J, Hobbs A. Safety culture. In: Reason J, Hobbs A, editors. Managing maintenance error: a practical guide. Hampshire: Ashgate Publishing Company; 2003. p. 145–8.
22. Rosero EB, Joshi GP, Minhajuddin A, Timaran CH, Modrall JG. Effects of hospital safety-net burden and hospital volume on failure to rescue after open abdominal aortic surgery. J Vasc Surg. 2017;66(2):404–12.
23. Salas E, Wilson K, Burke S, Wightman E, Howse W. A checklist for crew resource management training. Ergon Des. 2006:6–15.

24. Silber JH, Williams SV, Krakauer H, Schwartz JS. Hospital and patient characteristics associated with death after surgery: a study of adverse occurrence and failure to rescue. Med Care. 1992:615–29.
25. Smith P. The true story behind the deadliest air disaster of all time. The Telegraph. 2017. https://www.telegraph.co.uk/travel/comment/tenerife-airport-disaster/.
26. Taenzer AH, Pyke JB, McGrath SP. A review of current and emerging approaches to address failure-to-rescue. Anesthesiol: J Am Soci Anesthesiol. 2011;115(2):421–31.
27. Wachter RM. The evolution of patient safety in surgery. Patient Safety Network. 2017, December 1. Retrieved from https://www.psnet.ahrq.gov/perspective/evolution-patient-safety-surgery.
28. Weick KE, Sutcliffe KM. Managing the unexpected, vol. 9. San Francisco: Jossey-Bass; 2001.
29. Weller J, Boyd M, Cumin D. Teams, tribes and patient safety: overcoming barriers to effective teamwork in healthcare. Postgrad Med J. 2014;90(1061):149–54.
30. Weller J, Boyd M. Making a difference through improving teamwork in the operating room: a systematic review of the evidence of what works. Curr Anesthesiol Rep. 2014;4:77–83.
31. Young-Xu Y, Fore AM, Metcalf A, Payne K, Neily J, Sculli GL. Using crew resource management and a "read-and-do checklist" to reduce failure-to-rescue events on a step-down unit. AJN: Am J Nurs. 2013;113(9):51.
32. Yule S, Flin R, Patterson-Brown S. Non-technical skills for surgeons in the operating room: a review of the literature. Surgery. 2006;139:139–40.

Index

R. Gilani, J. L. Mills Sr. (eds.), *Vascular Complications of Surgery and Intervention*, https://doi.org/10.1007/978-3-030-86713-3

GPSR Compliance

The European Union's (EU) General Product Safety Regulation (GPSR) is a set of rules that requires consumer products to be safe and our obligations to ensure this.

If you have any concerns about our products, you can contact us on ProductSafety@springernature.com

In case Publisher is established outside the EU, the EU authorized representative is:

Springer Nature Customer Service Center GmbH
Europaplatz 3
69115 Heidelberg, Germany

Batch number: 10732090

Printed by Printforce, the Netherlands